International Medical Guide for Ships

3rd edition

Including the ship's medicine chest

World Health Organization

WHO Library Cataloguing-in-Publication Data

International medical guide for ships: including the ship's medicine chest. 3rd ed.

1. Naval medicine. 2. Ships. 3. Sanitation. I. World Health Organization. II. Title.

ISBN 978 92 4 154720 8 (NLM classification: WT 500)

ISBN 978 92 4 068231 3 (electronic version)

ISBN 978 92 4 154738 3 (paperback version)

Contents

Preface xv

Acknowledgements xvii

Introduction xix

How to use this guide xix

1 First aid 1

First aid on board 1

A basic life support sequence 3

Choking 9

Bleeding 10

2 Shock 13

3 Pain management 17

4 Head injuries 27

Anatomical note 27

General note on head injuries 27

Skull fractures 28

Traumatic brain injury (brain damage) 28

Post-concussion syndrome 30

5 Eye injuries and diseases 33

Eye injuries 33

Red flags 34

A blow on or near the eye 35

Corneal abrasion 36

Loose foreign bodies 36

Foreign bodies embedded in the eye 37

Wounds of the eyelids and eyeball 37

Chemical burns 38

Arc eyes ("welder's flash") 38

Noninfectious eye diseases 39

Subconjunctival haemorrhage 39

Cataract 39

Glaucoma 39

Infectious eye diseases 40

Blepharitis 40

Conjunctivitis 41

Keratitis 42

Hordeolum 42

Sudden painless loss of vision 42

6 Bone, joint, and muscle injuries 43

General treatment of injuries 43

Specific injuries 43

Strains and sprains 43

Compound fractures 44

Skull fractures 44
Nose, jaw, and face fractures 44
Neck (cervical spine) injuries 45
Collar bone (clavicle) injury 46
Shoulder injury 47
Injury to the upper arm (humerus) and elbow 48
Wrist and forearm fractures 49
Hand and finger injuries 50
Rib fractures 52
Fractures of the pelvis, hip, and femur 52
Knee injuries 52
Shin (tibia and fibula) fractures 54
Ankle injuries 54
Fractures of the foot and toes 56
Splints and slings 56

7 Abdominal and chest injuries **59**
Abdominal injuries 59
Blunt abdominal injuries 59
Penetrating abdominal injuries 61
Chest injuries 61
Simple rib fracture 62
Flail chest 63
Pneumothorax 64
Spontaneous pneumothorax 64
Tension pneumothorax 64
Penetrating chest wounds 65

8 Wounds **67**
Wound healing 67
Red flag wounds 68
How to close a wound 69
Using adhesive skin closures 69
Using skin adhesive (liquid stitches) 70
Suturing a wound 71
Local anaesthesia 74
Special wounds 74
Lips 74
Tongue 75
Ears and nose 75
Eyelids 75
Puncture wounds of the soles of the feet 76
Wound infection 76
Dressing wounds that cannot be closed 77

9 Burns, chemical splashes, smoke inhalation, and electrocution **79**
Clothing on fire 79
Heat burns and scalds 79
Infection of a burn 83
Respiratory tract burns 83

Electrical burns and electrocution 83
Chemical splashes 85
Flash burns (arc eye) *86*
Smoke inhalation 86

10 Heat stroke and other heat disorders **87**
Heat stroke 87
To prevent heat stroke 88
Stoker's cramps *89*
Heat exhaustion (or "heat collapse") *89*

11 Poisoning **91**
Poisoning with ingested drugs and chemicals 91
Red flags *93*
Common poisoning agents 93
Paracetamol (acetaminophen) *93*
Acetylsalicylic acid (Aspirin®) *94*
Methanol and ethylene glycol *94*
Organophosphate and carbamate insecticides *95*
Anticoagulants (warfarin, rat poison) *96*
Petroleum products *96*
Caustics *97*
Disinfectants and bleach *97*
Dangerous prescription drugs *97*
Poisoning from exposure to common gases or vapours 98
Carbon monoxide *98*
Cyanide *99*
Irritant gases – phosgene, chlorine, ammonia *99*
Carbon dioxide *100*
Flammable liquid vapours *100*
Freons *100*
Hydrogen sulphide ("Rotten egg gas", "Sewer gas") *100*
Bites and stings 101
Rat bites *101*
Snake bites *101*
Jellyfish stings *102*
Venomous fish *102*
Sea urchins *103*
Scorpions and spiders *103*

12 Examination of the patient **105**
Introduction 105
Consent 105
Privacy and confidentiality 107
The physical examination 109

13 Paralysis, strange behaviour, unconsciousness **113**
Stroke 113
Transient ischaemic attack (TIA) *115*

Headache 116
Red flags *117*
Seizures and epilepsy 118
Types of epileptic seizure *118*
Red flags *120*
Drugs that can precipitate seizures *121*
Loss of consciousness 121
Sudden loss of consciousness (syncope) *121*
Finding an unconscious person *122*
Diabetes mellitus and coma *123*
Diabetic ketoacidosis *124*
Hypoglycaemia *125*
Bell's palsy 125
Mental illness 126
Psychosis *126*
Forms of psychosis *127*
Depression *129*
Violent or threatening behaviour *130*
Suicide *130*
After an unsuccessful suicide attempt *131*
Post-traumatic stress disorder *132*

14 Chest pain and other disorders of the heart and circulation 133
Angina pectoris 133
Complications of myocardial infarction *135*
Palpitations *136*
Blocked arteries in the legs *137*
Deep vein thrombosis *138*

15 Respiratory diseases 139
Bronchitis 139
Bronchitis due to infection *139*
Bronchitis due to cigarette smoking *139*
Bronchiectasis 140
Common cold 140
Pleurisy 141
Pneumothorax *141*
Pneumonia 141
Lobar pneumonia *141*
Empyema *143*
Aspiration pneumonia and lung abscess *143*
Sinusitis 144
Hay fever 144
Asthma 145

16 Gastrointestinal and liver diseases 149
Abdominal pain – general points 149
Red flags in abdominal pain *151*

Severe abdominal pain 152
Appendicitis 152
Pancreatitis 153
Bowel obstruction 155
Diarrhoea 156
Foodborne illness 156
Dysentery 158
Traveller's diarrhoea 158
Food poisoning from marine toxins 159
Inflammatory bowel disease (colitis) 160
Ulcerative colitis 160
Crohn's disease 161
Antibiotic-associated colitis 162
Indigestion and pain related to meals 163
Gastro-oesophageal reflux disease 163
Peptic ulcer 163
Red flags 164
Heavy bleeding from the gastrointestinal tract (gastrointestinal haemorrhage) 165
Heavy upper gastrointestinal bleeding 165
Heavy lower gastrointestinal bleeding 167
Anal fissure 168
Haemorrhoids (piles) 168
Anal pruritis (anal itch) 169
Hernia 169
Inguinal (groin) hernia 170
Liver and biliary disease 171
Jaundice 171
Liver failure 172
Alcoholic liver disease 172
Gallstones 174

17 Kidney and other urinary disorders 177
Disorders of the kidney 177
Acute renal (kidney) failure 177
Chronic renal failure (Bright's disease) 179
Kidney stones (renal colic) 179
Other urinary disorders 180
Red urine 180
Urinary tract infection 181
Urinary tract infection in women 181
Urinary tract infection in men 181
Prostatitis 181
Chronic pelvic pain in men 182
Benign prostatic hyperplasia (BPH, enlarged prostate) 182
Acute urinary retention 183

18 Pregnancy and childbirth 185
Pregnancy 185
Drugs in pregnancy 185

Vaginal bleeding during pregnancy or suspected pregnancy 185
Ectopic pregnancy 186
Miscarriage 186
Salpingitis (inflammation of a fallopian tube) 188
Pruritus vulvae (external genital itching) 188
Childbirth 188
Preparing for the birth 188
Managing the early stages of childbirth 190
Managing the birth 190
Caring for the baby after delivery 191
Caring for the mother after delivery 192
Post-partum haemorrhage 193
Other possible problems after childbirth 193

19 Sexually transmitted infections 195
Urethritis 196
Urethritis in women 197
Gonococcal proctitis 198
Gonococcal pharyngitis 198
Genital ulcers 198
Acute pain in the scrotum 200
Epididymitis 200
Testicular torsion 200
Trauma to the scrotum 201
Testicular inflammation (orchitis) 201
Balanitis 201
Lymph node swelling in the groin 202
Vaginal discharge 203
Bacterial vaginosis 203
Vaginal candidiasis 203
Trichomoniasis 203
Pelvic inflammatory disease 204
Ano-genital warts 205
Pubic lice 205
Acquired immunodeficiency syndrome (AIDS) 205
Later stages of HIV and AIDS 206
Treatment of HIV infection 206
Post-exposure prophylaxis 207

20 Skin diseases 209
Questions to ask a patient 209
Barber's rash 209
Folliculitis 210
Pseudofolliculitis (also called "razor bumps") 210
Tinea barbae 211

Acne 211
Chaps 211
Dermatitis 212
Irritant contact dermatitis 212
Eczema (atopic dermatitis) 213
Allergic contact dermatitis 213
Fungal skin infections 214
Tinea pedis (athlete's foot) 214
Tinea corporis (ringworm) 214
Tinea cruris (Jock itch, Dhobie itch) 215
Bacterial skin infections 215
Impetigo 215
Carbuncles and furuncles (furunculosis) 216
Skin abscess 216
Pediculosis (lice infestation) 219
Scabies 220
Shingles (herpes zoster and varicella zoster) 221
Urticaria (hives) 221
Cellulitis and erysipelas 221
Cellulitis arising from wounds exposed to estuary or seawater 222

21 Bone, joint, and muscle disorders 225
Joint inflammation 225
Gout 225
Septic arthritis 226
Rheumatoid arthritis 226
Osteoarthritis 227
Problems in specific joints 227
The knee 227
The shoulder 228
The back 229
Red flags 230
The neck 230
Red flags 231

22 Tobacco, alcohol, and drug use 233
Four main questions to consider 233
Alcohol intoxication 234
Alcohol withdrawl 235
Minor withdrawal ("the shakes") 235
Major withdrawal (delirium tremens, DTs) 235
Cannabis intoxication 238
Opioids, opiates, and related drugs 239
Heroin intoxication 239
Heroin overdose 240
Infection in heroin users 240
Heroin withdrawal 241

Other opioids 242

Cocaine ("coke", "snow", etc.) 242

Amphetamines 243

Hallucinogen intoxication 244
Lysergic acid diethylamide (LSD) 245
Phencyclidine ("PCP", "angel dust") 245
Plant hallucinogens 245

"Flashbacks" 245

Kava kava 246

23 Infectious diseases 247

Infectious agents 247

How infections spread 247

Common terms used in connection with infections 249
Onset 249
Fever 250
Rash 250

Management of infectious diseases – general principles 251
Isolation 251
Needle-stick injuries 252

Treating infectious diseases 253
Food 253

Some common or important infections that could occur on board 254
Anthrax 254
Chickenpox and shingles (varicella-zoster virus) 254
Cholera 257
Dengue 258
Diphtheria 259
Ear infections 260
Hand infections in seafarers and fishers 262
Infectious mononucleosis (glandular fever) 262
Influenza 263
Malaria 265
Meningitis and meningococcal infection 269
Mumps 270
Plague 271
Rabies 272
Rubella (German measles) 273
SARS (severe acute respiratory syndrome) 273
Sore throat 274
Red flags 274
Tetanus (lockjaw) 275
Tuberculosis 275
Typhoid and paratyphoid fever 277
Viral hepatitis (hepatitis A, B, and C) 278
Whooping cough (pertussis) 280
Worms 281
Yellow fever 284

24 Dental problems 287

Some common dental problems 287

Tooth decay (caries) 287

Pulpitis and peri-apical abscess 287

Periodontal disease (gum inflammation) 287

Pericoronitis 287

Red flags 288

Lost fillings and broken teeth 288

A bleeding socket 288

Lost teeth 289

25 External assistance 291

Medical advice 291

Evacuation by helicopter 293

Ship-to-ship transfer of doctor or patient 295

Referral information to accompany evacuated patients 296

26 Nursing care and medical procedures 297

Nursing care 297

Preparing sick-quarters 297

First steps on a patient's arrival 297

Basic principles of nursing care 298

Caring for the bed-bound patient 299

Monitoring the vital signs 302

Bodily functions 308

Examining faeces, urine, sputum, and vomited matter 311

Mentally disturbed patients 313

The unconscious patient 314

Medical procedures 317

Applying cold 317

Applying heat 318

Catheterizing the urinary bladder 319

Surgical dressings 322

Administering medicines - basic principles 323

Routes of administration 323

Injections 324

Eye medication 329

Ear medication 330

27 Death at sea 333

Signs of death 333

Examining a dead body 334

Disposal of the body 335

Burial at sea 336

28 Medical care for survivors at sea 339

Abandoning ship 339

Surviving in a survival craft 340

Near-drowning 341

Generalized hypothermia due to cold water immersion 343

Cold exposure injuries 344
Frostnip 345
Frostbite 345
Immersion foot (trench foot) 346
Other medical problems aboard survival craft 347
Seasickness 347
Sunburn 347
Dehydration and malnutrition 347
Heat exposure 348
Contamination with oil 348
Food and water for rescued survivors 348
Medical resources on a lifeboat 349

29 Environmental control and hygiene **351**
Ventilation 351
Lighting 352
Food hygiene 353
Food-handlers 353
Food service facilities 354
Food storage 354
The galley (ship's kitchen) 356
Toilet and washing facilities 357
Liquid transport and potable water 357
Potable water sources 358
Potable water transport system 358
Potable water storage 359
Taking water on board 359
Disinfection of potable water 359
Disposal of liquid and solid wastes 360
Combating disease vectors 360
Rodents 360
Insects 362
Flies 363
Mosquitoes 363
Cockroaches 364
Bedbugs 364
Sanitary inspection 365

30 Preventing disease and promoting health in seafarers **367**
Preventing communicable diseases 367
Isolation 367
Immunization 367
Hepatitis A and hepatitis B 367
Other infections 367
Preventing other diseases 368
Stopping smoking 368
A balanced diet 368
Personal hygiene 369
Sleep 370
Preventing illness from exposure to extremes of temperature 370

Sunburn and skin cancer 370
Lifting heavy weights 370
Foot Injuries 371
Lack of exercise and boredom 371
Preventing ill-health from seafaring work 371
General principles of promoting safety on board ship 371
The Health and Safety Committee 372
Briefing for new tasks 372
Work place assessment 373
Provision of good medical care 373
Seafarers' lifestyles 373

31 Anatomy and physiology **375**
Cells 375
Tissues 375
Organs 375
Note on anatomical terms and descriptions 375
The skeletal system 376
The muscular system 377
The circulatory system 379
The respiratory system 379
The digestive system 381
The urinary system 386
The nervous system 386
The endocrine system 387
The blood 388
Blood and anaemia 388
The immune system 389
Allergy 390

32 International Health Regulations **393**
International Health Regulations (2005) 393
Part I – Definitions, purpose and scope, principles and responsible authorities 393
Part IV – Points of entry 398
Part V – Public health measures 400
Part VI – Health documents 405
Part VII – Charges 407
Annex 1 – B. Core capacity requirements for designated airports, ports and ground crossings 409
Annex 2 – Descision instrument for the assessment and notification of events that may constitute a public health emergency of international concern 410
Annex 3 – Model ship sanitation control exemption certificate/ship sanitation control certificate 413
Annex 4 – Technical requirements pertaining to conveyances and conveyance operators 415
Annex 5 – Specific measures for vector-borne diseases 416
Annex 6 – Vaccination, prophylaxis and related certificates 417
Annex 7 – Requirements concerning vaccination or prophylaxis for specific diseases 419
Annex 8 – Model of maritime declaration of health 420

33 The ship's medicine chest 423
Introduction 423
Basic rules for managing the medicine chest 423
Anaphylaxis 425
Drug rash and other drug-related skin problems 425
Controlled drugs 426
Ships carrying dangerous goods 427
Specific categories of medicines 427
Fluids for intravenous infusion 428
List of recommended medicines and equipment 430
Annex A: Forms for case reporting, referral, and evacuation 455
Ship master's report form 456
Ship's identity and navigational status form 458
Patient health status form 459
Primary physician's report form 460
Index 463

Preface

Seafaring has always been a dangerous occupation. Long voyages, extreme weather conditions, illnesses and accidents can take a heavy toll on the health of crew members. Not only are they exposed to greater risk, seafarers are also isolated from the usual sources of medical care and assistance available to people on shore.

WHO has consistently strived to improve the health of people at their place of work. When people also live in their work environment – as seafarers must – they face particular risks to their health. Practical guidance is essential for those who must provide assistance when seafarers fall ill or are injured. Since its first publication by WHO in 1967, the *International Medical Guide for Ships* has been the standard source of such guidance.

The second edition, written in 1988, was translated into more than 30 languages, and has been used in tens of thousands of ships. This, the third edition, contains fully updated recommendations aimed to promote and protect the health of seafarers. This edition is also consistent with the latest revisions of both the *WHO Model List of Essential Medicines* and the *International Health Regulations (2005)*.

The International Labour Organization (ILO) *Maritime Labour Convention 2006* stipulates that all ships shall carry a medicine chest, medical equipment and a medical guide. The *International Medical Guide for Ships* supports a main principle of that Convention: to ensure that seafarers are given health protection and medical care as comparable as possible to that which is generally available to workers ashore, including prompt access to the necessary medicines, medical equipment and facilities for diagnosis and treatment and to medical information and expertise.

The Convention states that ships carrying 100 or more persons and ordinarily engaged on international voyages of more than three days' duration shall carry a qualified medical doctor who is responsible for providing medical care. Ships which do not carry a medical doctor shall be required to have either at least one seafarer on board who is in charge of medical care and administering medicine as part of their regular duties or at least one seafarer on board competent to provide medical first aid. Persons in charge of medical care on board who are not medical doctors shall have satisfactorily completed training in medical care that meets the requirements of the *International Convention on Standards of Training, Certification and Watchkeeping for Seafarers*. The *International Medical Guide for Ships* is a standard reference for these training courses, and is designed for use by all crew members charged with providing medical care on board.

The *ILO Maritime Labour Convention 2006* stipulates that the competent authority shall ensure by a prearranged system that medical advice by radio or satellite communication to ships at sea is available 24 hours a day – the *International Medical Guide for Ships* explains when it is essential to seek such advice.

By carrying this guide on board ships, and following its instructions, countries can both fulfill their obligations under the terms of the *Maritime Labour Convention 2006*, and ensure the best possible health outcomes for their seafaring population. WHO is pleased to be able to contribute to this goal by presenting the third edition of the *International Medical Guide for Ships*.

Maria Neira
Director, Department of Protection of the Human Environment

Acknowledgements

The third edition of the *International Medical Guide for Ships* could not have been completed without the advice and support of the International Transport Workers' Federation (ITF), the International Shipping Federation (ISF), and the International Maritime Health Association (IMHA). The International Transport Workers' Federation funded content development for this edition.

WHO thanks the International Labour Organization and the International Maritime Organization (IMO) for their collaboration on the revision of this essential text.

WHO also wishes to acknowledge the following individuals who wrote and/or reviewed early draft chapters: F. Amenta, W. Baumeier, X. Baur, D. Becker, K. Benedict, M. Biekart, H. Buma, T. Carter, E. Dahl, M. Daoud, T.E. Harrison, B.M. Jaremin, E. Kazakevitch, Y. Walid Khalil, A. Lobenko, E. Lucero-Prisno III, O. Lyngenbo, Ngueng Truong Son, N. Nikoli, P. Sabro Nilson, H.I. Saarni, B.F. Schepers, R. Sucre, G. Tarling, H. Thouard, R. Van Cleempoel, M. Van Hall, K. Verbist, P. Verhaert, L.A. Viruly, V.J. Yelland, and L. Zvyagina.

Ural Cagirici, Marcos Castrol, Alf Magne Horneland, Suresh Idnani, Rossen Karavatchv, Nebojsa Nikolic, Morten Vinter, and Jon Whitlow jointly reviewed and endorsed the revised guide.

S.A.J.J. Rikken and R.C. Verbist compiled and edited the content of an earlier version of this edition, and coordination of the revision process was originally done at WHO by Carolyn Allsop, David Bramley, Greg Goldstein, and Deborah Nelson, and at ILO by Dani Appave, Joachim Grisham, Jean-Yves Legouas, and Elizabeth Tinoco.

Suzanne Hill advised on the compilation of the medicine chest. Content for the third edition was written and edited by John Maurice and Les Olson.

Tim Carter of the International Maritime Health Association, Tom Holmer of the International Transport Workers' Federation, and Natalie Shaw of the International Shipping Federation supervised the tripartite review of the final text.

Representatives of the International Transport Workers' Federation and the International Shipping Foundation endorsed this text at a joint ILO/WHO meeting on the revision of the International Medical Guide for Ships held in Geneva, 25–26 July 2007.

Sophie Guetaneh Aguettant was the graphic designer and Diana Hopkins was the proofreader for this edition. Gerry Eijkemans and Laragh Gollogly were managing editors.

Introduction

How to use this guide

The *International Medical Guide for Ships* is easy to read and understand. It tells you how to diagnose, treat and prevent health problems in seafarers, with a focus on the first 48 hours after injury.

It should be kept in the ship's medicine chest, and you should familiarize yourself with the content before a medical emergency occurs. This way, when there is a case of illness or injury on board, you can immediately turn to emergency medical advice on the topic at hand.

Chapters 1–24 follow this structure:

- general description of symptom or disease
- explanatory notes when necessary
- signs and symptoms
- key questions to ask
- what to do
- what not to do.

These chapters also contain information on how to prevent specific injuries or illness, by action that can be taken on board. General prevention and health promotion is covered in Chapter 30.

Since immediate response is essential for life-threatening conditions, the first 11 chapters cover the principals of first aid, and how to respond to choking, bleeding, shock, pain, injuries, wounds, burns, and poisoning.

Chapter 12 outlines the general principles of physical examination and the necessity of obtaining consent for examination and treatment.

Chapter 25 describes how to use external assistance and seek medical advice by radio, and includes a general recommendation on the use of digital photographs to assist in obtaining diagnostic and treatment advice in this context. It includes a form for obtaining and transcribing such advice.

Chapter 32 contains the relevant articles of the revised *International Health Regulations (2005)*.

Chapter 33 lists the necessary medicines for stocking the ship's medicine chest, including those which should only be used with radio medical advice. This list is consistent with WHO's essential drugs list, and provides indications, doses, and specific precautions for each entry.

Annex A contains medical referral and evacuation forms which should be copied and stored with the medical supplies.

This guide is designed to be used in conjunction with the most recent versions of the *Guide to Ship Sanitation*, and the IMO's *Medical First Aid Guide* and *Emergency Procedures for Ships Carrying Dangerous Goods*.

First aid

FIRST AID ON BOARD

First aid is treatment aimed at preventing the death or further damage to health of an ill or injured person perceived to be in a life-threatening condition. All crew members should receive training in first aid.

Step 1 Assess the situation: what do think happened and is there still danger?

(a) If giving first aid will expose you to danger, do not do it: call or go for help.

(b) If a person is still in danger, remove the danger or the person before giving first aid.

(c) If bystanders are in danger, warn them.

Step 2 If you are alone, shout for help.

Step 3 Choose the best place for first aid.

(a) On the spot?

- Not if fire is present.
- Not if there are potentially dangerous gases in the atmosphere.
- Not if there are other risks at the site of the accident.

(b) In the ship's infirmary (sick-bay) or in a cabin?

- Not if the delay in moving the person is dangerous.

Step 4 If there are several injured people, prioritize.

(a) Attend first to any unconscious person.

(b) If there is more than one unconscious person:

- check each for pulse and breathing;
- begin resuscitation of a person who is not breathing or has no detectable heart beat (see below, *Cardio-pulmonary resuscitation*).

(c) Attend to conscious patients:

- treat bleeding by applying pressure to the wound;
- wait until the patient has been moved to the sick bay before dealing with other injuries, **UNLESS** you suspect spinal injury (see below**,** *What to do in the case of spinal injury*).

✗ *What not to do when giving first aid*

- DO NOT GIVE FIRST AID if you have doubts about your ability to do so correctly.
- DO NOT ENTER AN ENCLOSED SPACE unless you are sure it is safe.
- DO NOT MOVE THE PERSON without checking for:
  - spinal injuries
  - fractured long bones.
- DO NOT GIVE THE PATIENT ANYTHING TO EAT OR DRINK (especially alcohol).

THE ABC SEQUENCE OF BASIC LIFE SUPPORT

Note

- **Basic life support** is a sequence of actions aimed at resuscitating a person whose life is in danger.

- **A person's life is in danger** when one or more of the two vital functions – breathing (respiratory function) and blood circulation (cardiac function) – have ceased or are about to cease and death is likely if proper action is not taken immediately.
- Basic life support restores the two vital functions: breathing and blood circulation. It uses an **"ABC" sequence** of actions to ensure an open **A**irway aimed at restoring **B**reathing and blood **C**irculation.
- **Cardio-pulmonary resuscitation (CPR)** is the main component of basic life support: it consists of artificial respiration and external cardiac compression.

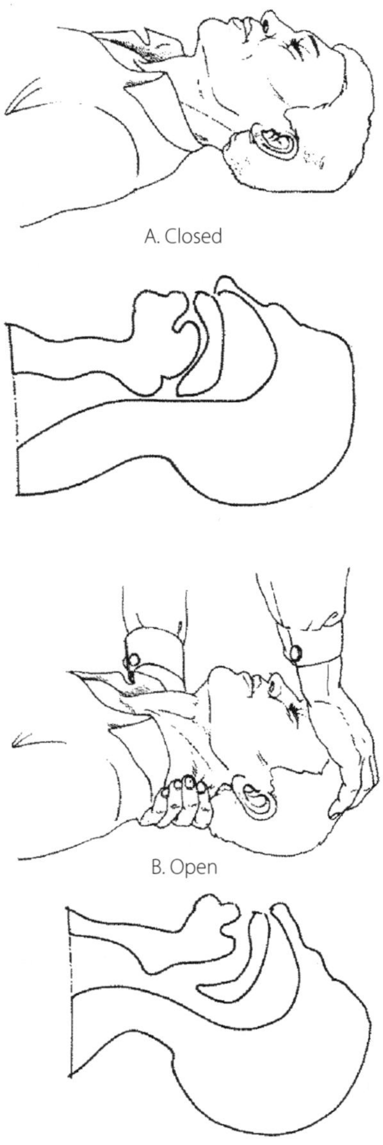

Figure 1.1 Establishing an open airway.

SHAKE AND SHOUT

- Before starting basic life support, shake the patient vigorously by the shoulder or leg and at the same time shout or call the patient's name if you know it.

AIRWAY – IF BLOCKED, OPEN IT

- Remove any loose-fitting dentures.
- Check for obvious spinal injury.
- Tilt the patient's head back by exerting pressure on the upper forehead with one hand (Figure 1.1).
- Use two fingers of the other hand to raise the chin.
- If spinal injury is suspected, tilt the head back, but only enough to keep the airway open, and pull the lower jaw forward rather than raising the chin.
- Prepare for the possibility of mouth-to-mouth rescue breathing by making sure the thumb and index finger of your hand that is on the patient's forehead are free to pinch the patient's nose.
- Use your fingers to remove any visible obstructions from the patient's mouth and throat.

BREATHING – IF STOPPED, RESTART IT

- Nook, listen, and feel for signs of regular breathing:
  - **nook** for chest movements;
  - **listen** for sounds of breathing at the patient's mouth (Figure 1.2);
  - **feel** for exhaled air on your cheek.
- If there are no signs of regular breathing:
  - send or shout for help;
  - give two rescue breaths (see below).
- If normal breathing resumes:
  - place the patient in the recovery position (Figure 1.3).
- If normal breathing does not resume:
  - check again for obstruction to the airway;

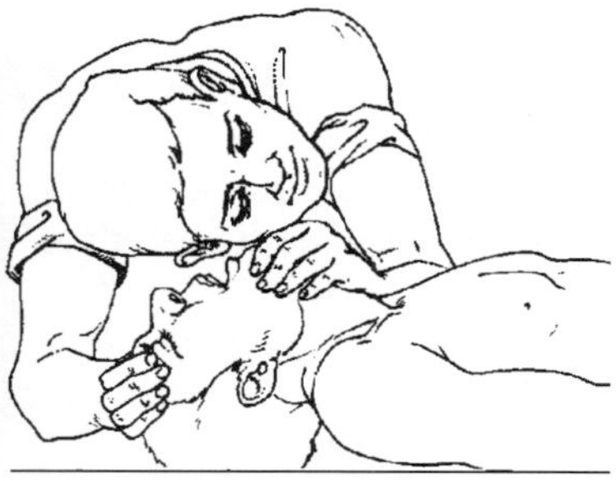

Figure 1.2 Unconscious patient: listen for breathing.

- check that the head is tilted enough and the chin raised enough;
- try again to restore breathing with two strong rescue breaths (see below).

- If normal breathing still does not resume, check the blood circulation (see next section).

CIRCULATION – IF STOPPED, RESTART IT

- Check the patient's pulse (Figure 1.4).
- If there is no detectable pulse, give chest compressions and rescue breaths (see below).
- When giving chest compression, do rescue breathing at the same time, since breathing stops when the heart stops.

Note

- **Once breathing and circulation have been restored, place the patient in the recovery position** (see below).

A BASIC LIFE SUPPORT SEQUENCE

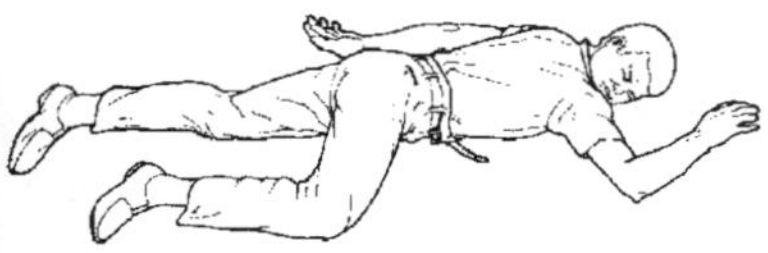

Figure 1.3 The recovery position for an unconscious patient.

- RESPONDS TO SHAKE AND SHOUT – NO.
- BREATHES – YES.
- HEART BEATS – YES:
  - put patient in recovery position (Figure 1.3)
  - check for other life-threatening conditions.
- RESPONDS TO SHAKE AND SHOUT – NO.
- BREATHES – NO.
- HEART BEATS – YES:
  - clear airway
  - apply rescue breathing.
- RESPONDS TO SHAKE AND SHOUT – NO.
- BREATHES – NO.
- HEART BEATS – NO:
  - apply cardio-pulmonary resuscitation (CPR).

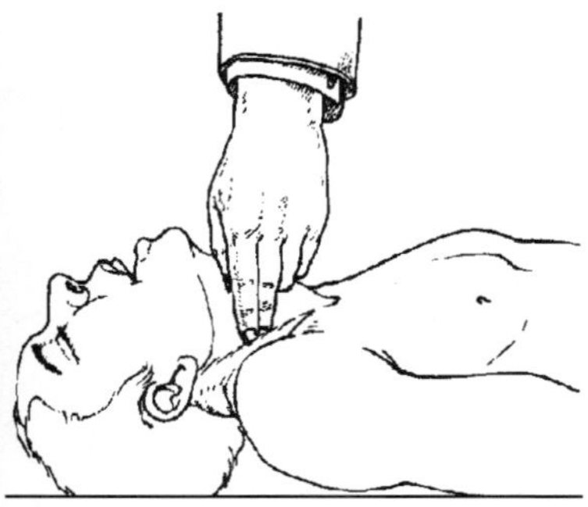

Figure 1.4 How to feel the carotid pulse.

➭ *How to perform rescue breathing (artificial respiration)*

MOUTH-TO-MOUTH RESCUE BREATHING

- With one hand under the patient's neck, keep the patient's head tilted as far back as it will go – unless you suspect spinal injury, in which case use minimal tilt.
- Place the heel of your other hand on the patient's forehead with the thumb and index finger facing towards the nose.
- Pinch the patient's nostrils with your thumb and index finger to prevent air from escaping.
- Open the patient's mouth, take a deep breath, then form a tight seal with your lips over and around the patient's mouth (Figure 1.5).

- Use a Guedel airway if available.
- Insert the Guedel airway between the patient's jaws with the concave curve facing upwards (towards the patient's head).
- Push the airway gently into the mouth while rotating it 180° so that the concave curve faces downwards and the airway points towards the patient's lungs. Leave the airway flange outside the teeth.
- If it is not possible to open the patient's mouth or to form a seal around it with your mouth, apply mouth-to-nose rescue breathing (see below).
- Breathe into the patient's mouth at a rate of one breath every five seconds or 12 breaths a minute, completely refilling your lungs after each breath.
- Continue until the patient's chest rises and falls with each rescue breath and you feel the patient's exhaled breath on your cheek (Figure 1.6).
- If you feel no air on your cheek, check if there is a foreign body in the patient's throat and, if so, remove it with your fingers before resuming rescue breathing.

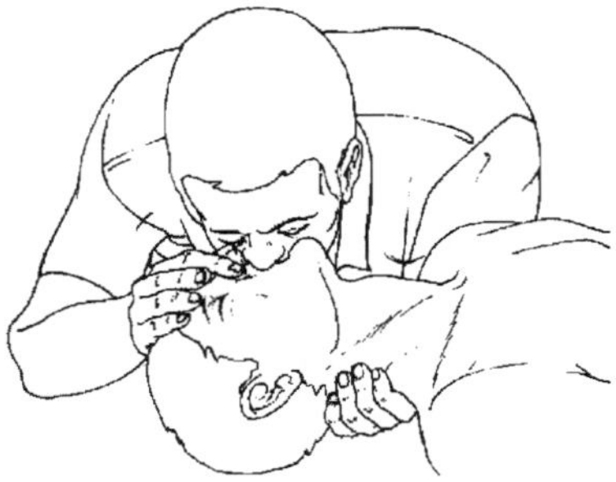

Figure 1.5 Mouth-to-mouth rescue breathing: form a tight seal around the patient's mouth and blow forcefully.

MOUTH-TO-NOSE RESCUE BREATHING

- Use mouth-to-nose rescue breathing if any one of the following conditions applies:
  - the patient's mouth cannot be opened;
  - a tight seal cannot be obtained around the patient's lips;
  - an obstruction cannot be removed from the patient's mouth;
  - the patient has been rescued from water and the rescuer needs to use one hand to support the body and is therefore unable to use that hand to close the nose for mouth-to-mouth rescue breathing.
- Keep the patient's head tilted back with one hand: use the other hand to lift the patient's lower jaw to seal the lips.
- Take a deep breath, seal your lips around the patient's nose and breathe into it forcefully and steadily until the patient's chest rises (Figure 1.7).
- Remove your mouth and allow the patient to exhale passively.
- Repeat the cycle 10–12 times per minute.

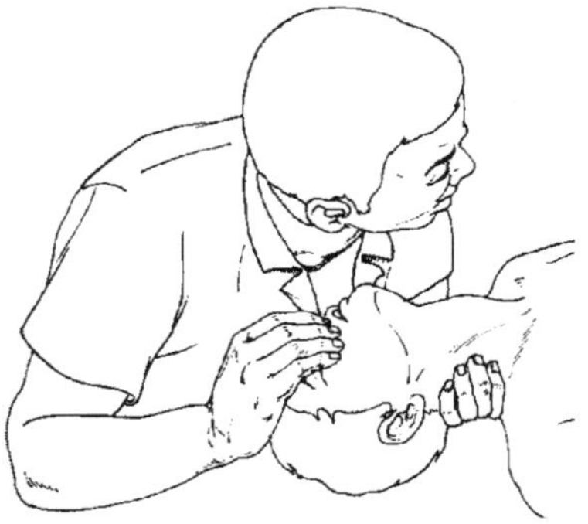

Figure 1.6 Mouth-to-mouth rescue breathing: remove your mouth and allow the patient to exhale.

USING A BAG AND MASK RESUSCITATOR

- A bag and mask resuscitator can be used for rescue breathing to replace mouth-to-mouth or mouth-to-nose breathing.
- The advantages of a bag and mask resuscitator are that a rescuer can use it for longer before becoming exhausted, and oxygen tubing can be attached to the bag.
- To use a bag and mask resuscitator:
  - lay the patient on his back;
  - check that the mask is approximately the right size for the patient;
  - insert a Guedel airway (see above);
  - send someone to bring an oxygen cylinder and attach oxygen tubing to the resuscitator: do not spend time doing this yourself, and do not wait until it has been done;
  - with one hand under the patient's neck, keep the patient's head tilted as far back as it will go – unless you suspect spinal injury, in which case use minimal tilt;

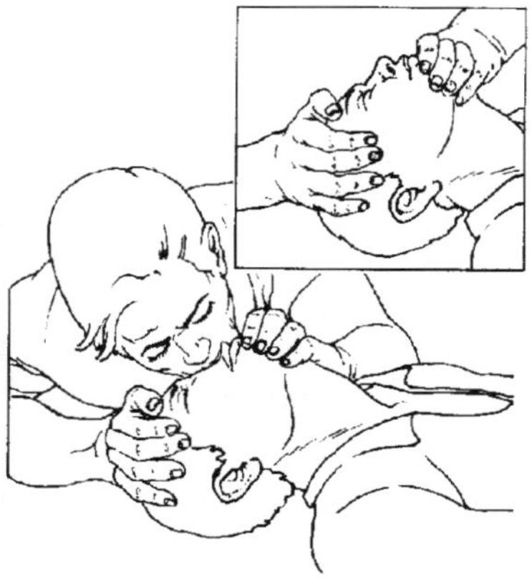

Figure 1.7 Mouth-to-nose rescue breathing.

- place the mask over the patient's nose and mouth;
- hold the mask in place with your right hand, by clamping your thumb over the mask and using your fingers to hook under the patient's jaw and pull it up towards the mask;
- use your left hand to compress the bag, forcing air into the patient's lungs;
- there is a valve which allows air to escape from the lungs when you release the bag: DO NOT take the mask off the patient's face between breaths;
- inflate the patient's lungs at a rate of about 12 per minute;
- check with each breath that there is little or no leak of air around the mask: common causes of a leak are the patient's head being turned to one side, and the jaw not being pulled upward firmly enough.

How to administer oxygen

- Note that:
  - oxygen is given to a patient who is breathing spontaneously but has difficulty breathing or has a disorder that impairs the uptake of oxygen into the lungs or the delivery of oxygen to the tissues;
  - spontaneous combustion can occur in the presence of oxygen: smoking, naked lights or fires must not be allowed where oxygen is being administered;
  - if an illness is serious enough to warrant the use of oxygen it is serious enough to seek medical advice;
  - oxygen delivered through valve and bag resuscitation kits – used primarily for victims who are not breathing – should be given only by trained personnel.
- Ensure that the airway is open.
- If the patient is unconscious, insert a Guedel airway (see above under *Mouth-to-mouth rescue breathing*).
- Check that the oxygen cylinder is not empty and that the regulator and flow meter are properly attached to the cylinder and turned off.
- Turn the main oxygen cylinder valve fully on.
- Fit the mask snugly over the patient's nose and mouth.
- Set the flow meter to the chosen rate.

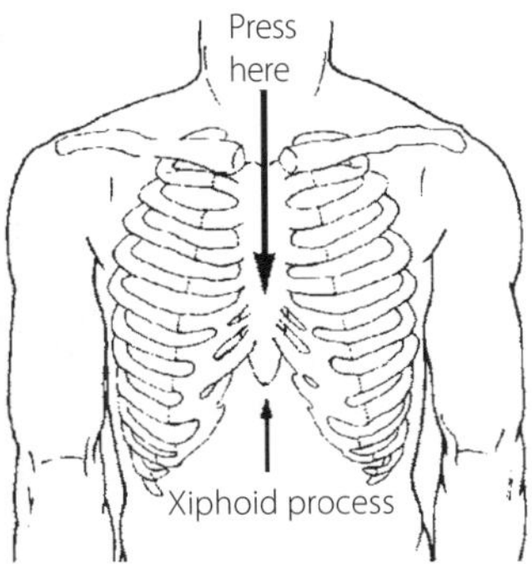

Figure 1.8 Where to press when doing chest compression.

How to perform chest compression

- Note that chest compression should always be performed in conjunction with rescue breathing: ideally, one rescuer gives chest compression and a second rescuer gives rescue breathing.
- Place the patient on a solid surface, if it is possible to do this without delay.
- Kneel at the patient's side and place your hand (**hand A**) that is closest to the patient's feet on the lower half of the patient's sternum (Figure 1.8).
- Keep the index and middle fingers of **hand A** together and with the middle finger locate the bottom edge of the lowest rib nearest to you.
- Slide both fingers medially (inwards) along this rib to the point where the rib joins the sternum.
- Place your middle finger on this point and your index finger on the sternum.

- Slide the heel of your other hand (**hand B**) down the sternum until it reaches the index finger of **hand A**: this should bring **hand B** to the middle of the lower half of the sternum or about 4 cm above the lower tip of the sternum (xiphoid process).
- Place the heel of **hand A** on top of **hand B**.
- Extend or lock together the fingers of both hands and lift them to check that you are not going to press on the patient's ribs.
- Rock forwards so that your shoulders are almost directly above the patient's chest.
- Keep your arms straight and push down on the sternum so as to depress it by 4–5 cm.
- Release the pressure but keep your hand in contact with the patient's chest.
- If you are the only rescuer, you should give 100 chest compressions per minute (one to two compressions a second) with two very quick rescue breaths after every 15 chest compressions (Figure 1.9).
- Count compressions aloud.
- Do not wait for the patient to exhale before resuming chest compressions.
- If there are two rescuers one should be at the patient's head giving one rescue breath after every five compressions, in which case chest compressions should be given at a rate of 60 per minute (if the victim is an adult): chest compressions should be continuous, with no pause for rescue breaths (Figure 1.10).
- Check the reaction of the patient's pupils:
  - if the pupils narrow (contract) when exposed to light (the light of a pocket lamp, for example), the brain is receiving adequate blood and oxygen;
  - if the pupils remain widely dilated and do not react to light, serious brain damage is imminent or has occurred.
- Check the carotid (neck) pulse after the first minute of heart compression/rescue breathing and every five minutes thereafter to see if the heart is beating spontaneously.
- If there are two rescuers they should change roles every few minutes.
- Look for other positive signs, such as:
  - expansion of the chest each time air is forced into the patient's lungs;
  - a detectable pulse each time the chest is compressed;
  - return of colour to the skin;
  - a spontaneous gasp for breath.

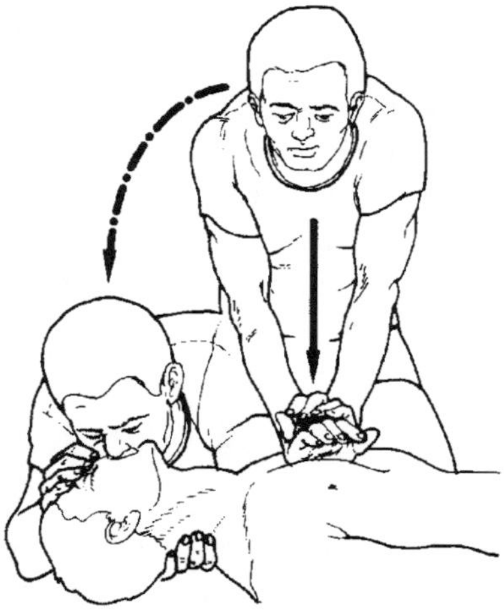

Figure 1.9 How to do chest compression with one rescuer.

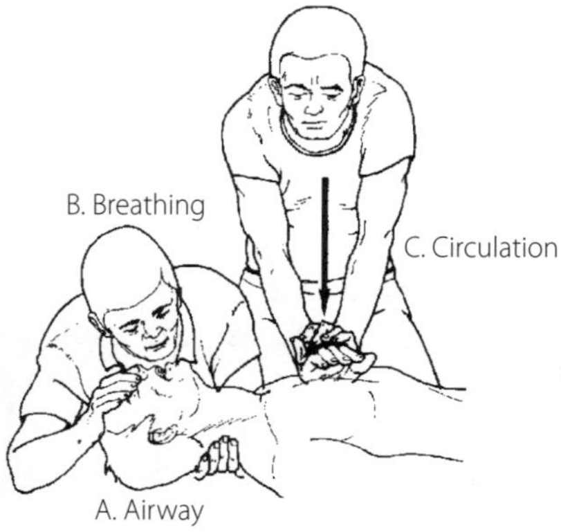

Figure 1.10 How to do chest compression with two rescuers.

✗ *What not to do when giving chest compression*

- **DO NOT START CHEST COMPRESSIONS** if the patient shows any evidence of a heart beat or pulse, even if the heart beat is very slow or very weak: in such cases, chest compression could cause dangerous abnormal heart rhythms and further complications.
- **DO NOT EXERT PRESSURE** on the lower tip of the sternum (xiphoid process) in case you tear the liver and cause severe internal bleeding.
- **DO NOT PRESS** on the patient's ribs: you risk causing rib fractures.
- **DO NOT STOP GIVING CHEST COMPRESSIONS UNTIL**:

- a physician tells you to; **OR**
- the patient's heart beat and breathing have returned; **OR**
- you are too exhausted to continue.

USE OF AUTOMATIC EXTERNAL DEFIBRILLATORS

Defibrillation is the use of a direct-current electrical shock to restore normal heart rhythm to a person whose heart has stopped pumping because it is in the abnormal rhythm ventricular fibrillation (cardiac arrest or sudden cardiac death). The Automatic External Defibrillator (AED) is a battery-powered device that detects the electrocardiogram of a person, uses a computer programme to determine whether the person's heart rhythm is ventricular fibrillation, then prompts the operator to trigger an electrical shock whose intensity is automatically adjusted by the AED.

AEDs can be used safely by people without medical training, and **if** used within 2 or 3 minutes of a cardiac arrest **and** followed up by hospital care, can improve short-term outcomes.

AEDs are not appropriate equipment for the majority of vessels. Vessels which often carry elderly passengers (who are much more likely to suffer cardiac arrest than younger people) and vessels whose operations expose crew to a risk of electrocution should consider carrying one or more AEDs. If AEDs are carried crew should be trained in their use, and in the care of patients surviving cardiac arrest.

✔ *What to do in the case of spinal injury* (for a more detailed action checklist see Chapter 6, Bone, joint, and muscle injuries, under Neck (cervical spine) injuries)

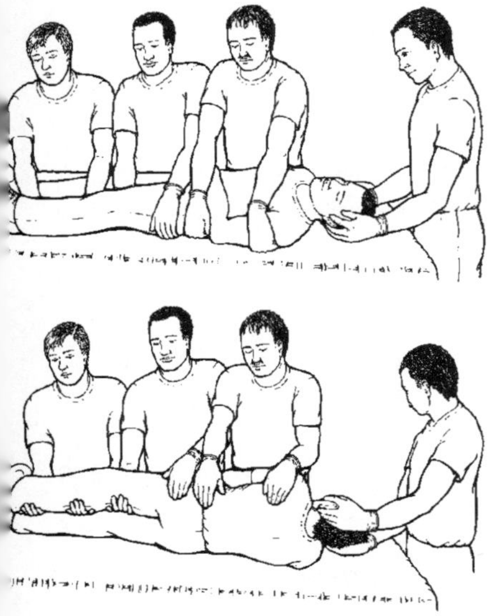

ure 1.11 How to move a patient with a spected spinal injury.

- Remember that in a patient whose spine is injured any movement, particularly extension of the neck, can cause permanent damage to the spinal cord.
- To move a patient with suspected spinal injury onto a stretcher, use the "log-rolling" manoeuvre: gently roll the patient onto the stretcher, keeping the patient's back and neck straight (Figure 1.11).
- Suspect a spinal injury if the patient meets any one of the following conditions:
  - is unconscious;
  - has fallen from a height of more than five metres;
  - has fallen on the head or heels;
  - has been struck on the head or neck;
  - has been rescued after diving into shallow water;
  - cannot move the toes when asked to;
  - complains of:
    - neck pain; **OR**
    - tingling or absence of sensation in the feet or legs.
- If any of the above conditions is met:
  - seek medical advice;
  - take particular care in handling and resuscitating the patient;
  - keep the patient's head, neck, and chest aligned;
  - use a spinal board and/or cervical collar, if available;

- keep the patient horizontal during the rescue procedure in order to minimize the consequences of low blood pressure, which is common in spinal injury.

How to apply the recovery position

- Use the recovery position for unconscious patients who are breathing and whose heart is beating: it prevents the tongue from blocking the airway and promotes drainage of fluids (blood or vomit) from the mouth, thereby reducing the risk of choking (see below).
- Make sure there are no pillows under the patient's head.
- Kneel at the side of the patient.
- Remove any fragile or potentially dangerous objects, such as glasses and loose-fitting dentures.
- Straighten the patient's legs.
- Take the patient's arm that is nearest to you and place it at right angles to the body, with the elbow bent and the hand with the palm facing up.
- Take the patient's other arm and place it across the chest so that the hand rests palm down on the cheek nearest to you.
- Place one of your hands on the patient's far shoulder, keeping the patient's hand on the cheek, and with your other hand grasp the patient's far leg just above the knee and roll the patient towards you.
- Adjust the patient's upper leg so that both the hip and the knee are bent at right angles (see Figure 1.3).
- Tilt the head back to make sure the airway remains open: use minimal tilt if you suspect a spinal injury.
- If necessary, adjust the position of the patient's hand under the cheek to keep the head tilted.
- Check regularly for breathing.
- Check blood circulation in the lower arm.
- To prevent bedsores, from time to time turn the patient gently onto the opposite side (see Chapter 26, *Nursing care and medical procedures*).
- After 12 hours of unconsciousness, administer fluid intravenously.
- Check now and again to ensure that all limbs are in mid-position – neither completely straight nor fully bent.
- Check that the eyelids remain closed at all times: if not, tape them shut to avoid damage to the eyeballs.
- Every two hours moisten the eyes with saline solution (0.9% sodium chloride) by opening the eyelids slightly and letting some saline solution drip gently into the corner of each eye.
- Every three hours moisten the mouth, cheeks, tongue, and teeth with a small swab moistened with water.

✗ What not to do when rescuing an unconscious patient

- DO NOT LEAVE THE PATIENT ALONE.
- DO NOT ALLOW THE PATIENT'S HEAD TO BEND FORWARDS with the chin sagging.

- DO NOT FORGET TO CHECK REGULARLY FOR BREATHING.
- DO NOT PULL, STRAIN, OR STRETCH ANY JOINTS.
- DO NOT GIVE ANYTHING BY MOUTH.

How to take the pulse

- Note that the best pulse to take in an emergency is the carotid (neck) pulse (see Figure 1.4).
- Use your index and middle fingers, not your thumb.
- To take the carotid (neck) pulse:
    - keep the patient's head tilted back and place your index and middle fingers on the larynx (Adam's apple);
    - slide your fingers down into the groove of the neck to the far side of the larynx.
- If you cannot feel the pulse for at least five seconds, there is too little or no blood circulation.

CHOKING

Choking is the result of an obstruction in the upper airway, either in the larynx (voice box) or trachea (windpipe). Choking prevents air from reaching the lungs and, as a result, oxygen from reaching the brain. Without immediate action, the patient loses consciousness. A complete obstruction of the airway is immediately life-threatening: if the obstruction or constriction is not removed, the patient will suffer brain damage and die within four to six minutes.

An obstruction of the upper airway may be caused by:

- a solid or semi-solid object, such as food, a foreign body, or a blood clot:
    - an inadequately chewed piece of meat is a very common cause of choking: in a third of cases the meat lodges above the vocal cords; in two thirds of cases it passes through the vocal cords and lodges in the trachea;
- an external constricting force, as in strangulation or hanging;
- swelling of the tissue lining the upper airway: this can be due to:
    - an allergic mechanism, as occurs with asthma or an insect sting;
    - the irritant or burning effect of gas fumes or smoke.

✔ *What to do*

- Suspect choking in a person:
    - whose skin turns blue or purple; **OR**
    - who cannot speak or breathe but only gasp; **OR**
    - who clutches the throat with one or both hands (a universal sign for choking), especially in mid-meal; **OR**
    - whose attempts to breathe in or out produce coughing or wheezing or whistling sounds.
- If you suspect that food or a foreign body is blocking the airway:
    - try to unblock the airway (see above, under *Basic life support*);
    - encourage the patient to cough;
    - if the patient cannot cough, perform the Heimlich manoeuvre (see below);

- do not attempt to hook the obstructing body out with a finger: you are likely to push it in further and worsen the obstruction.

How to perform the Heimlich manoeuvre (*abdominal thrusts*)

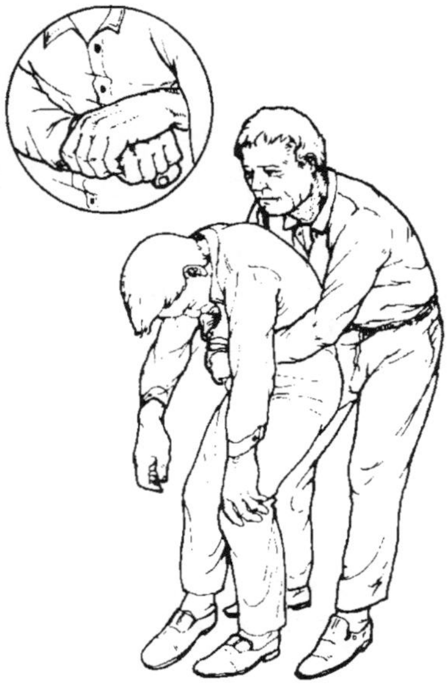

Figure 1.12 How to do the Heimlich manoeuvre on a standing patient.

IN A CONSCIOUS PATIENT

- Stand behind the patient and wrap your arms around the patient's waist.
- Make a fist with one hand and place it on the patient's abdomen between the navel and the rib cage (Figure 1.12).
- Grasp your fist with your other hand and bend the patient slightly forwards (if need be, using for support the back of a chair, corner of a table, or other protruding object).
- Keeping your arms away from the patient's rib cage, give four or five quick inward and upward thrusts to make the patient cough.
- Repeat these abdominal thrusts until the obstructing object is coughed out.

IN AN UNCONSCIOUS PATIENT

- Lay the patient down face up, head to one side.
- Kneel astride the patient's hips.
- Place one of your hands on top of the other, with the palm of the lower hand on the patient's abdomen, just above the navel (Figure 1.13).
- With the heel of the lower hand, make rapid inward and upward thrusts.
- Repeat this sequence until the obstructing object is ejected.

ON YOURSELF

- Put your fist on your upper abdomen, just above the navel.
- Grasp your fist with the other hand.
- Thrust your fist inwards and upwards; **OR**:
  - bend over a hard object with a protruding point (chair, wash-basin, etc.) and force your fist upwards into your upper abdomen.

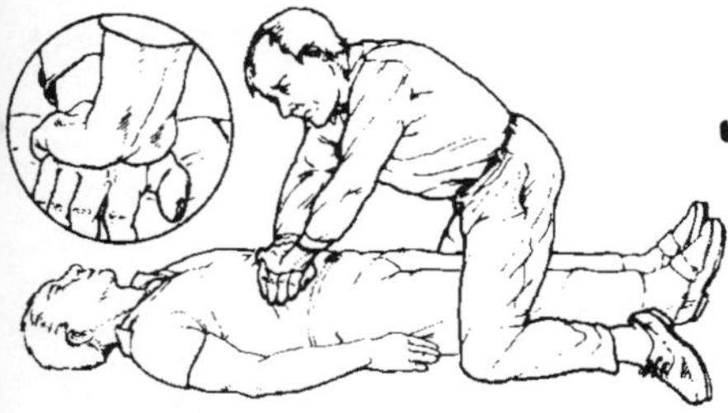

Figure 1.13 How to do the Heimlich manoeuvre on an unconscious patient.

✔ *What to do in a case of hanging or strangulation*

- Cut the rope and lay the patient on a firm, flat surface.
- If breathing has stopped, start cardio-pulmonary resuscitation (see above).
- Give oxygen, six litres per minute, using a non-rebreathing mask.
- Seek medical advice.

BLEEDING

Bleeding is the result of damage to blood vessels. The damage can be due to trauma or disease, such as peptic ulcer. Breaks in very small blood vessels occur all the time in healthy people and if the clotting system is abnormal there can be spontaneous bleeding.

KEY QUESTIONS

- Where is the bleeding coming from?
- What effect is the bleeding having on the patient?
- What can be done to stop the bleeding?

BLEEDING WOUNDS

✔ *What to do*

- Put on gloves and eye protection, if possible.
- Apply direct pressure to the wound with a dressing or piece of cloth or just the palm of your hand (Figure 1.14).
- Maintain the pressure for 10 minutes, the time it takes for the blood clotting process to produce a stable plug that stops the bleeding.
- If bleeding is from the arm or leg, elevating the limb above the level of the heart will slow the bleeding.
- When the bleeding has stopped, move the patient to a place with good lighting and facilities for closing and dressing the wound.
- Take the patient's pulse and blood pressure with the patient lying down and then standing up.
- If bleeding restarts, the blood clot has probably been displaced: reapply pressure and wait 10 minutes for more clot to form.
- Clean up the blood, and dispose of all contaminated personal protective equipment in an appropriate container marked for bio-hazardous waste.
- Seek medical advice if there is a rapid pulse that persists after the bleeding has stopped or a fall in blood pressure when the patient stands up: the patient may be developing hypovolaemic shock (see Chapter 2, *Shock*)
- Remember that faintness can be due to pain and fear as well as to blood loss.

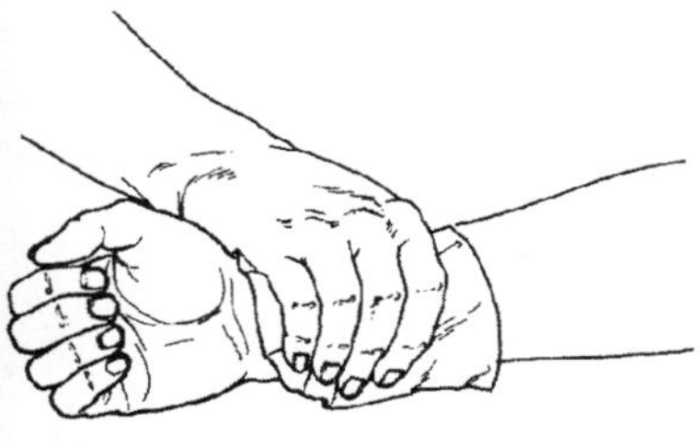

Figure 1.14 How to apply pressure to the wound.

✘ *What not to do*

- Do not stop pressing on the wound during the first 10 minutes to see if it has stopped bleeding.
- Do not remove a dressing if blood is seeping through it: place another dressing on top of the first one.
- Do not use a tourniquet or attempt to apply pressure to large arteries (at so-called pressure points).
- Do not attempt to clip bleeding arteries with forceps: you will not succeed in stopping the bleeding because the process of contraction that narrows the vessel also pulls it back into the wound and you are likely to damage surrounding structures, such as nerves.
- Do not try to estimate the volume of blood loss by looking at the puddle of blood: blood on the floor always looks alarmingly copious.

BLEEDING FROM THE NOSE

Although in most cases the diagnosis is obvious, in some cases, the blood from a nose bleed passes into the throat, is swallowed, and may be vomited.

Causes of nose bleed include:

- a blow to the face from a fist or blunt object;
- nose picking, usually in children;
- local infection and allergy;
- high blood pressure;
- hardening of an artery (arteriosclerosis) in older patients.

✔ *What to do*

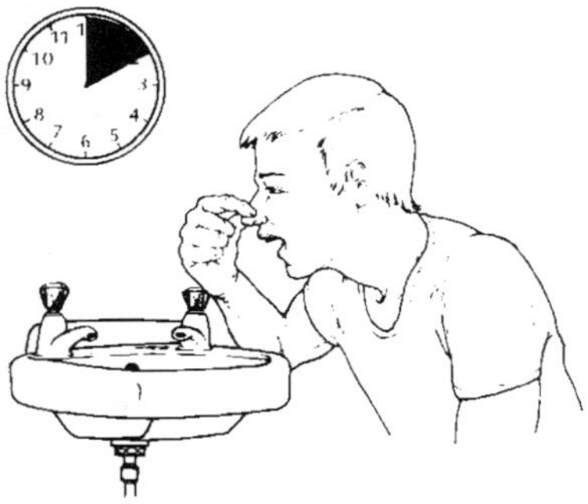

Figure 1.15 How to treat a nose bleed.

- Moisten a small gauze square with nasal decongestant spray and place it gently into the bleeding nostril.
- Have the patient compress the soft part of the nose firmly for 10 minutes without stopping: the fingers and thumb should cover the whole area below the bony parts (Figure 1.15).
- Have the patient sit bending forwards, so as not to swallow blood, and spit into a bowl any blood that drips into the throat.
- Seek medical advice if:
  - bleeding lasts more than 30 minutes; **OR**
  - bleeding is profuse; **OR**
  - bleeding cannot be stopped by the above measures; **OR**
  - the patient's blood pressure begins to fall; **OR**
  - the patient cannot sit up because of faintness.
- When the bleeding has stopped take the patient's blood pressure; if it is over 160 systolic seek medical advice.

Shock

In medicine, the term "shock" refers to a life-threatening condition affecting the body as a whole and involving a severe, long-lasting decline in the delivery of blood to the tissues. The reduction in blood flow to the tissues starves the cells of the nutrients carried in the blood, most critically oxygen and, if it continues long enough, the cells cease to function normally and eventually die.

The three main causes of shock are:

- a fall in blood volume to a critically low level (hypovolaemic shock):
  - hypovolaemic shock can be caused by bleeding (for whatever reason) or by dehydration: bleeding is likely to be the commonest cause on board ship;
- inadequate pumping of blood by the heart (cardiogenic shock):
  - cardiogenic shock can occur with any severe disease of the heart but myocardial infarction is by far the commonest cause;
- failure of the small blood vessels to provide adequate control of blood distribution to the tissues (distributive shock):
  - distributive shock is commonly due to:
    - severe infection (the commonest cause, in which case it is known as septic shock);
    - severe inflammatory disease, such as pancreatitis (see Chapter 16, *Gastrointestinal and liver diseases*);
    - anaphylaxis, which is a form of distributive shock that occurs very suddenly and its cause is usually obvious (see Chapter 31, *Anatomy and physiology*, and Chapter 33, *The ship's medicine chest*).

Note

- In medical terminology, "shock" does **not** (as it may in common usage) refer to:
  - a problem caused by blockage to major blood vessels;
  - a short-term drop in blood pressure, such as can occur in fainting;
  - a strong emotional response (e.g. fear) to danger.
- Low blood pressure does not necessarily mean that the patient is in shock: children and young, especially pregnant, women often have low blood pressure (as low as 90 mmHg systolic) although they are perfectly healthy.
- Cardiogenic and severe distributive shock are often fatal, even with the best modern hospital care.
- Hypovolaemic shock, in contrast, can often be reversed if treated early and vigorously.
- The body can deal with a degree of blood loss or severe infection, and, for a time, even with very severe blood loss or infection, especially if the patient is young and was previously healthy. This condition, in which the body's systems are under stress but still coping, is called "compensated shock". If blood loss continues or the infection is not treated the body's coping mechanisms are overwhelmed, and full-blown, or "de-compensated" shock can develop quickly.

Signs and symptoms

- In a case of compensated shock:
  - rapid pulse;
  - cool, pale skin (because the body is re-directing blood away from the skin towards the heart and brain);

- in some cases, normal or slightly low blood pressure (with the patient lying down, but blood pressure falls markedly when the patient is standing).

- In a case of full-blown shock:
  - very sick appearance;
  - low systolic blood pressure (typically less than 90 mmHg or, if it was previously high, more than 40 mmHg below the previous blood pressure reading);
  - cool and clammy skin;
  - low urine output (blood is shunted away from the kidneys);
  - confusion or delirium (as the body's attempts to maintain adequate blood flow to the brain begin to fail).
- In a case of distributive shock caused by infection:
  - low blood pressure;
  - pale, cool, and clammy skin;
  - low urine output;
  - fever;
  - evidence of the underlying infectious disease;
  - as shock progresses, reduced blood flow to many tissues produces:
    - confusion and delirium;
    - worsening failure of the heart, causing further falls in blood pressure and breathlessness, and of the kidneys, with further falls in urine output.

KEY QUESTIONS

- **Has there been blood loss? If so, suspect hypovolaemic shock**:
  - bleeding may be external and therefore readily visible;
  - a patient may vomit blood or pass blood rectally in the toilet during the night and be found next morning in bed in a state of shock;
  - always do a rectal examination to look for blood (see Chapter 16, *Gastrointestinal and liver diseases*).
- Is there evidence of heart disease? If so, suspect cardiogenic shock:
  - cardiogenic shock typically results from myocardial infarction, so the patient will normally be over 50 and will have been suffering from chest pain for over 30 minutes before developing shock;
  - check carefully for abnormal heart rhythm.
- Is there evidence of infection? If so, suspect septic shock:
  - the patient will normally have been very sick for 24–48 hours before the onset of septic shock, unless the infection is meningococcal (see Chapter 23, *Infectious diseases*), in which case shock can develop in a few hours: the presence of a rash suggests meningococcal infection;
  - fever will be present in the early stages but may be mild or absent once shock develops;
  - common sites of infection leading to septic shock are the urinary tract, the bowel and gallbladder, and the lungs.

✔ *What to do*

- In hypovolaemic shock:
  - note that you are very unlikely, on board, to save the life of a patient with cardiogenic or septic shock but with vigorous treatment you can save the life of a patient with hypovolaemic shock;
  - stop any external bleeding with pressure;
  - if the patient is conscious, to improve blood supply to the brain, have the patient lie flat with legs raised 25–35 cm;
  - if the patient is unconscious, place in the recovery, or coma, position (see Chapter 1, *First aid*);
  - give oxygen, six litres per minute, using a non-rebreathing mask;
  - insert an intravenous cannula (see Chapter 26, *Nursing care and medical procedures*);
  - give two litres of normal saline (0.9% sodium chloride solution) as rapidly as possible: this should take 20–30 minutes; if the fluid is flowing more slowly insert another cannula;
  - if there is severe pain from injuries, give morphine, 2.5–5.0 mg intravenously, at once, then after the first two litres of fluid – and **only then** – give 2.5 mg intravenously, every 10 minutes until pain is controlled;
  - seek medical advice **at this point** (but not before – your priority is to treat the patient) with a view to evacuating the patient;
  - until evacuation, continue giving normal saline at a rapid rate until blood pressure rises to 90 mmHg systolic; then give one litre every six hours.
- In cardiogenic shock:
  - sit the patient upright in bed, even if consciousness is impaired;
  - give oxygen at the highest possible flow rate, using a non-rebreathing mask;
  - give frusemide, 40 mg intravenously if possible, or intramuscularly;
  - give morphine, 10 mg intravenously if possible, or intramuscularly;
  - give aspirin, 150 mg orally;
  - seek medical advice at this point: over the next 30 minutes to one hour the patient will either improve or die, so no risks should be run to achieve urgent evacuation;
  - note that in a patient with cardiogenic shock, aggressive fluid replacement will usually worsen the condition: however, if you are treating a patient you believe to have hypovolaemic or distributive shock, do not withhold fluid replacement for fear of causing harm if the patient really has cardiogenic shock.
- In distributive shock:
  - if shock develops in the course of a severe established illness, such as an infection or pancreatitis, treat for that condition (see *What to do* section in the appropriate chapter); **IN ADDITION TREAT AS FOLLOWS:**
    - › insert an intravenous cannula;
    - › give two litres of normal saline (0.9% sodium chloride solution), as rapidly as possible, then one litre every four to six hours to keep blood pressure above 90 mmHg;

  - give ceftriaxone, 2 g intravenously, and then, beginning at 08:00 the next day, give ceftriaxone, 1 g intravenously, twice daily (if you are already giving other antibiotics for infection, stop them);
  - arrange for evacuation.
- If there is shock without apparent bleeding but with a rash or fever, treat as follows:
  - insert an intravenous cannula;
  - give ceftriaxone, 2 g intravenously, then, beginning at 08:00 or 20:00, whichever is first, give ceftriaxone, 1 g intravenously, twice daily;
  - give one litre of normal saline (0.9% sodium chloride solution) as rapidly as possible, then one litre every six hours;
  - give oxygen, six litres per minute, using a non-rebreathing mask;
  - seek medical advice with a view to evacuation.

✗ *What not to do in shock*

- Do not delay treatment.
- Do not under-treat because you are unsure of the diagnosis.
- Do not give sedatives or alcohol.
- Do not give anything by mouth to a patient with impaired consciousness.
- Do not give anything by mouth if surgery is likely to take place within the next six hours.

Pain management

Pain is the result of the way in which the brain – and consequently the mind or consciousness – interprets information about a sensation that the body is experiencing. The brain receives the information in the form of signals that travel via nerve pathways to the brain. The sensation itself may originate in a tissue such as the skin or a bone, or in an internal organ, or even somewhere along the nerve pain pathways. How the brain receives or reacts to these signals to produce the perception of "pain" can be affected by many factors; for example:

- stress or anxiety can make the mind more sensitive to pain, which is then experienced more intensely;
- inflammation of nerve pathways can make them more sensitive, again with the result that the pain is experienced more intensely;
- pain can be made worse by prolonged stimulation and consequent sensitization of the nerve pain pathways (this type of pain is sometimes called "wind-up pain"): in this situation, the pain is producing more pain.

There are two main types of pain: nociceptive pain and neuropathic pain:

- nociceptive pain, which arises from injury to tissues, is the more common type. nociceptive nerve endings (nociceptors) in the tissues respond to damage or inflammation. The pain signals from the nociceptors travel along the nerve pain pathways to the spinal cord and then to the brain.
- There are three types of nociceptive pain:
  - superficial nociceptive pain arising from skin;
  - deep nociceptive pain arising from deep tissues, such as bone;
  - visceral nociceptive pain arising from internal organs (viscera).
- Neuropathic pain arises from abnormal functioning of the nerve pain pathways without any injury to tissues.

See Table 3.1 for a schematic summary of the different types of pain.

Note on assessing the severity of pain

- Although there are cultural and individual differences in the way people react to pain, these differences should not be taken into account when assessing pain severity: the pain that needs to be managed is the pain that the patient complains of.
- A patient may have pain in more than one place, especially after an injury, and should be questioned about each pain separately: a diagram of the body with each painful place marked on it can help to keep track of different pains in an ill or injured patient.
- A patient who answers a question about the severity of pain should be asked to specify whether the answer refers to the pain being experienced at that moment in the present or to a time in the past when the pain was at its worst, or simply to the general severity of the pain.
- It may be helpful to know not only how severe the pain is but also how distressing or bearable it is to the patient or how bad it makes the patient feel. Words such as "excruciating", "cruel", or "agonising" are often used in cases of visceral pain, but less often by patients with pain from a fracture. Neuropathic pain is often experienced as particularly unpleasant and distressing and difficult to describe in words.
- To assess the severity of pain in children or patients whose mother tongue is not understood by anyone on board, the *FACES pain scale* (Figure 3.1) can be useful.

Table 3.1 The characteristics of different types of pain.

	Superficial nociceptive pain	Deep nociceptive pain	Visceral nociceptive pain	Neuropathic pain
Arising from	■ skin ■ lining of mouth ■ anus ■ urethra	■ bones ■ joints ■ muscles ■ ligaments ■ linings, such as pleura and peritoneum	■ solid or hollow internal organs	■ pain pathways
Described as	■ sharp ■ hot ■ stinging	■ dull ■ aching ■ throbbing	■ dull ■ aching ■ cramping	■ burning ■ shooting ■ pins-and–needles ■ pain in numb areas
Localized	■ very clearly defined ■ never spreads to other areas	■ well-defined but spreads to other areas	■ poorly defined and spreads to other areas	■ well-defined but does not usually spread to other areas
Movement	■ has no effect on pain	■ makes pain worse, so patient lies still	■ may relieve pain	■ does not affect pain unless movement stretches the nerve and then makes the pain worse
Tenderness	■ marked	■ marked	■ not usually present	■ not present, but normal stimuli may provoke pain
Nausea, vomiting, sweating	■ do not occur	■ occasional, if pain is severe	■ common	■ uncommon

✔ *What to do – in general*

- Develop a strategy that takes into account the patient's needs and that may well go beyond the administration of analgesics to include alternative or additional options, such as:
  - application of local heat, which can reduce the severity of pain associated with inflammation;
  - application of icepacks to a painful injury within the first 48 hours of its occurrence:
    - › apply icepacks for 10 minutes every two hours (but **NEVER** directly on the skin) then firmly bandage and have the patient elevate the injured part.

- Use analgesic drugs for severe injuries, such as fractures, and for painful illnesses (see section below, on individual analgesics).
- Administer doses of analgesic by the clock, i.e. in accordance with the decided dosage schedule: the aim is to avoid the pain becoming severe before the next dose of analgesic is administered.
- In choosing an analgesic drug from the ship's medicine chest – acetylsalicylic acid (Aspirin®), paracetamol, ibuprofen, tramadol, and morphine (in order of increasing analgesic potency) – consider:
  - **how severe the patient's pain is** (see Fig. 3.1);
  - **how to achieve, for a given patient, the right balance** between relief of pain and unwanted drug effects; note:
    - complete relief of severe pain is not usually possible without unwanted effects, such as sedation (drowsiness), but in some cases a higher level of sedation may be acceptable to achieve better pain control, and in others more pain may be accepted by the patient in order to maintain alertness;
  - **what the mechanism of the pain is**; note:
    - if inflammation is a major factor in the cause of pain, paracetamol will be ineffective but ibuprofen may be effective alone and will increase the effectiveness of stronger analgesics;
  - **how long the severe pain is likely to last;** note:
    - severe pain usually lasts for two to three days after a major fracture;
  - **whether or not the patient can swallow medication**:
    - if the patient cannot swallow medication, morphine is the only option;
  - **whether there are contraindications** to using any of the available drugs; such as:
    - a known peptic ulcer (do not give aspirin or ibuprofen);
    - the likelihood of surgery (do not give aspirin);
    - current use of anti-depressant drugs (do not give tramadol).
- To assess the effectiveness of whatever method of pain relief you are using:
  - use the *Faces pain scale* (Fig. 3.1) or any similar scale; **OR**
  - ask the patient to grade pain as:
    - none
    - mild
    - moderate but bearable

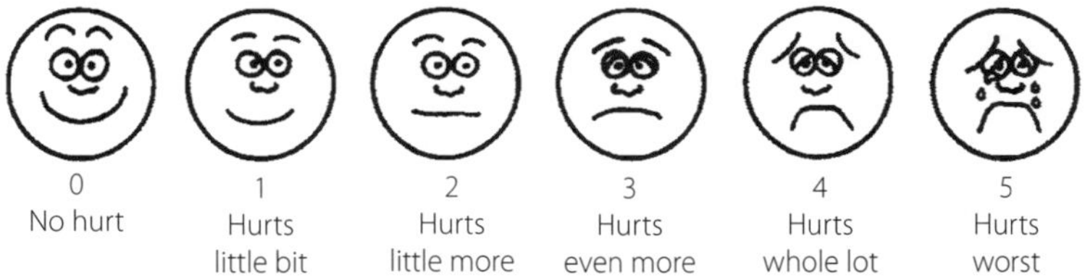
0
No hurt
1
Hurts little bit
2
Hurts little more
3
Hurts even more
4
Hurts whole lot
5
Hurts worst

Figure 3.1 FACES pain scale. In: Hockenberry MJ, Wilson D, Winkelstein ML. *Wong's Essentials of Pediatric Nursing,* 7th ed., St. Louis, Mosby Inc., 2005: 1259. Used with permission. Copyright, Mosby.

› severe
› unbearable.

- Note that "effective analgesia" or "control of pain" means a reduction of at least two levels in the patient's perception of the severity of pain.

✔ ***What to do in specific circumstances*** **(see section below on How to use the analgesics in the medicine chest, for details on individual analgesics)**

ANALGESIA IN CHILDREN

- Apply the same principles of analgesia as you would in adults: note that pain in children is often neglected or under-treated.
- Give morphine to a child if you would give it to an adult with the same injury or illness.
- Base the dose of analgesic, especially of morphine, on the child's body weight (see Table 3.2).
- Do not give acetylsalicylic acid (Aspirin®) to a patient under 18.

ANALGESIA IN PREGNANT WOMEN

- You can give morphine to a pregnant woman, although if you do so at a time close to delivery there is a risk of respiratory depression in the newborn baby:
  - to treat a baby with respiratory depression, give naloxone, 0.01 mg/kg body weight subcutaneously;
  - note that this dose is too small to be measured accurately using the naloxone ampoule available on board ship;
  - a naloxone ampoule contains 0.4 mg in 1ml: draw this up into a 5 ml syringe and add 3 ml water for injection; 1 ml of this solution contains 0.1 mg naloxone and the neonatal dose will then be about 0.3 ml.

Table 3.2 Starting doses of morphine given subcutaneously or intramuscularly for severe pain.

Patient's age (years)	Dose	Frequency
<16	0.05–0.1 mg per kg body weight	every 4 hours
16–39	7.5–12.5 mg	every 2 hours
40–59	5–10 mg	every 2 hours
60–69	2.5–7.5 mg	every 2 hours
>69	2.5–5 mg	every 2–3 hours

Small- and average-sized patients should first be given the dose at the lower end of the range, increasing to the higher end of the range if pain is not controlled after the second dose. Large patients should be given doses at the higher end of the range.

- Do not give tramadol to a pregnant woman: experience of its use in pregnancy is still limited.
- You can give ibuprofen to a pregnant woman or to a woman who is breast-feeding her baby but only for occasional or short-term use.

ANALGESIA IN OPIOID-DEPENDENT PATIENTS

- Note that opioid-dependent patients may require large doses of morphine if they have developed tolerance to the drug because of **current** use of **injected** opioid (see Chapter 22, *Tobacco, alcohol, and drug use*).
- You have no way of assessing in advance the degree of tolerance a patient may have developed to morphine: therefore, do not start with high doses, even if you think they may be necessary to control the pain.
- If possible, use the intravenous dose titration method to determine the dose of morphine required: give 5 mg intravenously, adding 5 mg increments every 10 minutes until pain is controlled. The total dose needed to control pain can then be given intramuscularly or intravenously every three to four hours.
- If it is not possible to determine the required dose, seek medical advice and begin treatment with intramuscular doses at the higher end of the recommended range (see Table 3.2).

✗ *What not to do*

- Do not delay treatment of patients with severe pain while you seek medical advice about the possible diagnosis: if you first do something to lessen the patient's pain you will learn much more about his illness and give the medical service a better chance of helping you reach a diagnosis.
- Do not start treatment with weak analgesics in a patient obviously suffering from severe pain.
- The starting dose for paracetamol or ibuprofen should be the normal full dose; if pain is not controlled after two doses switch to tramadol or morphine.
- Do not give the patient a dose of analgesic lower than the recommended dose unless the patient is too drowsy on the recommended dose.
- Do not increase the recommended intervals between doses of analgesic, especially when the patient is in severe pain and is on morphine (see below).
- Do not wait, after beginning treatment of a patient with severe pain, for the pain to become severe again before giving additional doses of analgesic.

How to use the analgesics in the medicine chest (see also Chapter 33, *The ship's medicine chest*)

DRUG COMBINATIONS (see section below on individual analgesics)

- For severe pain associated with inflammatory conditions (e.g. pleurisy) or with fractures, the most useful combination is ibuprofen plus morphine.

- For pain arising from solid organs, such as the liver, paracetamol plus morphine is sometimes useful but in patients in whom inflammation is contributing to the pain paracetamol will not help.
- Tramadol and morphine should not be given together.

PARACETAMOL

- Paracetamol is the first choice of analgesic for mild pain and for reducing fever.
- It is similar in analgesic efficacy to acetylsalicylic acid but generally preferred because it is less likely to cause bleeding from the stomach.
- The usual initial dose to relieve pain is two 500 mg tablets every six hours up to a maximum of 4 g per day.
- Pain relief is noticeable after 20 minutes.
- At normal doses unwanted effects are rare but giving a single dose of 10–15 g can cause fatal liver damage.

ACETYLSALICYLIC ACID (ASPIRIN®)

- Acetylsalicylic acid has long been used for the management of mild-to-moderate pain, such as headache, musculoskeletal pain, menstrual cramps, and for reducing fever, but paracetamol is usually a better choice (see preceding paragraph).
- The usual dose is 600–1000 mg every four hours.
- Unwanted effects at normal doses are generally mild: the most common include stomach irritation with slight blood loss, skin reactions in allergic patients, and increased bleeding time (i.e. the time it takes for bleeding from a small cut to stop).

IBUPROFEN

- Ibuprofen is a nonsteroidal anti-inflammatory drug (NSAID) but has fewer unwanted effects than other NSAIDs and can reduce both pain and inflammation.
- Ibuprofen is used in the treatment of mild-to-moderate pain, especially pain of musculoskeletal origin.
- The usual initial dose of ibuprofen is 800 mg three to four times daily up to a maximum of 3.2 g per day.
- Ibuprofen takes effect 30–40 minutes after taking a dose.
- The commonest unwanted effects of ibuprofen are nausea and vomiting.
- Other important unwanted effects are kidney failure, fluid retention (oedema), and allergic reactions.
- NSAIDs should not be given to patients with stomach problems or kidney disease without consulting a doctor.

TRAMADOL

- Tramadol is an opioid with a low potential for abuse.
- It is used for moderate pain, for which it is as effective as morphine; it is not as effective as morphine for severe pain.

- The usual initial dose of tramadol is 100 mg every eight hours up to a maximum of 400 mg per day.
- The unwanted effects of tramadol are typical of opioids – drowsiness, a sense of relaxation and dissociation, small pupils, reduced respiratory rate, slurred speech, impaired mental function – but the drug causes constipation less often than other opioids.
- Tramadol can cause dangerous respiratory depression in higher than recommended doses; note:
  - naloxone, the usual opioid antidote, reverses the respiratory depression caused by an overdose of tramadol but may precipitate fits.
- The effect of tramadol, which is noticeable about an hour after taking a dose, peaks at two to four hours and lasts six to eight hours.
- Tramadol should not be used in patients with epilepsy, in whom it can provoke fits.
- Tramadol should not be used in patients taking anti-depressant drugs.

MORPHINE (AMPOULES)

- Morphine is an opiate (i.e. extracted from the opium poppy) analgesic drug that is effective for severe pain.
- Morphine should not be used in a patient:
  - in coma, unless the patient is dying of a clearly-documented illness such as cancer;
  - with severe liver disease;
  - with severe respiratory disease, except for pneumonia or pleurisy causing severe pain.
- Morphine should not be used in a patient:
  - known to have epilepsy;
  - with a head injury;
  - in acute alcohol intoxication or withdrawal (see Chapter 22, *Tobacco, alcohol, and drug use*);
  - with asthma;
  - with shock, of whatever cause (see Chapter 2, *Shock*).
- The effect of morphine is intensified by simultaneous use of NSAIDs, such as ibuprofen (see above) but not if the pain arises from internal organs.
- Severe pain encountered on board ship is likely to remain severe for at least 12–24 hours and will require repeated doses of morphine: exceptions may be a dislocated shoulder (see Chapter 6, *Bone, joint, and muscle injuries*) which can be reduced, or an episode of biliary colic (see Chapter 16, *Gastrointestinal and liver diseases*).
- Morphine is more likely to be effective if small doses are given frequently than if large doses are given infrequently.
- There are several different salts of morphine (morphine sulfate, morphine tartrate, and morphine hydrochloride): the dose is the same for all.
- When morphine can be given:
  - orally: the effect is noticeable in about one hour and lasts about four hours:

  - 20 mg of morphine given orally is approximately equivalent to 10 mg given intramuscularly;
  - oral morphine is preferred to injections for patients who are eating or drinking normally, especially if the morphine is likely to be needed for more than two or three days;
- by intravenous injection: the effect is noticeable almost immediately and lasts two to three hours;
- by intramuscular injection: the effect is noticeable in 10–15 minutes and lasts two to three hours;
- by subcutaneous injection: the effect is noticeable in 10–15 minutes and lasts two to three hours:
  - subcutaneous injections are appropriate for long-term treatment in patients who cannot swallow but are not recommended for immediate pain relief.

Starting doses of morphine

- **Given by subcutaneous or intramuscular injection**, see Table 3.2 or use the intravenous dose titration method, as follows:
  - 5 mg of morphine should be given intravenously then 5-mg increments should be added intravenously every 10 minutes until pain is controlled; the total dose needed to control pain can then be given intravenously or intramuscularly every three to four hours.
- **Given orally,** every four hours, the starting dose of morphine should be about 50% higher than the three- to four-hourly intramuscular dose (see Table 3.2.) or than the dose determined by the intravenous dose titration method described above.

Assessing the effectiveness of morphine analgesia

- Use the sedation score (Table 3.3) to decide whether the morphine dose should be reduced.
- If, after the second dose, pain is relieved but not fully under control, ask the patient whether the effect is adequate 30 minutes to one hour after receiving the dose, even though the pain returns before the next dose is due.
- If the analgesic effect is adequate at 30–60 minutes but the pain returns before the next dose is due, the interval between doses should be reduced.
- If the analgesic effect is inadequate at 30–60 minutes, the dose should be increased.
- In a patient with a fracture, if the pain is well-controlled when the patient is resting but "breaks through" when the patient has to be moved, small "top-up" doses of morphine (e.g. 5 mg intramuscularly or intravenously) should be given 10–15 minutes before the patient has to be moved.

Unwanted or adverse effects of morphine

- Common unwanted effects of morphine are:
  - respiratory depression:
    - this is the most dangerous adverse effect of morphine;
    - counting the respiratory rate is not a reliable method of assessing respiratory depression; and

Table 3.3 The sedation score (adapted from the *Australian Medicines Handbook,* 2006).

- 0 – fully alert
- S – normal sleep: in assessing whether the patient is sleeping normally or is deeply sedated observe whether:
  - the patient's posture is that of normal sleep;
  - the time of day and the surroundings are conducive to sleep
- 1 – mild sedation: occasionally drowsy, easy to rouse
- 2 – moderate sedation: constantly drowsy (e.g. falls asleep while talking) but easy to rouse
- 3 – deep sedation: sleeping and difficult to rouse

The use of analgesics should aim to keep the score, ideally, at 1; if the score is 2, subsequent doses should be reduced by 25%; if the score is 3, the next dose should be omitted and subsequent doses reduced by 50%.

  - the likelihood of respiratory depression is best indicated by the degree of sedation, assessed using the sedation score (Table 3.3).
- constipation:
  - this occurs in all patients given repeated doses of morphine;
  - fluid intake and a diet rich in fruit and vegetables should be recommended, if the patient's illness makes this possible;
  - a patient likely to need more than two days of morphine should be given a stool softener and laxative as soon as swallowing is possible.
- vomiting:
  - vomiting is common with the first dose but tends to lessen with repeated doses;
  - ondansetron, 4 mg orally, can be given if vomiting is troublesome but should not be prescribed for regular use as it may not be needed more than once.

Head injuries

Injury, or trauma, to the head can damage the scalp, the skull, and the brain. Much of the damage caused by a head injury is due to the fact that the skull is a rigid box within which the brain floats like a peanut in its shell.

ANATOMICAL NOTE

The brain is surrounded and protected by:

- **three fibrous layers (meninges)**:
  - **the dura**, a tough fibrous layer that forms an inner lining to the skull;
  - **the arachnoid,** a second, thinner layer;
  - **the pia,** a fine layer that sticks closely to the brain;
- **the subarachnoid fluid,** which fills the subarachnoid space between the arachnoid and the pia.

General note on head injuries

- A blow to one side of the skull causes the brain on that side to be hit by the inside of the skull, then thrown across the cranium to be hit by the other side of the skull:
  - a single blow to one side of the head can thus damage several areas of the brain.
- A blow to the skull can cause parts of the brain, especially the upper, more mobile parts (vs. the more fixed lower parts), to move relative to one another:
  - this results in sheer stress on the nerve fibres.
- A skull fracture can tear the blood vessels that supply the meninges and that run along the inner surface of the skull between the dura and the skull:
  - the result can be an extra-dural haemorrhage, requiring life-saving surgery to remove the accumulated blood.
- A blow to the skull causing the brain to move inside the skull can tear the veins that run from the surface of the brain to the dura and that drain blood from the brain:
  - the result can be a subdural haemorrhage, which is often associated with severe brain injury.
- An increase in the volume of the brain can occur as a result of brain swelling (cerebral oedema) or bleeding inside the brain or bleeding between the brain and the skull:
  - as a result pressure inside the skull (intracranial pressure) increases;
  - if the intracranial pressure exceeds a critical level, it will squeeze the brain downwards into the foramen magnum – the only large hole in the skull, situated at the base of the brain;
  - the squeezed brain tissue will compress the brainstem, which passes through the foramen magnum, and will likely cause death.
- If intracranial pressure becomes so high that blood flow to the brain falls, the body responds by raising the blood pressure and slowing the pulse; this is a very bad sign, usually followed quickly by death.
- The skull is too small to hold much blood: if the blood pressure of a patient with a head injury is low or falling he may be bleeding somewhere else, most likely in the abdomen.

- **Closed head injury**:
  - a closed head injury occurs when the head receives a blow with a blunt object or strikes a hard, unmoving object (the ground, for example, in a fall);
  - if the blow is hard enough, the brain suffers damage from its impact with the skull;
  - the skull itself may remain intact or be broken.
- **Penetrating head injury:**
  - a penetrating head injury is the result of an object, such as a bullet, entering the brain;
  - penetrating head injuries are usually severe, and visibly so.

Skull fractures

There are two main types of skull fracture:

- **linear fractures**, in which there is a break in a cranial bone resembling a thin line, without splintering, depression, or distortion of the bone:
  - occur at the point of impact;
  - are not usually serious but signify that the head has suffered a heavy blow capable of causing brain injury;
  - can occur in a patient who has not suffered a brain injury and can be absent in a patient who has suffered a severe brain injury;
  - cause bruising and swelling from bleeding under skin and muscle: the swelling is soft and "boggy" and has poorly defined edges – unlike the "egg" swelling that occurs under the skin with less severe injuries; note:
    - the larger the area of swelling, the more likely it is that a skull fracture has occurred;
- **depressed fractures**, in which there is a break in a cranial bone or crushing of a portion of the skull, with an inward depression of the bone towards the brain; depressed fractures:
  - usually follow a blow from a relatively small object, such as a hammer, rather than from impact onto a flat surface;
  - require considerable force;
  - are more often associated with brain injury than are linear fractures;
  - are often compound fractures (see below).

A linear or depressed fracture can be simple or compound:

- in **a simple fracture:**
  - the bone is broken but the skin over it is undamaged;
- in a **compound fracture:**
  - the fracture communicates with the air;
  - this can happen when the skin over the fracture is broken or lost; **OR**
  - in the absence of a scalp wound, the fracture communicates with the ear or with the sinuses.

Traumatic brain injury (brain damage)

Signs and symptoms

- Loss or impairment of consciousness;
- confusion;

- loss of memory (amnesia) for the period around the time of the injury, which includes:
  - retrograde amnesia, for the period leading up to the injury;
  - antegrade amnesia, for the period after the injury; note
  - broadly, the more severe the injury the longer the period of both retrograde and antegrade amnesia.

Note

- If **any** of the above signs or symptoms is present at **any** time after a head injury, brain injury of some degree is present.
- Trauma can cause not only immediate brain injury but also progressive brain swelling or bleeding into the space between the brain and skull: the result is a gradual deterioration of the patient's condition over a period of hours after the injury.

✔ *What to do*

- Remember that:
  - multiple injuries, including injuries to the head, are likely to result from a fall from a height of more than four metres;
  - a brain injury is likely to result from a fall on the head:
    - from a height of more than one metre; **OR**
    - down four or more stairs.
- In a patient with a head injury, check for other injuries, especially of the neck or spinal cord (see Chapter 6, *Bone, joint, and muscle injuries*) and also for bleeding wounds (see Chapter 8, *Wounds*).
- Place an unconscious patient in the coma, or recovery, position, unless you suspect spinal injury.
- Check for an obvious compound skull fracture.
- Check the patient's tetanus immunization status if there is an open wound.
- Use the Glasgow Coma Scale (GCS) (see Table 26.3 in Chapter 26, *Nursing care and medical procedures*) to assess the degree of impairment of consciousness, which is the most important outcome of traumatic brain injury.
- If the Glasgow Coma Scale score is less than 13 when measured at 30 minutes after the injury:
  - seek medical advice with a view to urgent evacuation;
  - **do not** give anything by mouth;
  - **do not** give morphine unless there is severe pain from other injuries;
  - if you give morphine, note down that you have done so, together with the dose, time, and route of administration **both** in the patient's medical record **and**, using a waterproof indelible marker, on a conspicuous part of the patient's body away from major wounds (forearm, chest, or forehead).
- Seek medical advice about the advisability of evacuation even if the Glasgow Coma Scale score is 13 or more but:
  - the patient is over 65; **OR**
  - fell onto the head from a height of more than one metre or down four or more stairs.

- If the Glasgow Coma Scale score is 13 or more 30 minutes after the injury and there are no other injuries:
  - put the patient to bed;
  - give nothing by mouth except sips of water;
  - reassess the patient frequently;
  - two hours after the injury:
    - measure the Glasgow Coma Scale;
    - check for retrograde amnesia (Ask the patient: "What is the last thing you remember clearly **before** the accident?");
    - check for antegrade amnesia (Ask the patient: "What is the first thing you remember clearly **after** the accident?").
- Seek medical advice with a view to evacuation if **any one** of the following is present two hours after the injury:
  - a Glasgow Coma Scale score less than 15;
  - vomiting on more than once occasion;
  - a seizure (fit or convulsion);
  - retrograde amnesia about the period 30 minutes or more before the accident.
- If the Glasgow Coma Scale score is 15 (the maximum) two hours after the injury and none of the above warning signs are present:
  - put the patient to bed;
  - have an attendant monitor the patient's condition at least every two to three hours for the next 24 hours, waking the patient if need be.
- Have the attendant report immediately and seek medical advice with a view to evacuation, if the patient meets **any one** of the following conditions:
  - cannot be woken
  - has a severe headache
  - is confused
  - is unsteady when trying to stand
  - has a seizure (fit)
  - is incontinent of urine or faeces
  - has weakness or numbness of any part of the body.

Post-concussion syndrome

Post-concussion syndrome occurs in many patients who have suffered a traumatic brain injury, more frequently after a mild than after a severe brain injury. Post-concussion syndrome is also more common in women than in men and in older than in younger patients. The cause is unknown.

Post-concussion syndrome begins as the patient is recovering from the brain injury, peaks one to two weeks after the injury, and usually subsides and disappears about a month after the injury. Occasionally, the syndrome persists for several months or even years.

Signs and symptoms

- Headache, usually resembling a tension headache (see Chapter 13, *Paralysis, strange behaviour, unconsciousness)*;
- dizziness;

- personality change, typically irritability, intolerance of noise and crowds, a tendency to uncontrollable anger, and suspiciousness;
- poor memory and concentration;
- insomnia.

✔ *What to do*

- Adjust work tasks to a level of difficulty the patient can manage without stress.
- To treat headache, see Chapter 13, *Paralysis, strange behaviour, unconsciousness*.
- To reduce the risk of medication overuse headache, warn the patient not to take acetylsalicylic acid (Aspirin®) or paracetamol for more than three days in any week.
- If symptoms persist, have the patient see a doctor.

Eye injuries and diseases

EYE INJURIES

Eye injuries can result from a number of causes, including a foreign body, a direct blow to the eye, laceration, exposure to a chemical, and a burn. The first step in dealing with an eye injury is to record a full account of the circumstances of its occurrence followed by a careful eye examination.

KEY QUESTIONS TO ASK THE PATIENT

- Is your vision normal?
- Can you read ordinary print with the affected eye?
  - Note that if the patient can keep both eyes open comfortably and read normally, the eye problem is unlikely to be serious.
- Does it feel as if there is something in your eye that stops you from opening it or keeping it open?
  - If the answer is "yes" and there has not been a recent injury to the eye or a foreign body in the eye, there is probably a problem with the cornea.
- Does bright light bother you?
- Have you suffered an injury to the eye?
  - If the answer is "yes", ask if the patient has been grinding, hammering or drilling metal, since metal fragments produced by these activities can readily penetrate the eye.
- Have you been working with chemicals? Which?
- Do you wear contact lenses?
- Have you noticed any discharge from the eye?

How to examine the eye

- Have the patient lie down, with the head supported and slightly tilted back.
- Check that you have:
  - good lighting (an overhead light or strong daylight);
  - a powerful hand-held torch;
  - a magnifying glass (preferably a × 8 loupe);
  - soft paper tissues;
  - moist cotton wool swabs or buds;
  - fluorescein eye stain strips;
  - anaesthetic eye drops (0.5% solution of tetracaine hydrochloride):
    - never put more than one dose of anaesthetic into the eye;
  - antibiotic eye ointment (1% tetracycline hydrochloride ointment):
    - do not use the same tube of eye ointment for more than one patient or for more than one course of treatment.
- Compare the injured eye with the other eye, using a diagram to record your findings.
- Check if the patient can open the affected eye and can keep it open.
- Test for vision:
  - test for vision before any bright light is shone on the eye or any drops are used;
  - ask the patient to read from a newspaper or book;

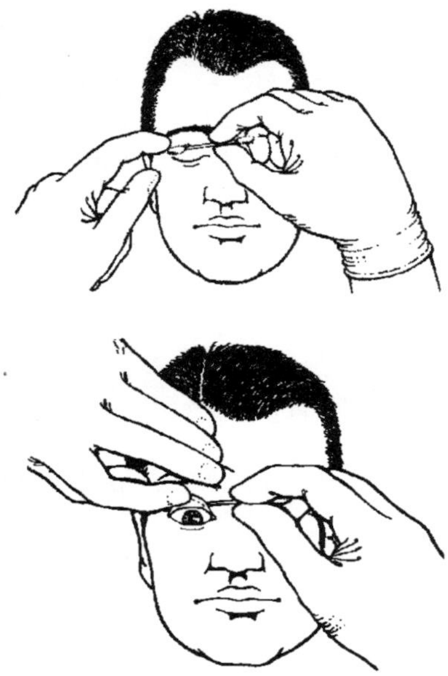

Figure 5.1 How to evert the eyelid.

- › if reading is not normal test with larger print, such as a newspaper headline or book title;
- › if the patient still cannot read print hold up two or three fingers and ask the patient to count them;
- › if counting fingers is not possible, check if the patient can tell light from dark.

- Use a darkened room to check the size of the pupil and its reaction to light:
  - if there is corneal damage, the pupil is often small (1–2 mm in diameter) and it can be hard to see it becoming smaller in response to light.
- Examine the sclera (the white of the eye) for damage or foreign bodies:
  - gently hold apart the eyelids with the fingers and ask the patient to look up, down, left and right;
  - make sure you see clearly into each corner of the eye.
- Inspect the inside of the lower lid by gently pulling it down, with patient looking up.
- Inspect the inner surface of the upper eyelid for damage or foreign bodies; to do this it is necessary to roll back the upper lid:
  - with the patient looking down, place the index finger of one hand or a matchstick across the upper lid while grasping the eyelashes firmly but gently between the index finger and thumb of the other hand (Figure 5.1);
  - pull gently upwards on the eyelashes, pressing down with your index finger or the matchstick and folding the eyelid back over it;
  - the lid will return to its normal position if the patient blinks once or twice.
- Inspect the cornea (the transparent front part of the eye that covers the iris, pupil, and anterior chamber) and surrounding area:
  - use the loupe, and slant light across the cornea, which will help show up any abnormality;
  - the cornea should be clear;
  - any area of cloudiness or opacity, or the presence of foreign bodies, should be noted;
  - the surrounding sclera may be reddish, indicating possible irritation of the cornea;
  - remove any obvious loose foreign bodies (see section below, *Loose foreign bodies*).
- Stain the eye with fluorescein to show up any damage to the cornea or conjunctiva:
  - with the patient looking up, draw the fluorescein paper strip gently across the pulled down lower lid;
  - have the patient blink a couple of times to spread the dye over the eye;
  - wipe away any excess dye from the eyelids;
  - areas of corneal or conjunctival damage will be stained green;
    - › note any such areas on a drawing of the eye in the patient's chart.

Red flags

Seek medical advice urgently in these cases:

- a patient who has suffered an eye injury and has:
  - a pupil that does not react to light;
  - an enlarged pupil;
  - an irregularly shaped pupil;
  - a pool of blood at the bottom of the iris (the coloured part of the eye).

- a patient with a painful red eye who:
  - normally wears contact lenses;
  - has impaired vision;
  - is bothered by bright light;
  - suffered an eye injury yesterday;
  - had a foreign body in the eye yesterday;
  - feels as though he has something in the eye but cannot remember anything entering the eye.

A blow on or near the eye

A blow on or near the eye can cause:

- complete or partial detachment of the retina (the innermost layer of the eye);
- bleeding into the eyeball;
- a fracture of the eye socket (blowout fracture);
- a fracture of the rim (orbit) of the eye.

Damage to the eyeball is most common eye injury and results from blows with objects, such as a golf ball, that fit neatly within the eye socket. Objects larger than the eye socket, such as fists, do not usually damage the eyeball. The orbit is very strong and usually only suffers impact injury in a motor vehicle accident or from heavy blows with an object, such as a baseball bat.

Signs and symptoms

- Usually (but not always) immediate discomfort or a feeling that there is something in the eye.
- In a case of blowout fracture:
  - pain
  - swelling
  - in many cases, inability to move the eye in one direction, most commonly upwards, due to trapping of an eye muscle in the fracture.
- In a case of retinal detachment:
  - a dark spot seen to be "drifting around" in the field of vision (visual floater).
- In a case of fracture of the rim of the eye socket:
  - pain
  - swelling
  - alteration in the shape of the orbit
  - a palpable "step" in the orbital rim.

✔ *What to do*

- Put the patient to bed.
- Seek medical advice.
- If you suspect retinal detachment, have the patient see an eye specialist as soon as possible.
- If there is a blowout fracture, the patient will need surgical treatment, but this is best done seven to 10 days after the injury.

- In the case of a fracture of the orbit, which is usually caused by a heavy blow, consider the possibility that other injuries of the eye, or of the face or brain, may have occurred requiring early surgical treatment.

Corneal abrasion

A scratch or abrasion on the cornea can be caused by:

- a foreign body under the eyelids;
- a fingernail touching the eye;
- using old or poorly cleaned contact lenses.

Signs and symptoms

- Vision may be normal or it may be impaired if the abrasion has been present for several hours.
- The pupil is often small.
- A large pupil which does not respond to light could indicate that the eye has been penetrated by a foreign body.
- A pool of blood behind the cornea (seen with the patient upright) suggests a penetrating injury.
- Green staining with fluorescein can identify areas of corneal abrasion.

✔ *What to do*

- Apply eye ointment along the inner surface of the lower lid (Figure 5.2) and ask the patient to blink several times to spread the ointment across the eye.
- To relieve pain, immobilize the eyelid by strapping an eye pad firmly to the eye for a maximum of 24 hours.
- The next day re-examine the eye with fluorescein stain:
  - if there is no sign of staining, stop the treatment;
  - if the cornea still stains, repeat the treatment every 24 hours until the staining ceases or the patient sees a doctor.
- If there is evidence of corneal abrasion in a patient who wears contact lenses and if there is no evidence of a foreign body (see section below, *Loose foreign bodies*), have the patient see a doctor urgently: contact lenses can cause corneal abrasions resulting in severe corneal infection.

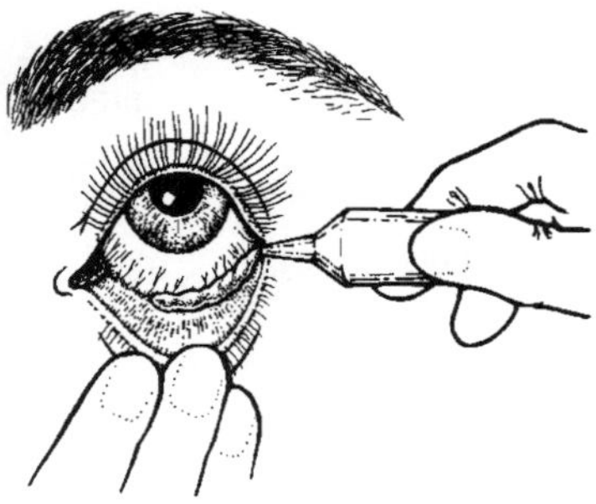

Figure 5.2 How to apply ointment to the eye.

✘ *What not to do*

- Do not use a local anaesthetic solution to relieve the pain of a corneal abrasion.
- Do not use an eye pad in a patient wearing contact lenses.

Loose foreign bodies

✔ *What to do*

- If the foreign body is under an eyelid or over the conjunctiva:
  - gently remove it using **moistened** cotton wool on a stick or a **moistened** cotton bud;

- stain the eye with fluorescein and mark any areas of staining on an eye diagram:
  - › If there is any staining, treat as for corneal abrasion (see above, *Corneal abrasion*).

- If the foreign body is lying on the cornea:
  - put three drops of anaesthetic into the eye and repeat three times at two-minute intervals;
  - after a few minutes, try to remove the foreign body with a moistened cotton bud;
  - have a doctor see the patient as soon as possible: metallic foreign bodies can stain the cornea ("rust rings").
- If you have managed to remove the foreign body, treat as for corneal abrasion (see above, *Corneal abrasion*):
  - cover the eye lightly with a dressing until the anaesthesia has worn off (while the anaesthesia is still active the patient will not be aware of another foreign body entering the eye).

✗ *What not to do*

- Do not attempt to remove a foreign body with a sharp instrument.
- If the foreign body does not move readily, abandon attempts to remove it.

Foreign bodies embedded in the eye

When very small pieces of metal, grit, etc. become embedded in the cornea or the sclera, or even penetrate the eyeball, it may be very difficult to see either the wound or the object, even with fluorescein staining. The patient may not have felt any pain. You should suspect such an accident if the patient has been hammering, chipping, milling, boring, or striking metal with a tool, or standing near someone who was doing so, or has rubbed the eyes after dirt has entered them.

✔ *What to do*

- Treat as for corneal abrasion (see above, *Corneal abrasion*) but:
  - apply tetracycline ointment repeatedly, at least once every six hours;
  - pad the eye.
- Have the patient see an ophthalmologist as soon as possible.
- Keep the pad on the eye until the patient is seen by an ophthalmologist.

✗ *What not to do*

- Do not attempt to remove the foreign body yourself.
- Do not allow the patient to rub the eye.

Wounds of the eyelids and eyeball

✔ *What to do*

- If the eyeball is cut and if the eye leaks fluid or a jelly-like substance, get medical advice at once.
- In the meantime, close the patient's eyelids or bring them as close together as possible.

- To keep the eyelid of the affected eye shut, cover it with a layer or two of sterile petroleum jelly gauze.
- Place an eye pad over the gauze and keep it in place with strips of adhesive tape or sticking plaster.

Chemical burns

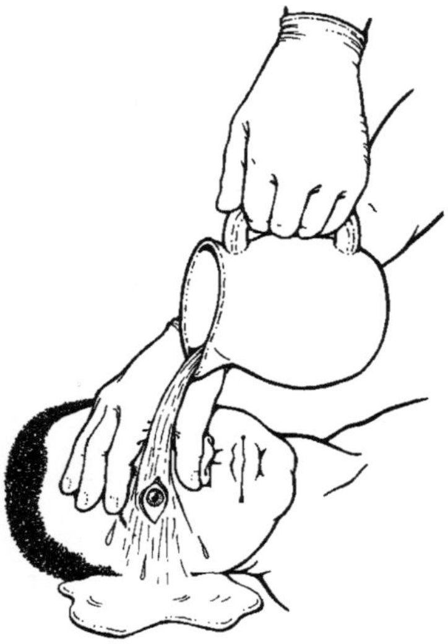

Figure 5.3 How to wash chemicals out of the eye.

✔ *What to do*

- Wash the chemical out of the eye with copious amounts of water for as long as necessary, usually at least 10 minutes (Figure 5.3).
- Stain the eye with fluorescein:
  - if there is marked staining of the eye:
    - › apply eye ointment copiously to prevent the eyelids sticking to the eyeball and cover the eye with petroleum jelly gauze and an eye pad;
    - › repeat every four hours;
    - › have the patient see a doctor as soon as possible;
  - if the staining is less marked:
    - › apply tetracycline eye ointment every four hours and cover the eye with petroleum jelly gauze and a pad;
    - › examine the eye each day, using fluorescein;
    - › after the eye is no longer stained by fluorescein but remains white continue treatment for 24 hours.

Arc eyes ("welder's flash")

The ultra-violet (UV) radiation in an electric arc can burn the surface of unprotected eyes.

Signs and symptoms

- Within 24 hours of the exposure, both eyes (rarely only one eye) feel gritty and appear red;
- bright light hurts the eyes.

✔ *What to do*

- Examine the eyes carefully for foreign bodies.
- Stain with fluorescein.
- If only one eye is affected you can probably rule out arc eye and suspect:
  - an embedded foreign body in the cornea; **OR**
  - an area of corneal damage (which shows up as a green stain on application of fluorescein).
- To relieve symptoms, bathe the eyes with cold water and apply cold compresses to the eyelids.
- To relieve the discomfort caused by light, have the patient wear dark glasses.
- To reduce the gritty feeling in the eyes, apply tetracycline eye ointment to the eyes every four hours.
- Advise the patient to avoid further exposure to welding and to wear dark glasses in bright sunlight until the eyes have fully recovered.

NONINFECTIOUS EYE DISEASES

Subconjunctival haemorrhage

This condition is caused by bleeding from tiny blood vessels between the conjunctiva (the transparent membrane covering the eye) and the sclera (the white of the eye). It often follows vomiting or straining.

Signs and symptoms

- The blood spreads over the sclera, producing a dramatic appearance of bright red blood over a large part of the white of the eye.
- Often noted by the patient on first getting up in the morning, or brought to the patient's attention by a shipmate.
- There is no pain, no feeling of something in the eye, and vision is normal.

✔ *What to do*

- Reassure the patient: although alarming, the condition is harmless; no treatment is needed, and the blood goes away in 1–2 weeks.

Cataract

A cataract is a clouding of the lens of the eye. It occurs typically in people over 60 but may affect younger people who have diabetes mellitus or have suffered an eye injury. It is caused by exposure to sunlight. Contributing factors include diabetes, smoking, and excessive alcohol consumption.

Signs and symptoms

- Impaired vision, especially distance vision and at night;
- worsening of pre-existing short-sightedness;
- intolerance of glare and bright light;
- absence of pain.

✔ *What to do*

- Have the patient see a specialist on shore for a complete eye examination whenever convenient.
- Delay surgical removal of the cataract – an operation that can restore vision – until visual impairment causes problems in everyday life: delaying treatment does not affect the outcome of surgery.

Glaucoma

Glaucoma is an eye disease in which the fluid in the eyeball is under higher pressure than usual. In some cases, glaucoma develops as a result of damage due to previous injury or inflammation of the eye. There are two main types of glaucoma: acute angle closure glaucoma and primary open angle glaucoma.

ACUTE ANGLE CLOSURE GLAUCOMA (also known as acute congestive glaucoma)

This is an extremely serious condition caused by a sudden increase in eye pressure. It requires immediate treatment by an eye specialist.

Signs and symptoms

- Feeling unwell;
- agonizing pain felt not in the eyeball itself but in the forehead or temple;
- in some cases, nausea and vomiting;
- redness of the eye;
- slight cloudiness of the cornea;
- no reaction of the pupil to light;
- impaired vision, with coloured haloes seen around bright lights.

✔ *What to do*

- Seek medical advice urgently: emergency surgery may be needed to lower the pressure in the eye and prevent irreversible loss of vision, which can occur within hours.
- To relieve the usually excruciating pain, give morphine, 10–15 mg intramuscularly, repeating every three to four hours, if necessary.

PRIMARY OPEN ANGLE GLAUCOMA

This is a common cause of loss of vision. It is unrelated to acute angle closure glaucoma. Loss of vision is gradual, first affecting the far edges of the field of vision. There are few or no symptoms and they only appear at a very late stage of the disease. Treatment requires specialized training and equipment, normally not available on board: it can be effective but must be given before visual loss has occurred.

INFECTIOUS EYE DISEASES

The most common eye infections encountered on board include blepharitis (infection of the eyelid margins), conjunctivitis (infection of the conjunctiva), styes (infection of the glands in the lid margins), and, more rarely, keratitis (infection of the cornea). Trachoma also occurs in some areas of the world.

Blepharitis

Blepharitis is an inflammation of the margins of the eyelids.

Signs and symptoms

- Redness and thickening of the eyelids;
- a dandruff-like crusting of the eyelids;
- itching;
- burning sensation;
- loss of the eyelashes;
- watering of the eyes;

- sensitivity to light;
- in some cases, shallow ulcers at the edges of the eyelids.

✔ *What to do*

- Recommend that, at night and on rising, the patient use a sterile applicator or clean fingertips to apply 1% tetracycline eye ointment directly to the lashes at the lid margins.
- Seek medical advice: if the condition persists, the patient should see an ophthalmologist at a convenient port of call.

Conjunctivitis

Conjunctivitis is an infection of the conjunctiva of the eye caused by viruses or, less often, by bacteria. Bacterial conjunctivitis and viral conjunctivitis are highly contagious and can spread rapidly among crew members. Viral conjunctivitis is spread through infected fingers, fomites, bedding, clothing, door-knobs, books, etc., or improperly sterilized ophthalmic instruments.

Signs and symptoms

- One eye affected in most cases of bacterial conjunctivitis.
- Both eyes affected in most cases of viral conjunctivitis.
- Redness of the whole conjunctiva.
- Discharge:
  - more copious and opaque, like pus, in bacterial conjunctivitis;
  - watery and less profuse in viral conjunctivitis.
- Watering of the eye.
- Occasionally, slight pain or sensitivity to light.
- Eyelids often stuck together in the morning, opening only after soaking in warm water.

✔ *What to do*

- Apply tetracycline eye ointment.
- To prevent the spread of conjunctivitis, isolate the patient for the duration of the illness and warn other crew members to:
  - maintain scrupulous personal hygiene;
  - use only their own towels or disposable towels;
  - wash their hands frequently.
- Have the patient return to work only when the discharge has ceased or at the earliest after 24 hours of antibiotic treatment.

✗ *What not to do*

- **Never use** corticosteroid preparations (such as hydrocortisone ointment) to treat a red eye.
- Do not make a diagnosis of conjunctivitis, if the patient:
  - normally wears contact lenses; **OR**
  - has impaired vision; **OR**

- has suffered a recent eye injury; **OR**
- has a foreign body in the eye;
- in these cases seek medical advice urgently.

Keratitis

Keratitis is an inflammatory condition affecting the cornea. It is more serious than conjunctivitis because scarring of the cornea may result in serious loss of vision. Keratitis may be due to primary or secondary infections from bacteria or viruses.

Signs and symptoms

- In many cases, a scratchy moderate-to-severe pain;
- redness of the eye;
- excessive watering of the eye;
- conjunctival discharge;
- blurred vision.

✔ *What to do*

- Seek medical advice.

✗ *What not to do*

- **Never use** corticosteroid preparations (such as hydrocortisone ointment) to treat keratitis without ophthalmologic supervision.

Hordeolum

Hordeolum is an inflammation of the eyelid caused by a bacterium, most commonly *Staphylococcus aureus*. The infection may be in a gland just on the inside of the eyelid or around an eyelash (stye).

Signs and symptoms

- Red, painful, tender swelling on the eyelid;
- in many cases, a visible bead of pus on the eyelid.

✔ *What to do*

- Apply an antibiotic ointment four times daily for seven days.
- If there is no improvement in one to two days, have the patient see a doctor at the next port of call.

SUDDEN PAINLESS LOSS OF VISION

This problem is more often due to a disorder in blood supply to the retina or the brain than to an eye disease. It is a type of transient ischaemic attack (see Chapter 13, *Paralysis, strange behaviour, unconsciousness*) and typically lasts for a few seconds to a few minutes.

✔ *What to do*

- Give aspirin, 150 mg (half a standard tablet) daily.
- Have the patient see a doctor at the next port with good medical facilities.

Bone, joint, and muscle injuries

Injuries to bones, muscles, or joints are common on board ship. All require careful investigation. In the case of a major injury, such as a fracture of the spine, pelvis, or a long bone, medical advice should be sought immediately with a view to urgent evacuation of the patient to an onshore facility. Some injuries, such as those of the collar bone, rarely cause major problems; while in other sites, such as the thumb, wrist or knee, even apparently minor injuries can cause severe, long-term problems.

GENERAL TREATMENT OF INJURIES

The basis of treatment of joint and muscle injuries is "**RICE**": **R**est, **I**ce, **C**ompression, **E**levation, plus pain relief.

Rest of the injured part should continue until it can be used without pain. Activity within the limits of pain should be encouraged but patients should not return to normal activity if that activity causes pain.

Ice can be applied as a cold pack (see Chapter 26, *Nursing care and medical procedures*) or by putting the injured part, such as a foot or ankle, in ice-water for 15 to 20 minutes four times daily for the first 48 hours or until the injury heals.

Compression should be applied with a firm elastic bandage, unless the injury is in a part of the body where compression is not possible, as in the case of a shoulder injury.

Elevation of the injured part above the level of the heart can reduce swelling and speed recovery.

TO RELIEVE PAIN

- If the patient does not have a fracture, apply the RICE routine and give ibuprofen 400 mg orally, every six hours.
- In the case of a fracture, particularly of a bone such as the femur or tibia that is difficult to immobilize fully on board ship, you may have to give tramadol, 50–100 mg orally, three times daily or morphine, 10–20 mg orally, every three to four hours for the first three days or so.

SPECIFIC INJURIES

Strains and sprains

A strain or sprain is an injury in which a tendon (the cord that attaches muscle to bone) or a ligament (the cord that holds bones together) is partly or completely torn. A sprain can occur after a single injury or after repeated minor injuries, and can render the affected joint unstable. Tendon and ligament damage can occur with the same injuries that cause fractures but in some cases, such as a knee injury, damage to a ligament is common and a fracture uncommon. In other cases, such as an ankle injury, ligament damage and fracture can occur at the same time.

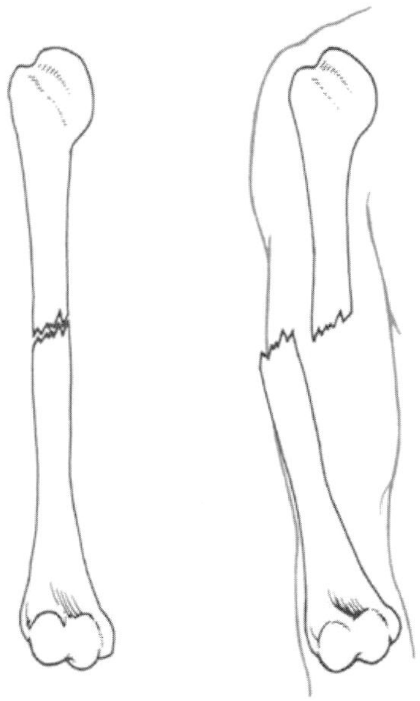

Simple Compound

Figure 6.1 Simple and compound fractures.

Compound fractures (see also Chapter 8, *Wounds*)

Compound fractures are fractures associated with a wound, such that the fracture communicates with the air (Figure 6.1). Compound fractures are nearly always serious and require evacuation.

✔ *What to do*

- Seek medical advice at once with a view to evacuation.
- If evacuation is impossible or likely to be delayed, give amoxycillin/clavulanate, 875/125 mg orally, twice daily.
- If the patient is allergic to penicillin, give azithromycin, 500 mg orally, twice daily.
- Do not suture the wound: cover it with a clean, dry dressing and inspect it daily for signs of infection, such as increasing heat, redness, swelling, and the appearance of pus.
- If the patient has a fracture of an arm or leg, check sensation and pulse in the hand or foot: occasionally, fractures can damage nerves or arteries that run near them.
- Seek medical advice urgently if:
  - sensation is abnormal; OR
  - pulses are absent or weaker on the injured side than on the unaffected side.

Skull fractures (see Chapter 4, *Head injuries*)

Nose, jaw, and face fractures

THE NOSE

A nose fracture is usually caused by a direct blow, as in a fight. No treatment is needed unless the alignment of the fractured nose is cosmetically unacceptable to the patient, in which case correction can be delayed until a convenient time.

THE LOWER JAW (MANDIBLE)

A fracture of the mandible is usually caused by a direct blow, as in a fight or fall: in a fight, the fractured mandible is often the only injury but in a fall, head or neck injuries are usually also present.

✔ *What to do*

- Remember to wear gloves when examining the patient: there are often bleeding wounds inside the mouth.
- Look and feel for swelling, tenderness, wounds, and bruising, both outside and inside the mouth.
- Ask the patient to clench the teeth: if this is painful, suspect a fracture.
- Ask the patient whether the upper and lower teeth meet as they usually do: if they feel out of alignment, suspect a fracture.
- If you suspect a fracture of the mandible in a patient with no evidence of a wound that

might indicate a compound fracture, and if the patient's jaw is not out of alignment, treat for pain and have the patient see a doctor at the next port.

- If there appears to be a compound fracture or, if the jaw is out of alignment, seek medical advice.

THE UPPER JAW (MAXILLA) AND FACE

Fractures of the upper jaw occur only with very high-impact injuries and are, therefore, usually associated with other severe injuries, including brain trauma. A fracture of the cheek bone can be caused by a direct blow, as in a fight, but such blows are seldom strong enough to displace bone fragments.

✔ *What to do*

- If you notice a difference between the two sides of the patient's face, the fracture is probably displaced and needs to be treated surgically: surgery is best done a week or so after the injury, by which time the swelling should have subsided and the surgeon can see whether surgery has achieved the proper alignment.
- If the patient cannot move the eyes normally or sees double, seek medical advice with a view to urgent evacuation for possible surgery.
- Suspect a compound fracture if the cheek or eye socket is fractured AND there is bleeding from the nose.

Neck (cervical spine) injuries

There are seven vertebrae in the neck, numbered C1 to C7 from the top down. Most severe injuries occur between C4 and C7. Fractures most often arise when the neck is forcibly bent backwards, as in a fall on the head or from a heavy blow to the front of the head when the body is held immobile. A neck injury is often associated with a brain injury, making diagnostic assessment difficult.

In a spinal cord injury, a fracture can make the vertebral column unstable, so that one vertebra moves forwards or backwards relative to an adjacent vertebra.

✔ *What to do*

- If the mechanism of injury makes a neck injury possible or likely, immobilize the neck with a rigid collar and board before attempting to move or examine the patient.
- Use the Glasgow Coma Scale (see Chapter 26, *Nursing care and medical procedures*, Table 26.3) to determine the patient's level of consciousness: if the score is 15:
  - ask the patient to move all four limbs in turn;
  - ask if the patient feels tingling or pins-and-needles in the arms or legs.
- If the Glasgow Coma Scale score is less than 15, reassess in 30 minutes: if the score is 15, assess the neck injury then.
- You cannot assess a neck injury in a patient with impaired consciousness: leave the neck immobilized with rigid collar and board until the patient's consciousness returns to normal.

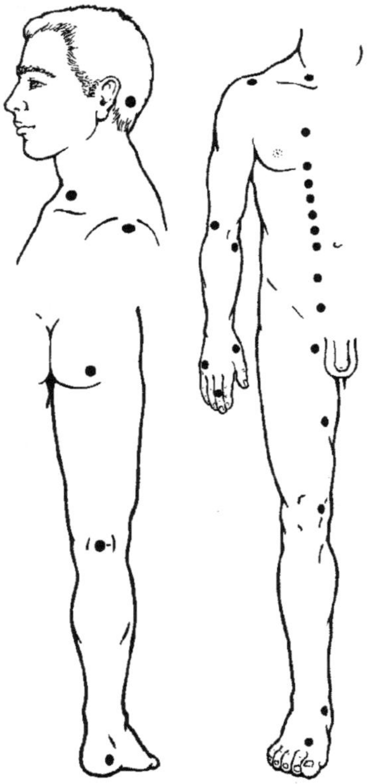

Figure 6.2 Where to check for sensation. Sensation should be tested only once with a sharp object at each point.

- To check for sensation, prick each of the points shown in Figure 6.2 with a pin or other sharp object:
  - each time you prick a point, ask: "Do you feel that?":
    - if the answer is "Yes" ask: "Does it feel sharp or blunt?";
  - use the nipple and the belly-button (navel) as landmarks along the trunk.
- Seek medical advice with a view to evacuation if there is:
  - weakness of the arms or legs;
  - numbness or tingling or any areas the patient cannot feel when you test for sensation.
- Note down carefully any deficits in sensation and have this information available when you call for medical advice.
- If sensation and movement are normal, move the patient to the sick bay or ship's hospital for a more complete examination.
- Designate four crew members to assist you:
  - have one assistant hold the patient's head in line with the neck, making sure **THE HEAD DOES NOT MOVE** on the neck;
  - at the same time, have the three remaining assistants roll the patient onto one side.
- Remove the rigid collar carefully, **BUT DO NOT REMOVE THE COLLAR IF**:
  - the patient expresses anxiety about your doing so: this often indicates a fracture;
  - you cannot assemble four reliable assistants.
- Gently examine the neck for tenderness and muscle spasm.
- Gently feel down the line of the vertebrae looking for tender points and irregularity.
- If you find local tenderness on the back of the neck, seek medical advice with a view to evacuation.
- While awaiting evacuation, replace the patient's collar and leave it in place.
- If there is no tenderness at all, or even slight tenderness or muscle spasm in the neck, ask the patient to rotate the neck to the right and to the left: if the patient is reluctant to do this, **DO NOT INSIST** – it could be a sign of a fracture.
- You can be almost sure there is no serious injury if all three of the following conditions are met:
  - movement and sensation normal;
  - no tenderness, or even slight tenderness, on the back of the neck;
  - the patient can rotate the neck 45° to both right and left.
- If the first two conditions are met but the third is not, leave the patient's collar on and give ibuprofen 400 mg orally, every six hours.
- If there is no improvement 24 hours later, seek medical advice.

Collar bone (clavicle) injury

The clavicle is commonly fractured in falls onto an outstretched hand. Because the bone is close to the skin, the diagnosis is usually obvious. Complications are rare.

✔ *What to do*

- Apply a sling and swathe (Figure 6.3) or Velpeau bandage (Figure 6.4).
- Give ibuprofen, 400 mg orally, every six hours.
- Note that it will take three to four weeks before the patient can use the arm normally.

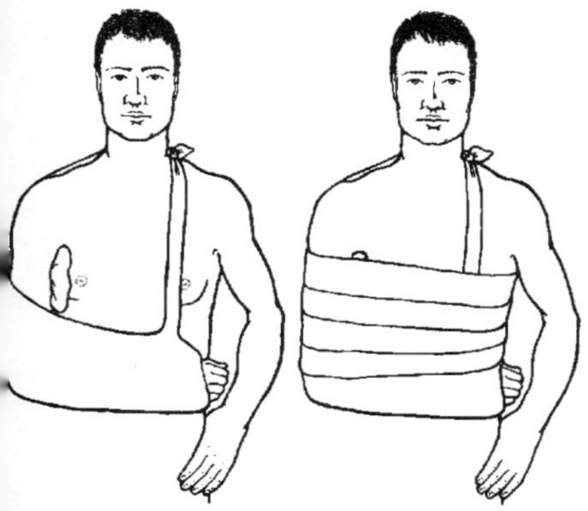

igure 6.3 How to apply a sling and swathe.

powdered pad is placed in the armpit to revent skin maceration. The sling, or swathe, is eeded to limit movement of the shoulder.

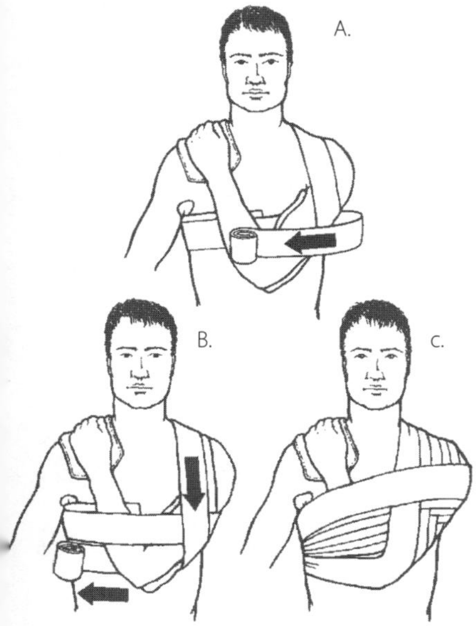

gure 6.4 How to apply a Velpeau bandage.

Start at A and repeat B and C until several layers of bandage are applied. The weight of the arm is supported by looping the stockinet over the shoulder and around the elbow.

Apply as for the sling and swathe splint but the hand is held higher and the forearm lies against the chest. The choice is determined by whichever is more comfortable for the patient.

Shoulder injury

SHOULDER DISLOCATION

A shoulder dislocation occurs when the ball (head) at the top end of the upper arm bone (humerus) slips out of the relatively shallow socket (glenoid fossa) of the shoulder blade (scapula). The dislocation (Figure 6.5) usually causes the head of the humerus to lie in front of the glenoid (anterior dislocation).

Common causes of shoulder dislocation include:

- a fall on the outstretched arm;
- a direct fall on the point of the shoulder;
- a forceful effort to throw, lift, or hit (usually in patients with previous damage to the shoulder).

Signs and symptoms

- Pain, often severe.
- Abnormal shoulder contour: the outside of the shoulder is flattened and there is often a dip instead of a bulge over the deltoid muscle.

✔ *What to do*

- Use the gravitational technique to reduce the dislocation (Figure 6.6), as follows:
  - give morphine, 10 mg intramuscularly, and wait 30 minutes;
  - place the patient face down on a table, with the arm hanging down;
  - pad the armpit;
  - secure approximately seven to eight kilograms of weight to the hand;
  - reduction will occur once the shoulder muscles have become fatigued, usually within 30 minutes;
  - if reduction does not occur, seek medical advice.
- Following reduction, apply a sling and swathe splint (Figure 6.3) or Velpeau bandage (Figure 6.4) used for shoulder and upper arm (humeus) injuries, to be worn for three weeks.

SHOULDER SPRAIN

A shoulder sprain involves the joint (acromio-clavicular or A–C joint) between the collar bone (clavicle) and the shoulder blade (scapula). It is often the result of a fall onto the shoulder when the arm is at the side. Chronic sprains may arise after work that requires the patient to reach across the chest or upwards above the head.

Signs and symptoms

- Pain in the front of the shoulder, made worse by pulling the arm across the chest;

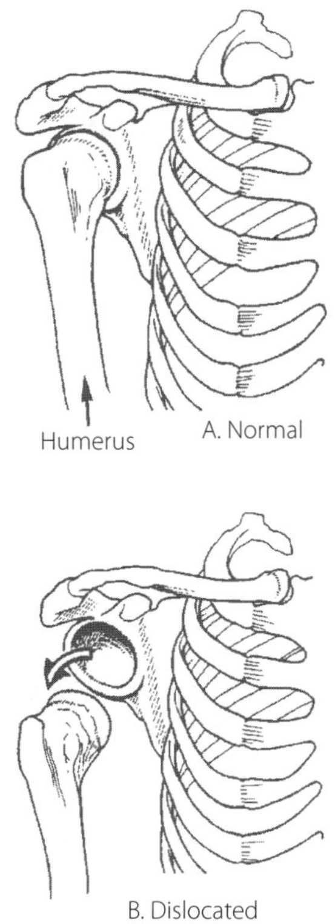

Figure 6.5 A dislocated shoulder.

- tenderness over the outer end of the clavicle;
- swelling, usually slight: obvious swelling indicates severe injury.

✔ *What to do*

- Avoid using a sling, which tends to worsen the pain.
- To diminish the risk of pain at night, have the patient sleep face up or face down but not on the side.
- Ensure that the patient's work does not involve having to use the affected arm to lift more than a few kilograms.
- If the pain does not subside and shoulder function does not return over a week or so, or if there is considerable swelling or obvious deformity of the joint, have the patient see a doctor at the next port.

Injury to the upper arm (humerus) and elbow

FRACTURE OF THE UPPER END OF THE HUMERUS

Fractures of the upper end (head) of the humerus are uncommon. When they occur, they are usually in individuals over 80 years of age.

FRACTURE OF THE MID-SHAFT OF THE HUMERUS

Fractures of the mid-shaft of the humerus usually result from a forceful throwing movement. Because of the twisting force, the fracture does not occur straight across the bone but obliquely or in a spiral.

Signs and symptoms

- Sudden, severe pain at the site of the injury;
- bruising and swelling soon after.

✔ *What to do*

- Seek medical advice: hospital treatment is usually required, because the oblique or spiral break means that the ends of the bone tend to slip past one another, shortening the arm.
- Since the nerves of the arm can be damaged by the fracture as they run near the humerus, check the strength the patient can apply to:
  - straightening the wrist and fingers;
  - spreading the fingers apart with the wrist and fingers straight;
  - applying a pincer grip between the thumb and ring finger.
- While awaiting evacuation, apply a sugar tong splint (Figure 6.7) with support for the arm at the wrist (**do not** support the elbow).

ELBOW FRACTURE OR DISLOCATION

Falling on the outstretched hand can cause a fracture or dislocation of the elbow but much less often than a shoulder dislocation. Fracture and dislocation of the elbow often occur together.

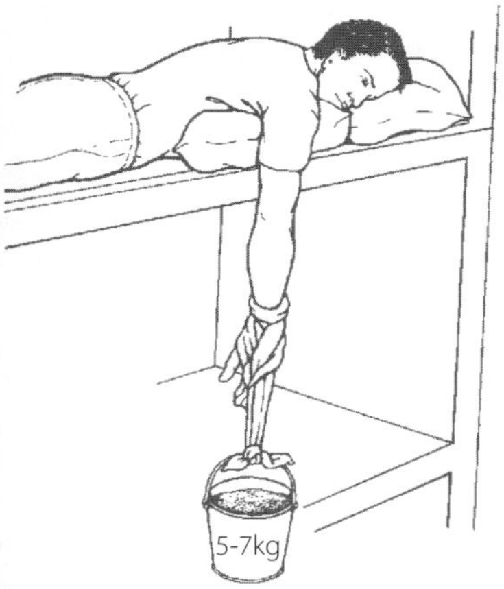

Figure 6.6 How to reduce a shoulder dislocation using gravity.

Signs and symptoms

- Pain
- obvious deformity
- inability to move the elbow.

What to do

- Seek medical advice with a view to evacuation: reducing the dislocation requires anaesthesia.
- Meanwhile, place the arm in a sling and give an analgesic, such as tramadol, 100 mg orally, every six to eight hours.

Wrist and forearm fractures

In children, a fracture of the mid-section of a forearm bone shaft can be caused by a fall but in adults it is usually one of several injuries caused by a major trauma. In young adults, a fall on the outstretched hand commonly causes a fracture of the lower extremity of the radius (Colles' fracture), which results in significant displacement of the bones and obvious deformity at the site of the fracture. In some cases, there is also injury to nerves and blood vessels in the wrist.

What to do

- Check for sensation in the fingers.
- Check for circulation: push gently on the finger pulps so that they go pale; if circulation is normal, colour should return in about two seconds.
- If there is no evidence of injury to the nerves or arteries supplying the hand, evacuation can be delayed for up to 24 hours.
- If the nerves or arteries are damaged, immediate evacuation is necessary.
- While awaiting evacuation, place the arm in a sling and give an analgesic, such as ibuprofen, 400 mg orally, every six hours, or tramadol, 100 mg orally, every six to eight hours.
- If there is evidence of nerve or artery injury and evacuation cannot be arranged immediately, you may have to reduce the fracture on board ship in order to relieve the compression of the artery. In this case:
  - give morphine, 15 mg intramuscularly, and wait 30 minutes;
  - with an assistant holding the patient's upper arm and elbow, take the patient's hand **exactly** as if you were shaking hands, then pull steadily but forcefully in the alignment of the forearm until the wrist straightens;
  - apply a splint (Figure 6.8).

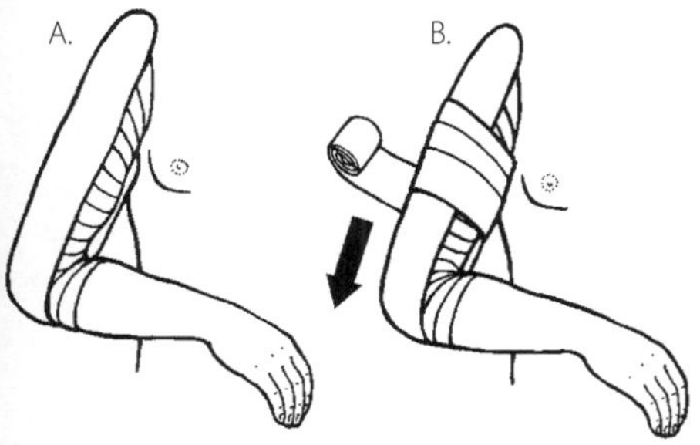

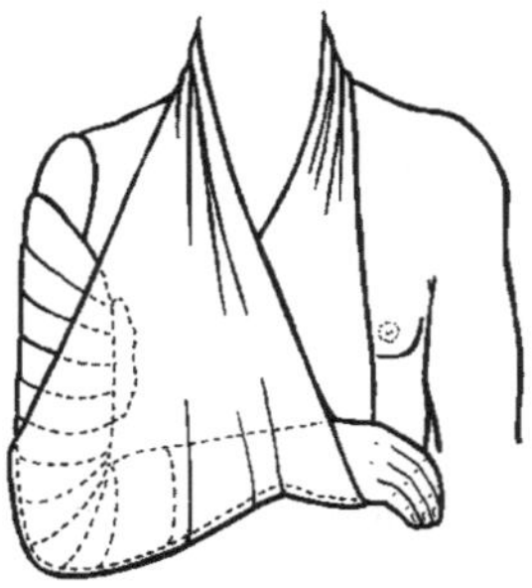

igure 6.7 How to apply a sugar tong splint for the humerus.

Position the plaster (A); secure the splint in place (B).

The plaster is applied from the armpit to around the elbow and up the arm on the other side to armpit level.

Used for upper arm (humeral) fractures.

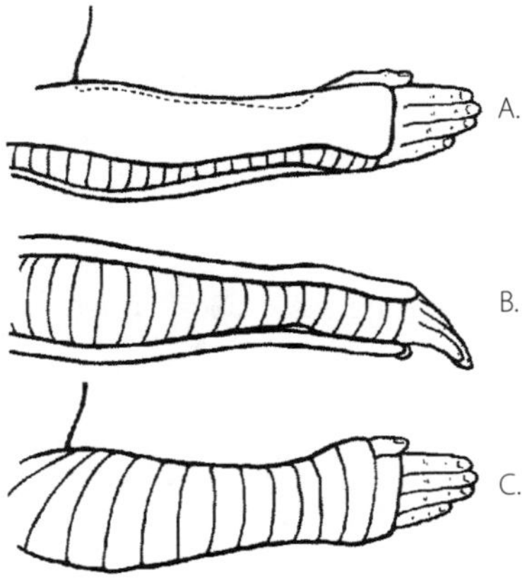

Figure 6.8 How to apply a splint for the forearm.

- Used for wrist and lower forearm fractures.
- A and B show the position of the plaster and C the finished splint:
  - the plaster extends from the knuckles (metacarpophalangeal joints) then along the forearm, then wraps around the elbow and reaches down to the middle of the palm of the hand;
  - the patient should wiggle the fingers from time to time to prevent finger stiffness.
- A double sugar-tong splint, that combines the proximal and distal sugar-tong splints, is used for elbow and forearm fractures.
- A reverse sugar-tong splint, which wraps around the hand and between the thumb and fingers instead of around the elbow, is used for stable injuries of the elbow area or forearm and for Colles' (wrist) fractures.

Hand and finger injuries

Hand injuries are common. Even apparently minor injuries can lead to serious disability – the loss of a thumb can be more disabling for a worker than the loss of an eye. The first three centimetres of the hand below the wrist are occupied by the eight carpal bones, arranged in two rows.

SCAPHOID FRACTURES

The scaphoid, a small bone in the wrist just below the extremity of the radius, is often injured in a fall onto the hand.

Signs and symptoms

- Pain in the wrist;
- tenderness on the outside of the wrist in the hollow at the base of the thumb (the "anatomical snuff-box");
- minimal or absent swelling and bruising;
- reduced grip strength and pain on attempting to grip, although ability to move the wrist is more or less normal.

✔ *What to do*

- If there is tenderness over the scaphoid after a fall, seek medical advice: this type of injury may require prolonged treatment and can cause serious long-term problems.
- If you suspect a scaphoid fracture, apply a thumb spica splint (Figure 6.10) until an X-ray can be taken.

METACARPAL FRACTURES

The metacarpal bones connect the wrist to the fingers and make up the arch of the hand. They can be fractured by a blow to the hand from a weight or a hammer or by an end-on blow when the patient hits someone or something with a closed fist or falls while carrying an object in the fist. The fifth (little finger) metacarpal is especially likely to fracture in this way. The main problem with metacarpal fractures is twisting of the far end, so that the attached finger is out of alignment and overlaps adjacent fingers when the patient makes a fist. This can cause long-term interference with gripping.

✔ *What to do*

- Ask the patient to keep the fingers straight but to bend the joint between the hand and fingers as far as possible: the fingernails should be lined up neatly in a straight line when you look at them end on.
- If the alignment of the fingers is normal, apply a gutter splint (Figure 6.11) and give ibuprofen, 400 mg orally, every six hours.
- If the fingers are rotated, have the patient evacuated with a view to reduction and surgical repair of the fracture, which should be done within three to four days.

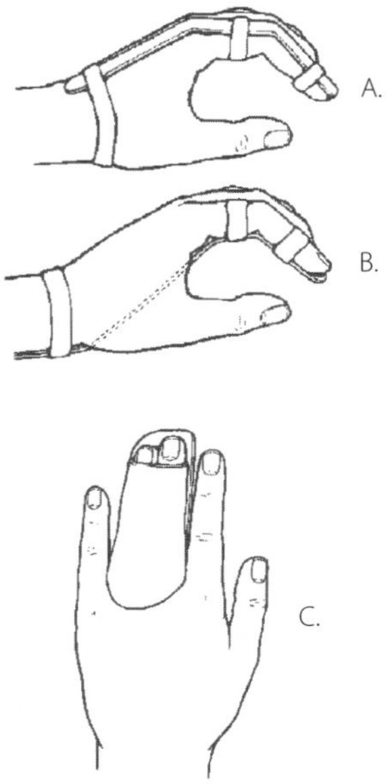

Figure 6.9 How to apply a volar splint.

- Used for fractures of the fingertips (distal phalanges) and the middle and top knuckles (interphalangeal joints).
- Commercial splints shown at A, B and C show a "buddy splint", using a healthy finger to immobilize the fractured finger.
- Splinting should be done with the middle knuckle bent at an angle of 15° to 20°.

- If the patient has punched an opponent in a fight and there are signs of skin damage on the fingers caused by contact with the opponent's teeth, you should suspect a compound metacarpal fracture: arrange for evacution, since the risk of infection is high.
- Meanwhile, give amoxycillin/clavulanate, 875/125 mg orally, twice daily.
- If you suspect a closed finger fracture, apply a volar buddy splint (Figure 6.9) and give a mild analgesic, such as ibuprofen, 400 mg orally, every six hours.
- In the case of a finger dislocation due to forced extension of the finger, reduce the dislocation by firm traction and downward pressure and then apply a buddy splint (Figure 6.9).

THUMB FRACTURES

The thumb is often injured in fights or by falls that force the thumb away from the hand. Many thumb fractures involve the joint at the base of the thumb. If these fractures are not treated by surgery, serious loss of thumb function can occur.

✔ *What to do*

- Apply a thumb spica (Figure 6.10) or gutter splint (Figure 6.11) to the wrist and thumb.
- Give ibuprofen, 400 mg orally, every six hours.
- Arrange for evacuation within two to three days in order to preserve long-term hand function.

CUTS ON THE HANDS AND FINGERS

Cuts may damage nerves or tendons in the hands and fingers and the damage is unlikely to heal without surgery. Closing finger cuts with sutures can also damage nerves and **should never be attempted on board ship**.

Note

- The tendons of the fingers slide through sheaths on the upper and lower sides of the fingers.
- Cuts on the palm or fleshy parts of the hand do not often damage tendons.
- Cuts on the back of the hand, which could damage-tendons, are relatively uncommon.
- Cut tendons can usually be seen in the wound once bleeding has stopped, although if the cut occurred when the fingers were bent but is examined with them straight the cut in the tendon may be pulled away from the wound.

The nerves most prone to cuts are:

- **the ulnar nerve**, which enters the hand along the little-finger side of the wrist;
  - **the ulnar nerve** is close to the skin surface at the fold of the wrist and may easily be cut by wounds at this point;
  - the patient will be unable to straighten the fourth (ring) and fifth (little) fingers.
- **the finger (digital)** nerves, which run along both sides of each finger;

- cutting a finger nerve will cause loss of feeling along the side of the finger;
- if the index or little finger is affected, gripping can be difficult.

✔ *What to do*

- If the patient has a cut nerve or tendon, arrange for immediate evacuation with a view to surgical treatment to reconnect the cut nerves or tendons.

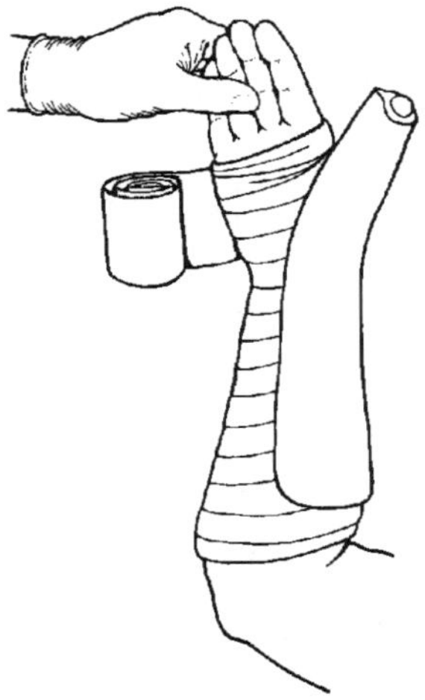

Figure 6.10 How to apply a thumb spica.

- Used for wrist fractures, particularly of the scaphoid bone, just under the thumb.
- The splint is placed on the thumb side of the forearm and wraps the thumb onto the forearm and hand.

Rib fractures (see Chapter 7, *Abdominal and chest injuries*)

Fractures of the pelvis, hip, and femur

In young adults, fractures of the pelvis, around the hip joint, and of the femur usually occur in conjunction with other injuries caused by major trauma. There is marked blood loss from these fractures and hypovolaemic shock can occur: maintaining adequate blood volume until evacuation can take place is the key to treatment on board ship. Hip fractures, i.e. fractures of the upper end of the thigh bone (neck of the femur), occur mainly in elderly women with thinning of the bones (osteoporosis). Occasionally, fractures of the neck of the femur occur in men who have osteoporosis because of a medical illness that requires long-term use of cortisone or similar medications.

Signs and symptoms

- In the case of fractures arising in relatively minor falls:
  - pain in the hip, often mild;
  - inability to stand or walk in most cases, although in some cases the patient can stand;
  - shortening of the injured leg by 2–5 cm relative to the other leg;
  - foot turned outwards.

✔ *What to do*

- Arrange for evacuation with a view to early surgery, although blood loss is not substantial and evacuation need not take place urgently.
- While awaiting evacuation, give an analgesic, starting with tramadol, 100 mg orally, every eight hours, or morphine, 10–20 mg orally, every three to four hours.

Knee injuries

The knee is the largest joint in the body. It is also the most mechanically complex joint and the one most susceptible to injury and wear-and-tear. The knee is a hinge joint between the thigh bone (femur) and the larger of the two shin bones (tibia). The smaller shin bone (fibula) and the knee cap (patella) are not part of the knee joint. The knee joint also has four main ligaments: two (collateral ligaments) outside the joint, one on each side, and two (cruciate ligaments) inside the joint, of which the anterior cruciate ligament, which runs from the front of the tibia to the back of the femur, is more often injured. There are also two crescent-shaped cartilage pads (menisci) inside the joint, one on the inner half and one on the outer half.

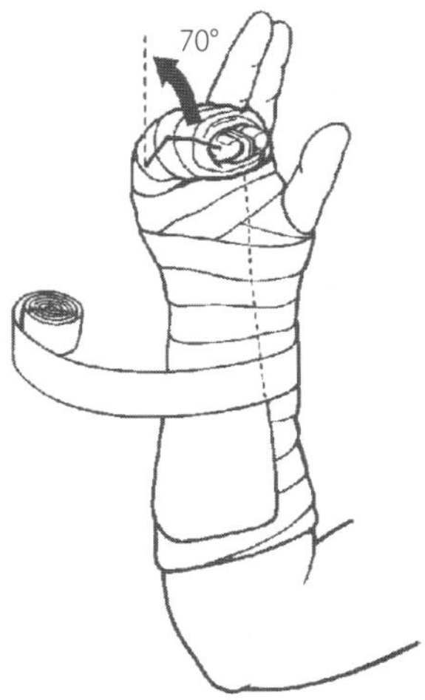

Figure 6.11 How to apply a gutter splint.

- Used for hand (metacarpal) and finger (phalangeal) fractures.
- Can be used to immobilize the index and long fingers (radial splint) or the ring finger and little finger (ulnar or boxer splint).
- To avoid finger stiffness, the fingers should be splinted with the knuckles (metacarpophalangeal joints) bent at an angle of 70°, the finger joints nearer the hand (proximal interphalangeal joints) at an angle of 20° to 30°, and the end finger joints (distal interphalangeal joints) at an angle of 5° to 10°.
- To prevent skin irritation, gauze should be placed between the fingers before application of the splint.

Fractures around the knee are uncommon but ligament damage is very common, especially when a twisting force or blow is applied to a bent knee.

How to assess a knee injury

- Check if there is a difference in the size of the thigh on one side: severe injury to the knee can cause loss of muscle bulk in the thigh in a few days and the difference is usually evident.
- Check if the hollows around the knee are rounded out, indicating the presence of fluid in the joint and thus more severe injury.
- Ask the patient to walk: if walking appears normal, have the patient walk heel-to-toe along a line.
- If walking along a line is not a problem, have the patient squat as far down as pain allows: the patient should keep the back straight, holding onto a table edge if necessary, and then stand up again.
- If walking and squatting present no problem, ask the patient to move forward while squatting ("duck-waddle").
- There are four diagnostic possibilities:
  - there is no injury or abnormality of the knee if the patient:
    - can walk, squat and duck-waddle;
  - the injury is minor if the patient:
    - can walk and squat but not duck-waddle; AND
    - has little or no fluid in the knee;
  - there may be significant injury, but further evaluation can wait until the next port, if the patient:
    - walks with a limp; AND/OR
    - cannot squat; AND/OR
    - has swelling of the knee; BUT
    - pain is absent or mild;
  - there may be serious injury requiring early treatment if the patient:
    - cannot walk; OR
    - has severe pain; AND
    - has a large amount of fluid in the knee.

✔ What to do (in the case of 3 or 4, above)

- Have the patient avoid:
  - walking more than required for self-care and eating;
  - standing for long periods;
  - squatting.
- Note that confinement to bed is not necessary.
- Apply the RICE steps described above.
- Advise the patient to exercise the thigh muscles twice daily, as follows:
  - place several heavy objects (cans of food, for example) totalling about 5 kg in weight. in a cloth or strong plastic bag;

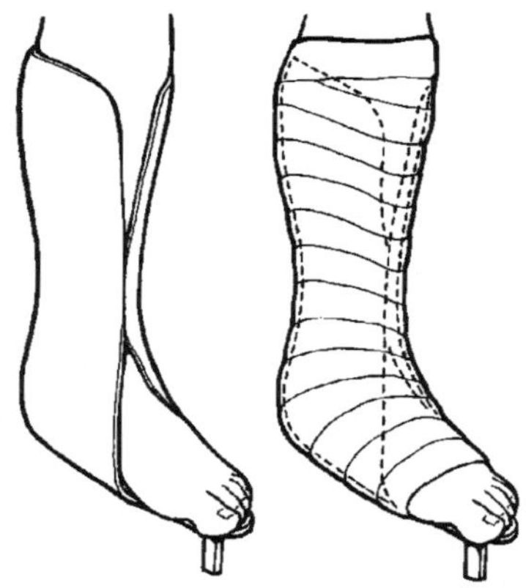

Figure 6.12 How to apply a posterior leg or ankle splint.

- Used for fractures of the lower leg, ankle, and foot, reduced (realigned) dislocations, and severe sprains.
- A plaster splint extends from midfoot (metatarsals) to the top of the calf bone (fibular neck).
- Used in combination with the stirrup splint to increase stability: the posterior splint should be applied first.

- have the patient sit on a high stool or the edge of a bunk;
- hook the cloth or bag over the patient's foot and have the patient straighten the knee 10–15 times, then rest for one minute, then repeat the sequence of 10–15 movements three times.

Shin (tibia and fibula) fractures

The tibia is the main weight-bearing bone of the lower leg. It forms the flat, hard surface of the shin. The fibula is more slender and forms the outer side of the lower leg. Fractures of the tibia and fibula require large forces and on board ship are most likely to result from falls from a height or crush injuries to the leg. Because the tibia is immediately under the skin, compound fractures are common.

COMPLICATIONS

Swelling due to the fracture, with an increase in pressure in the leg great enough to block off the blood supply, resulting in:

- pallor of the skin
- loss of circulation (pulse) in the foot
- worsening pain
- weakness and numbness in the foot and ankle.

This is an emergency: the leg may be lost if pressure is not relieved quickly.

✔ *What to do*

- Seek medical advice with a view to evacuation.
- While awaiting evacuation, give morphine, 10–15 mg intramuscularly, every four hours, and apply a posterior leg splint (Figure 6.12).
- Do not cover the toes with the splint, and check their colour and sensation every 30 minutes: if pallor or numbness appear seek medical advice **again**.
- Give only water by mouth.

Ankle injuries

The ankle is a mortise joint formed by the foot and the two shin bones. The ends of the shin bones on either side of the ankle are called the medial malleolus and lateral malleolus, on the inner and outer side, respectively, of the ankle. The malleoli are joined to the foot bones by ligaments. The ankle is often injured in trips and falls, and also in falls onto the heels from a height.

TRIP-AND-FALL ANKLE INJURIES

Note

- An ankle sprain most often involves the outer side of the ankle and occurs when the foot is forced medially (inward) while flexed (downward), as when a patient trips on the right foot and falls forwards and to the right.
- The same injury may cause a tear of the ligament or a fracture of the lateral malleolus: it is not easy to tell whether it is the bone or the ligament that has broken but the long-term outcome is the same.

- A less common injury occurs when the ankle is forcibly flexed upwards and/or outwards, as in an impact against the front part of the sole of the foot or a trip-and-fall with the foot turned outwards, causing either a sprain or a fracture of the medial malleolus.

How to assess the severity of a trip-and-fall injury

- Ask these questions:
  - How did the injury occur?
  - Could you walk immediately after the injury?
  - Can you put weight on the ankle?
  - Have you injured this ankle before? (A repeat injury is likely to cause joint instability.)
- If only the lateral (outer) side of the ankle is affected, the injury is unlikely to cause serious problems.
- Look for swelling and bruising:
  - if you find neither swelling nor bruising, there is unlikely to be a fracture or ligament tear;
  - if you find both swelling and bruising, there is very likely to be either a fracture or a ligament tear.
- Feel the whole foot and leg, up to and including the knee, for tenderness, which might suggest a fracture: pay particular attention to the back of the leg near the ankle and the tips of the tibia (inner leg bone) and fibula (outer leg bone).
- Gently move the ankle inwards, outwards, up and down: if this causes no pain, the injury is unlikely to be serious.
- Watch the patient walking: if the patient could walk immediately after the injury and can walk four steps now (even with a limp), the injury is unlikely to be serious.

What to do

- If the medial (inner) side of the ankle is affected or if both sides are affected seek medical advice: these injuries could be serious.
- Otherwise, apply the principles outlined above, under *General treatment of injuries*.
- Bandage the ankle firmly.
- Have the patient begin ankle exercises on the day of injury:
  - use the big toe to "draw" in the air, twice every hour, all the letters of the alphabet (or the thirty or so most common characters, if the patient's mother tongue is Chinese).
- Have the patient bear weight on the ankle as soon as this is possible.
- If the ankle is unstable or "gives way", the patient may need surgical treatment, but this should be delayed until healing is complete.

ANKLE INJURIES CAUSED BY A FALL FROM A HEIGHT

Ankle injuries due to a fall from a height are often severe and generally affect both sides of the ankle as well as the heel bones and bones in other areas of the body, such as the knee, hip, and spine.

What to do

- Seek medical advice with a view to evacuation.

Fractures of the foot and toes

The bones of the foot below the ankle are arranged in much the same way as the hand bones, with two rows of small bones (tarsal bones) immediately below the ankle joint, five long bones (metatarsal bones), and the bones of the toes.

- Fractures of the tarsal bones are uncommon and usually occur in conjunction with other fractures caused by major trauma.
- Fractures of the metatarsal bones can be caused by a blow, such as when a heavy object falls on the foot, or by a fall from a height with the patient landing on the feet.
- The metatarsal bones can also fracture after repetitive bouts of stress to which the patient is not accustomed:
  - such fractures are sometimes called "march fractures", because they are common in military recruits;
  - "march fractures" cause obvious swelling and bruising and localized tenderness.
- Toe fractures are caused by direct trauma, such as from a blow or a heavy weight or forceful end-on trauma (usually toe-stubbing).

✔ *What to do*

- If the patient has a closed fracture of a single metatarsal bone or a march fracture:
  - advise rest;
  - give a mild analgesic, such as ibuprofen, 400 mg orally, every six hours;
  - apply a firm bandage to the foot and ankle.
- In the case of a metatarsal fracture with extensive crushing of tissues or of a compound fracture, arrange for evacuation:
  - meanwhile, give amoxycillin/clavulanate, 875/125 mg orally, twice daily.
- In the case of a simple toe fracture, i.e. not a compound fracture or crush injury, and not involving the big toe, apply buddy taping (Figure 6.14) and give a mild analgesic, such as ibuprofen, 400 mg orally, every six hours.
- Fractures of the big toe, which is important for walking and balance, require careful treatment: if the fracture is closed and an extensive crush injury has not occurred, surgical treatment can be delayed; meanwhile:
  - give ibuprofen, 400 mg orally, every six hours;
  - apply a posterior leg splint (Figure 6.12);
  - have the patient see a doctor as soon as practicable.

SPLINTS AND SLINGS

Splints support and protect injured bones and soft tissue. They reduce pain, swelling, and muscle spasm, and immobilize the injured area while it is healing, making it easier to transport the patient.

SPLINTS

- A splint is a long, narrow slab of rigid material applied with elastic tape to prevent movement of a fractured bone or dislocated joint. Air (inflatable) splints provide less support than rigid splints but are quicker and easier to apply.

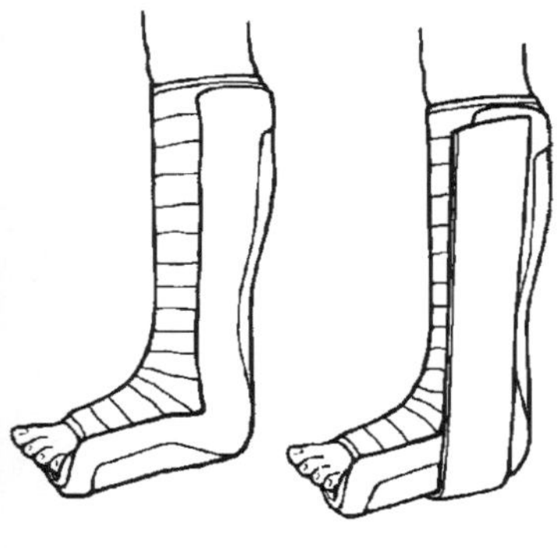

Figure 6.13 How to apply a stirrup splint.

- Used for fractures of or near to the ankle, sometimes in combination with the posterior leg splint (see above), which should be placed first.

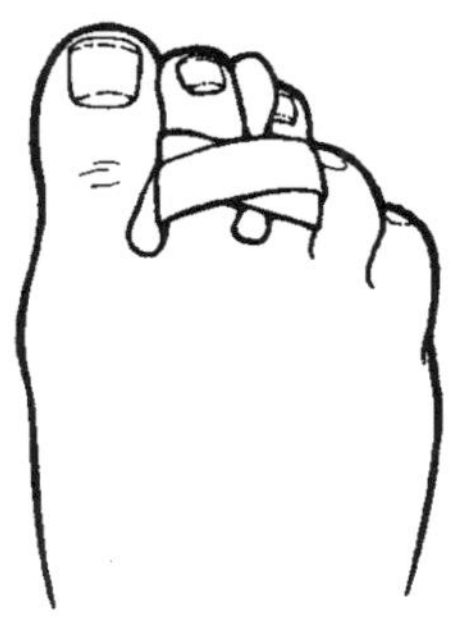

Figure 6.14 How to do buddy taping for toe fractures.

- Used for fractures of the toes:
  - the fractured toe is secured to the adjacent toe with adhesive strips;
  - a small sheet of wadding is placed between the toes to prevent maceration.

- Splints should not completely encircle the limb: they should allow for expansion if the injured area swells.
- A splint consists of a layer of stockinet, a layer of cotton-wool padding, and several layers of plaster (or pre-padded fibre glass) arranged parallel to the limb. A final layer of cotton or elastic bandage is wrapped around the plaster or fibreglass to hold everything in place. Makeshift splints can be made from cardboard or any other malleable, semi-rigid material that can be found on board.

How to apply a splint

- Expose the extremity completely and clean and dress skin wounds before applying the splint.
- Test for nerve or artery damage before and after applying a splint: check the five "**Ps**":
  - Pallor at or below the fracture;
  - Pain in the hand or foot below the fracture;
  - Paraesthesia (pins-and-needles or loss of sensation) below the fracture (for example, the wrist or fingertips, for an arm fracture; the ankle or toes, for a leg fracture);
  - Pulselessness – no pulse felt at a point below the fracture (inner elbow, wrist, ankle);
  - Paralysis – patient unable to wiggle fingers or toes.
- If any of these "Ps" is present, seek medical advice urgently.
- Pad heels or elbows and all bony prominences with padded cotton bandage.
- If fingers or toes are included in the splint, place padding between the patient's fingers and toes and extra padding over the fracture site.
- To prevent stiffness and loss of function, splint affected joints as far as possible in their normal resting positions.
- To reduce swelling, apply an ice bag (or a bag of frozen vegetables) to the fracture site for not more than 20 minutes and have the patient keep the extremity elevated.
- To apply a plaster splint follow these steps:
  - cut the plaster strips to a little more than the required length so that they can be folded back on themselves to create a smooth edge;
  - cut a generous length of stockinet (too long is better than just enough): stretch it and smooth it over the extremity so that it extends beyond the upper and lower edges of the area to be splinted;
  - **loosely** bandage the area to be splinted with cotton wool or padded bandage, beginning from the fingers or toes and bandaging upward;
  - dip the plaster strips in water at room temperature and place them on an open towel to remove excess water and enable the plaster to be smoothed;
  - apply the plaster strips to the extremity, moulding them to the extremity – approximately 8 to 10 layers are necessary for an upper extremity splint and 12 to 14 layers for a lower extremity splint; **BUT**
  - **DO NOT** squeeze the edges – there must be no visible finger impressions;
  - fold back the upper and lower ends of the strips to form a smooth edge and fold the stockinet over the edge of the plaster;

- wrap an elastic bandage around the extremity, starting at the bottom and moving upwards: the bandage must not be tight; **DO NOT** stretch it at any point;
- secure the plaster to the extremity with tape: the final layer should not be wrapped too tightly;
- have the patient keep the limb in the desired position until the plaster hardens.

- To apply a fibreglass splint, follow the manufacturer's instructions, which usually involve the following steps:
  - cut the splint to the required length, i.e. slightly longer than necessary, so that you can fold it back on itself to create a smooth edge;
  - apply stockinet and cotton wool or padded bandage as for a plaster splint;
  - dip the fibreglass splint in water at room temperature and place it on an open towel to remove excess water;
  - when the outside of the splint feels dry, apply it to the extremity and mould it to the desired shape;
  - stretch the stockinet over the upper and lower ends of the splint to prevent sharp edges;
  - wrap an elastic bandage around the extremity, starting at the bottom and moving upwards; the bandage must not be tight; **DO NOT** stretch it at any point.
- Check the five Ps (**P**allor, **P**ain, **P**aresthaesia, **P**ulselessness, and **P**aralysis) six hours after applying the splint, then every 24 hours: if you find a single P, remove the splint at once and seek medical advice.
- As swelling lessens, the splint may become loose: rebandage it more firmly or replace it if it does not provide a good fit.
- Tell the patient to report any worsening of pain, difficulty moving fingers or toes, or numbness or pins-and-needles: if any of these symptoms occur remove the splint at once.
- If the symptoms disappear at once, reapply the splint more loosely.
- If the symptoms do not disappear at once, seek medical advice.

COMPLICATIONS OF SPLINTING

- Sores from pressure of a poorly padded splint;
- abrasions from loose or badly-fitting splints;
- nerve or blood vessel problems from tight-fitting splints.

Abdominal and chest injuries

ABDOMINAL INJURIES

There are two main types of abdominal injury:

- blunt injuries, which are caused by crushing forces and blows from blunt objects;
- penetrating injuries, such as those caused by knife or gunshot wounds.

Either type of abdominal injury can be life-threatening, as a result of:

- rupture and bleeding of solid organs in the abdomen, especially the liver, spleen, and kidneys:
  - bleeding can be immediate, resulting in death within minutes or hours, or delayed, causing death after several days or weeks;
- damage to major blood vessels;
- penetration of the bowel, leading to infection of the peritoneum (the thin membrane covering the organs within the abdominal cavity), and death within hours or days.

Blunt abdominal injuries

A blunt abdominal injury occurs when a person is crushed by a heavy object or struck by a blunt object or falls from a height (usually of more than five metres). In all these circumstances, major trauma to the chest, head, or limbs is often associated with abdominal trauma. Detecting even major damage to organs in the abdomen can be difficult after blunt injuries. Always seek medical advice when a crew member falls from a height or suffers a crush injury, however minor the injury appears.

✔ *What to do*

- If the patient has been injured in a way likely to have caused damage to abdominal organs, such as by a crush injury to the abdomen or a fall of more than five metres, assume that damage has occurred to abdominal organs and have the patient evacuated.
- Evacuate any patient who shows evidence of blood loss, namely any one of the following signs:
  - persistently rapid pulse
  - low or falling blood pressure
  - pallor.
- To assess the likelihood of serious injury, determine:
  - whether the patient fell from a height and, if so, from what height;
  - whether a crush injury occurred, by what means, and at what speed the causative object was moving;
  - whether the patient was hit by something, on what part of the body, and with what force.
- Check the vital signs (see Chapter 1, *First aid*):
  - airway

- breathing
- blood circulation
- level of consciousness.

- If there is bleeding, apply pressure.
- Check for obvious fractures.
- Check for obvious head injury.
- Check if the chest moves on both sides when the patient breathes in.
- Check and make a record of:
  - pulse rate
  - blood pressure
  - level of consciousness
  - movement of all four limbs
  - pupil size.
- Seek medical advice at this point: it may be obvious that there are, or are likely to be, major injuries; if so:
  - prepare for evacuation of the patient;
  - insert an intravenous cannula, and give normal saline (0.9% sodium chloride), one litre over six hours, or more as advised by a doctor.
- If there is severe pain, give morphine, 10 mg intravenously or intramuscularly.
- If there are no obvious major injuries:
  - move the patient to a suitable place on board where you can carry out a more complete examination (see Chapter 12, *Examination of the patient*).
- Check the vital signs again (airway, breathing, blood circulation, level of consciousness) and note down the findings.
- Remove all the patient's clothing and examine the whole body thoroughly and systematically for wounds, bruising, and tenderness.
- Look especially for the following **red flag signs**:
  - bruising and tenderness over the lower ribs: lower rib fractures are often associated with damage to the spleen (on the left) or the liver (on the right);
  - blood visible at the opening of the urethra, suggesting damage to the urethra;
  - generalized tenderness or distension of the abdomen;
  - absence of bowel sounds;
  - pain in the shoulder not explained by injury, suggesting bleeding in the upper abdomen;
  - a "new" pain in the abdomen, suggesting a ruptured bowel or damage to the pancreas;
  - fever, suggesting peritonitis due to a ruptured bowel.
- Check and record the vital signs again: a rising pulse rate is the first and most reliable indication of continuing blood loss.
- Ask if the patient can pass urine:
  - if the patient can pass urine, test the urine for blood each time the patient passes urine: a positive result may be due to damage to the kidney or urethra;
  - if the patient has not passed urine over a six hour period, rupture of the urethra may have occurred.

- If no significant injury is apparent, keep the patient in bed and reassess the patient's condition frequently.
- Give nothing by mouth unless advised by a doctor.
- **Remember: evacuate any patient with evidence of serious injury AND any patient in whom the circumstances of an injury suggest that it is likely to be serious.**

Penetrating abdominal injuries

Penetrating abdominal injuries, whether the result of a stab, gunshot, or other accidental event, require evacuation of the patient. Evacuation should not be delayed, even if the patient does not think that a wound has penetrated the abdominal wall.

Note

- Signs of blood loss – rapid pulse, falling blood pressure, pallor – in the first minutes or hours after an injury may be due to damage of the liver or spleen or a major artery.
- Fever with increasing abdominal pain and distension suggests that the patient has peritonitis, which usually takes hours or days to develop.

✔ *What to do*

- Seek medical advice and prepare the patient for evacuation.
- Insert an intravenous cannula and give normal saline (0.9% sodium chloride), one litre over six hours or as advised by a doctor.
- Give ceftriaxone, 1 g intravenously, twice daily.
- To relieve pain, give morphine, 10–15 mg intramuscularly or intravenously, every three to four hours.
- Give nothing by mouth.

✔ *What to do in case of an open abdominal wound with protrusion of gut*

- Seek medical advice and prepare for evacuation of the patient.
- In addition to the measures recommended above for penetrating abdominal injuries:
  - apply sterile dressings moistened with sterile normal saline (0.9% sodium chloride);
  - use a loose binder to keep the dressings in place;
  - cover the dressings to retain warmth.

✗ *What not to do in a case of an open abdominal wound with protrusion of gut*

- Do not apply direct pressure to the protruding gut.
- Do not attempt to push the gut back into place.

CHEST INJURIES

The chest cavity contains several vital organs, such as the heart, lungs, and great vessels (including the aorta). Chest injuries should, therefore, always be regarded as serious. Internal bleeding and respiratory failure can cause death in minutes. Crush injuries of the chest are nearly always more extensive than they seem at first sight and they are always serious.

✔ *What to do*

- Seek medical advice, but before doing so be prepared to answer these questions:
  - How did the injury occur?
  - Are there, or are there likely to be, other injuries?
- If you suspect head injury, what is the Glasgow Coma Scale score (see Chapter 26, *Nursing care and medical procedures*, Table 26.3)?
  - What are the pulse rate and blood pressure?
- If the injury is not obviously severe, before seeking medical advice:
  - check for wounds:
    - if there is a wound, put your ear close to it: if you hear a "sucking wound" with air going into the wound as the patient breathes, it means that the wound has penetrated the chest (see section below, *Penetrating chest wounds*);
    - feel for tenderness;
    - marked tenderness is usually a sign of a rib fracture (see next section);
  - listen with a stethoscope to both sides of the chest:
    - absence of breath sounds on one side is a sign of a serious injury.
- If the injury appears to be minor, look for rib fractures by "springing" the chest, that is:
  - put one hand on each side of the rib cage and give a brief inward push: if there is a rib fracture;
  - the patient will feel pain at the site of the fracture.

Simple rib fracture

A simple rib fracture is one that does not affect the structural integrity of the chest wall or inflict damage on any internal organ. The cause of a simple rib fracture is usually a blow to the chest wall, not a crush injury. Complete healing of the fracture can take up to six weeks but most patients can return to work after three or four weeks.

Note

- In a patient with a rib fracture caused by a blow to the lower chest, there may be damage to the liver if the blow was on the right side of the chest or to the spleen if it was on the left side of the chest (see section above, *Abdominal injuries*).
- If a direct injury to the chest fractures a patient's clavicle (collar bone) the blow must have been very heavy and probably caused multiple rib fractures.
- A patient with three or more rib fractures or with fractures on both sides of the chest should be evacuated: there is a real risk of severe damage to the heart, lungs, liver, or spleen.
- Because of pain, a patient with a rib fracture will tend to lie still, breathe shallowly, and avoid coughing: as a result, secretions and mucus remain in the lungs and infection is likely: to avoid infection, therefore, adequate pain relief should be provided from the start.

Signs and symptoms

- Chest wall pain, especially with movement, coughing, laughing, or breathing;
- marked tenderness at the site of the fracture;
- bone crepitus (crackling, crinkly sensation), sometimes felt on palpation of the rib cage;
- shallow breathing.

What to do

- If the patient can breathe in fully and can cough, give ibuprofen, 400 mg orally, every six hours.
- If pain prevents the patient from taking in a full breath **AND** from coughing, give:
  - morphine, 20 mg orally, every four hours; **OR**
  - 10 mg intramuscularly, every three to four hours; **AND**
  - ibuprofen, 400 mg orally, every six hours.
- If necessary, adjust the morphine dose at frequent intervals in order to keep the patient free enough of pain and awake enough to move around, breathe deeply, and cough: consider giving smaller doses more frequently if drowsiness occurs.
- Reassess the need for morphine at 24 hours and then daily.

Flail chest

Flail chest occurs after a major chest injury (on board ship, usually a crush injury) that has fractured multiple ribs in more than one place, resulting in one part of the chest wall being disconnected from the rest. The result is "paradoxical" chest motion: with every breath, one section of the chest moves in, instead of out, preventing adequate inflation of the lungs. Bruising of the lung underneath the injured area is nearly always present. Rapid action is required to avoid progressively severe breathing difficulties that can cause a life-threatening fall in blood oxygen concentration.

Signs and symptoms

- Severe chest wall pain, especially with movement, coughing, or breathing;
- bone crepitus (crackling, crinkly sensation) felt on palpation of the rib cage;
- breathing rapid, shallow, and gasping;
- retraction (instead of expansion) during inspiration of part of the chest wall;
- bluish or purplish discoloration of skin (cyanosis), due to deficient oxygenation of the blood.

What to do

- Seek medical advice and prepare for evacuation of the patient.
- Administer high-flow oxygen with a non-rebreathing mask.
- Check for possible injuries to heart, lungs, and abdominal organs.
- To relieve pain, give morphine, 10 mg intramuscularly or intravenously.
- Keep the patient under close observation for possible pneumothorax (see below).

- Do not give the patient anything to eat or drink if evacuation is imminent: emergency anaesthesia may be required.
- Insert an intravenous cannula, even if pulse and blood pressure are normal.

Pneumothorax

Pneumothorax occurs when air accumulates between the two thin membrane sacs (pleurae) surrounding the lungs and lining the inside of the chest wall, respectively. The lung retains its normal size and position because the pressure in the pleural space is less than the atmospheric pressure: the resulting suction effect holds the lung up against the rib cage. This mechanism requires the pleural space to be sealed. When the pleura is pierced the seal is broken, air enters the pleural space, and the lung collapses. A pneumothorax may occur in healthy people (spontaneous pneumothorax) or may result from a penetrating wound or a broken rib segment that penetrates the pleura or the lung, allowing air to enter the pleural space (traumatic pneumothorax).

Spontaneous pneumothorax

Spontaneous pneumothorax occurs when small bubbles or blebs on the surface of the lung burst. These bubbles or blebs form in the lungs of some cigarette smokers, especially those who are tall and thin. Spontaneous pneumothorax occurs predominantly in men under the age of 40.

Signs and symptoms

- Sudden chest pain in a young man;
- pain when breathing in;
- shallow breathing as a result of pain;
- crepitus under the skin, which may develop after a few hours or days, usually around the neck but not over the chest wall;
- in many cases, diminished breath sounds on the affected side, but breath sounds may be normal if the pneumothorax is small.

What to do in a case of spontaneous pneumothorax

- In most cases, no treatment is required: serious breathing problems are rare and the air in the pleural space is generally absorbed in a few days.
- Warn the patient not to travel by air or to scuba dive until a doctor confirms that the pneumothorax has resolved.
- People who have had one spontaneous pneumothorax are prone to further episodes, even if they recover fully from the first episode: advise the patient to see a doctor at the end of the voyage with a view to having surgery to prevent further episodes.

Tension pneumothorax

A tension pneumothorax is a potentially life-threatening chest injury. It is nearly always a consequence of a traumatic pneumothorax and is only rarely associated with spontaneous pneumothorax. Tension pneumothorax occurs when air leaks into the pleural space and the tissues surrounding the point of leakage form a one-way valve trapping the air inside the pleural space. Every time the patient breathes in air is sucked into the pleural space but it cannot escape when the patient breathes out. The pressure builds up in the pleural space and displaces the heart, great vessels, and the other lung towards the opposite side of the chest cavity. When the pressure of the trapped air reaches a critical level – and it can do so very soon after the injury – the return of blood to the heart stops and, in the absence of treatment, the patient dies.

Signs and symptoms

- In a patient with a chest injury onset, over a few minutes, of:
  - apprehension and agitation
  - increasing difficulty breathing
  - swollen neck veins
  - rapid, faint pulse
  - low blood pressure
  - diminished or absent breath sounds on the affected side
  - bluish skin discolouring (cyanosis)
  - displacement of the windpipe (trachea) away from the affected side, detected by placing a finger in the notch at the top of the breast bone and pushing gently: if the finger slips to one side, the trachea has shifted to the other side.

What to do

- Seek medical advice **but do not delay treatment**.
- To relieve pressure inside the pleural space, insert a large-bore needle into the chest (Figure 7.1) through the space between the second and third ribs half way along the clavicle (collar bone): there will be a rush of air out of the chest and the patient will turn pink:
  - you can improvise a one-way valve by passing the needle through the end of a latex glove finger;
  - do not take the time to do this if the patient is blue: release the air from the pleural space first;
  - note that the patient is now in the same situation as a patient with spontaneous pneumothorax and should not have difficulty breathing, provided there are no other injuries;
  - if the patient's condition does not improve, suspect bleeding into the membrane that surrounds the heart – this cannot be treated on board ship.
- Check for other injuries.
- Arrange for evacuation of the patient: the needle in the pleural space will prevent spontaneous resolution of the pneumothorax but if you remove it, another tension pneumothorax may form.
- Administer high flow oxygen.

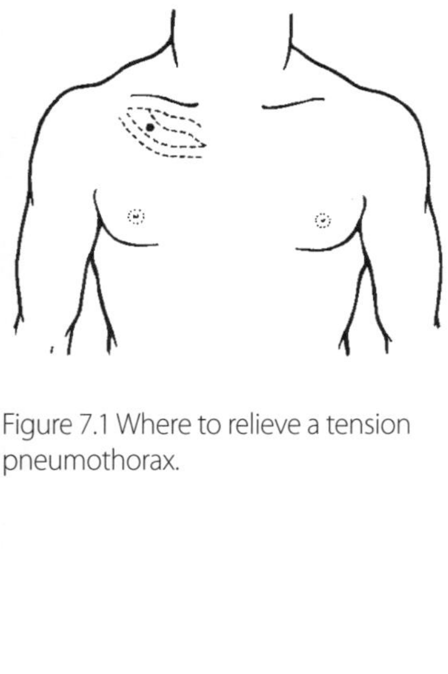

Figure 7.1 Where to relieve a tension pneumothorax.

Penetrating chest wounds

A penetrating chest wound can be life-threatening. It is usually caused by a gunshot or a stab wound or, more rarely, a fall onto a protruding object, such as metal scaffolding. The chest wall is about three to four centimetres thick, so that even short objects forced

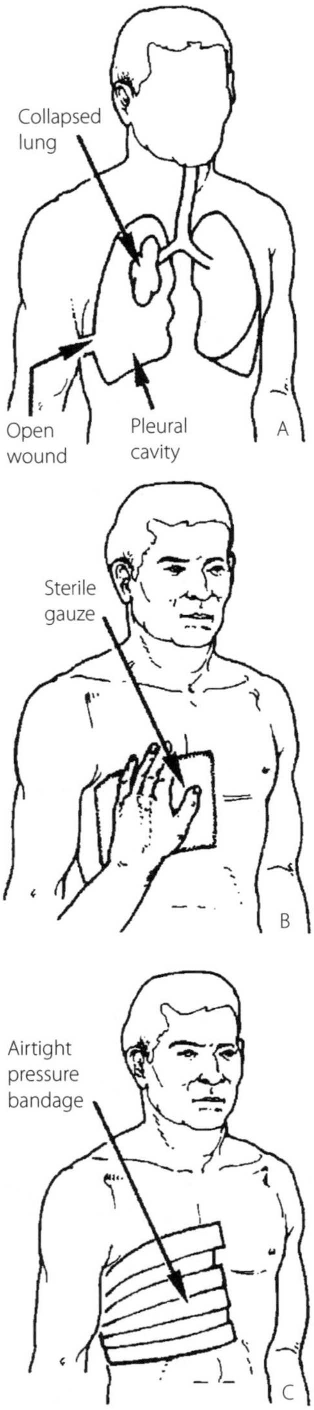

Figure 7.2 How to cover a large chest wound.

through it may penetrate the lung. Even if the lung, heart, or major vessels are not damaged there are fairly large arteries running between the ribs and damage to them can cause severe bleeding.

✔ *What to do*

- Seek medical advice with a view to urgent evacuation.
- Note that the patient can die quickly from bleeding from a major blood vessel or if both lungs are punctured (bilateral pneumothorax).
- If there is an open wound through which you can hear air entering the chest when the patient breathes in, seal the wound with a large wad of gauze and tape (Figure 7.2).
- Treat external bleeding with direct pressure.
- Give oxygen at high flow rates.
- Insert an intravenous cannula, and give normal saline (0.9% sodium chloride), one litre every four to six hours.
- Position the patient so that the uninjured, or less injured side, is downwards.

Chapter 8

Wounds

WOUND HEALING

There are two main types of healing:

- **healing by primary intention**: occurs in a wound whose edges are in contact (either naturally or after treatment) and in which there is neither infection nor damage to tissues on either side;
- **healing by secondary intention**: occurs when the edges of a wound remain apart or there is infection of, or damage to, the tissues around the wound. The wound is gradually filled from the bottom up by "granulation tissue", which is made up of new blood vessels and collagen.

KEY QUESTIONS

- What caused the wound?
  - If the wound was caused by a cut from a sharp, clean knife:
    - tissue around the wound is not likely to be damaged;
    - the wound is not likely to become infected.
  - If the wound was caused by a stab from a knife, dagger, or blunt object:
    - damage to important organs is likely, depending on the depth of the wound.
  - If the wound was caused by a blunt edge or flat surface, as in falling and striking the head against a bulkhead:
    - the skin may be torn;
    - the wound is usually irregular;
    - there may be extensive bruising and crushing of surrounding tissues;
    - the wound is likely to become infected;
    - on healing, scarring is likely.
  - If the cause was a bite:
    - tissue around the wound usually suffers crushing and bruising;
    - infection is likely, especially if the bite was from human teeth.
- Did the wound come into contact with dirt, soil, manure, or water from the sea or a river?
  - The circumstances in which the wound was caused should make this point clear.
  - Infection is likely.
- How deep is the wound and what is underneath it?
  - The base of the wound may be near or over a joint or tendon.
  - There may be damage to important structures.
- Could there be a foreign body in the wound?
  - Foreign bodies increase the risk of wound infection.
  - There may still be a foreign body even if it is not visible.
  - Glass fragments in the wound are likely if the patient has been stabbed with a glass shard, has stepped on glass, or has been injured by flying glass.
- Could a tendon or nerve be injured?

- Hand wounds (see Chapter 6, *Bone, joint, and muscle injuries*) are likely to involve nerve and tendon injuries.
- Nerves close to the surface that can be injured by relatively minor cuts are found on:
  - the little-finger side of the elbow – a cut nerve prevents straightening of the ring and little fingers and causes numbness of the little finger;
  - the outside of the leg immediately below the knee – a cut nerve causes "foot drop", which is an inability to bend the ankle upwards towards the shin;
  - the face, just in front of the ear – a cut nerve may prevent frowning, raising an eyebrow, opening or tightly closing the eye, or smiling.

- Is the patient fully immunized against tetanus? (see Chapter 30, *Preventing disease and promoting health in seafarers.*)

RED FLAG WOUNDS

In the following cases, seek medical advice **urgently** with a view to evacuation:

- stab wound:
  - if you are not absolutely certain that the wound is too shallow to have affected major organs or nerves or blood vessels, assume that the patient has suffered a serious injury.
- wound associated with major or extensive crush injury:
  - example: a hand trapped in a machine roller;
- wound near a suspected fracture:
  - it is safest to assume that any wound near a fracture represents a compound fracture: the consequences of an inadequately treated compound fracture can be severe;
- wound caused by injection of grease or paint under pressure:
  - the skin wound is often small but there can be extensive tissue destruction;
  - if a hand is involved, as is often the case with such wounds, the outcome can be catastrophic.

✔ *What to do*

- Wash your hands.
- Put on gloves and eye protection.
- Inspect the wound for:
  - foreign bodies and dirt;
  - nerve and tendon damage (especially if the wound is over a tendon);
    - if you examine a finger that was cut while it was bent, you will not see the cut tendon under the wound if you examine the finger while it is straight;
  - you may have to use a local anaesthetic before you can make a thorough inspection (see section below, *Local anaesthesia*);
    - if so check again for nerve damage before injecting the anaesthetic;
  - if you suspect that there is a glass fragment in the wound, arrange for the patient to see a doctor at the next port with a view to having an X-ray and any fragments removed.

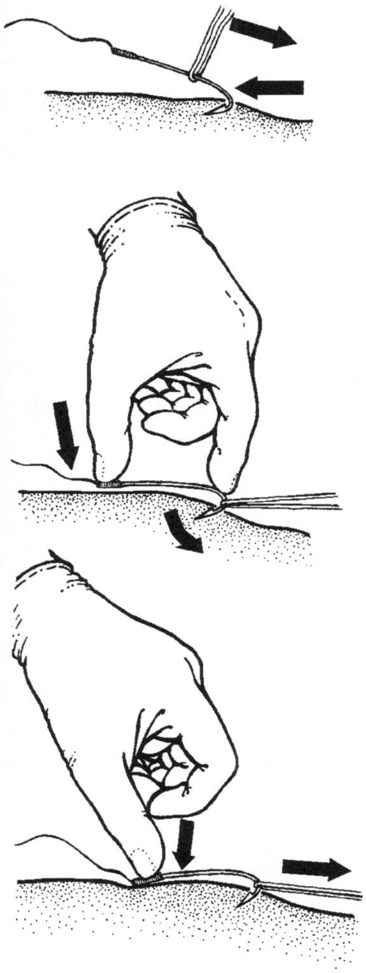

Figure 8.1 How to remove a fishhook.

- If you can see a foreign body, remove it with forceps. Figures 8.1 and 8.2 show how to remove fishhooks.
- If you suspect a foreign body but cannot see or feel it and if the circumstances suggest it is clean glass or metal, it is usually better to leave the wound alone than to tamper too much with it.
- To stop the wound bleeding:
  - apply direct pressure with a gauze pad for 10–15 minutes;
  - wait for 10 minutes before checking if the wound has stopped bleeding;
  - if blood continues to spurt from the wound, reapply pressure;
  - DO NOT attempt blind clamping of bleeding points;
  - if a major artery has been cut, surgical repair is needed and the patient should be evacuated to a hospital;
  - if a minor artery is bleeding from the skin, apply pressure and suture the wound (see section below, *Suturing a wound*).
- To wash out the wound:
  - use a 50-ml or 60-ml syringe with a 19-gauge needle, preferably a blunt ("drawing up") needle, because high pressures and large volumes are needed for efficient cleansing;
  - add one volume of povidone-iodine to 10 volumes of potable water (do not use chlorhexidine or hydrogen peroxide);
  - flush the wound with a strong jet from the syringe: this should remove dirt, fragments of tissue, blood clots, and bacteria;
  - flush repeatedly, using a total of 200–500 ml of liquid;
  - take care to avoid splashing liquid contaminated with blood into your eyes: WEAR EYE PROTECTION.
- If the circumstances of the injury suggest that there may be foreign bodies in the wound or that the wound may have caused injury to a tendon, inspect the wound once more after cleaning it out.
- Decide how to close the wound (see section below, *How to close wounds*).

✗ *What not to do*

- Do not shave the hair around a wound: you risk infecting the wound or leaving hair fragments in it:
  - clip the hair or wet it and comb it away from the edges of the wound.
- Do not shave or even clip eyebrows: they may not grow back.

HOW TO CLOSE A WOUND

Using adhesive skin closures

With small, clean cuts you may be able to use "butterfly closures", which consist of two adhesive patches joined by a narrow non-adhesive bridge. Butterfly closures work best when the skin is elastic, as in young people, or when it adheres tightly to the underlying tissue, as on the face.

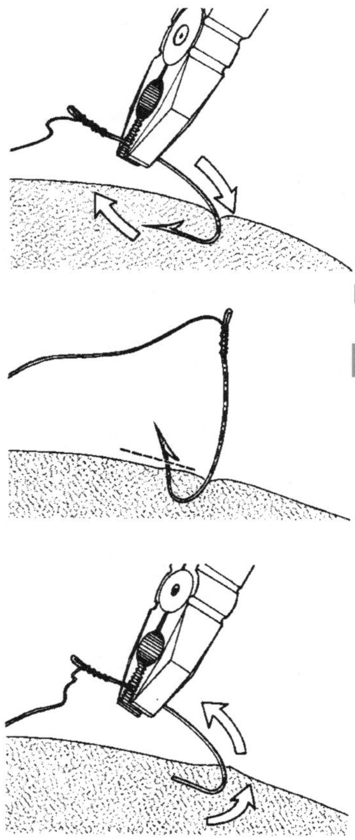

Figure 8.2 Alternative method of removing a fishhook.

✔ What to do

- Make sure the edges of the wound are dry (Figure 8.3).
- Remove the butterfly closure from its envelope and strip off the protective backing.
- Bring the edges of the wound together by fixing the closure on either side of the wound so that the non-adhesive bridge lies across the wound (Figure 8.4).

Using skin adhesive (liquid stitches)

Note

- Cyanoacrylate skin adhesive compounds are as effective as, or more effective than, sutures for closing wounds (except for the wounds listed below, under section, *Special wounds*).
- Skin adhesive is especially useful:
  - when it is difficult to keep the wound dry;
  - for small wounds whose edges can be brought together easily without tension.
- Skin adhesive also:
  - avoids the need for additional dressings;
  - is waterproof;
  - requires no local anaesthesia.
- The main risk with skin adhesive is that it may enter an eye, or glue fingers together, or glue gauze strips or instruments (especially plastic forceps) to the wound.
- Skin adhesive should not be used with a wound that:
  - will be moved a lot, such as a wound that lies across a joint;
  - is on the inside of the mouth, because moisture prevents the adhesive sticking to the skin;
  - is dirty;
  - involves severe bruising of surrounding tissues;
  - involves damage to surrounding skin.

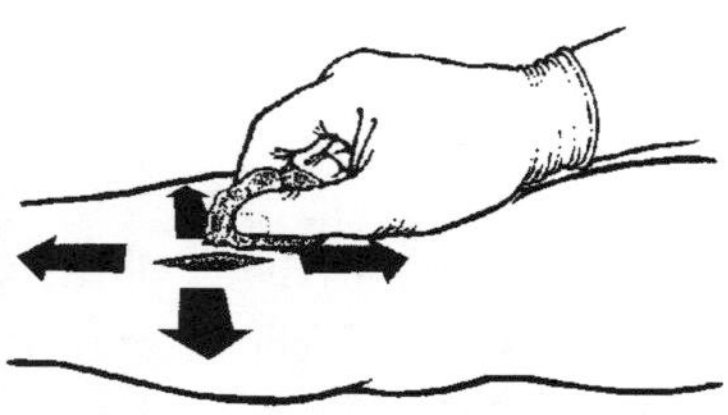

Figure 8.3 Drying the area around a wound.

✔ What to do

- Wash and inspect the wound.
- Warn the patient that the adhesive gives off heat as it dries.
- Have the patient or an assistant place their fingers 2 cm or so away from the wound and press inwards towards the wound so as bring the wound edges together (taking care not to get adhesive onto their fingers, because they will stick to the skin).
- Make sure bleeding has stopped and that the skin is dry (blood from the wound or wet skin will prevent the adhesive from sticking).

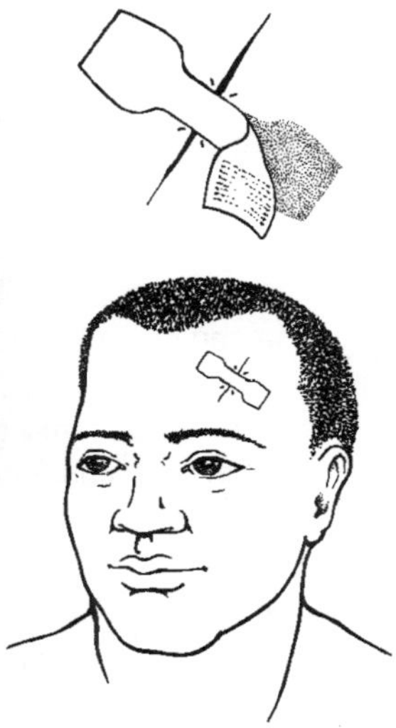

Figure 8.4 Applying a butterfly strip skin closure.

- Spread the skin adhesive gently across the wound with a smooth continuous motion, so as to cover the wound area and 5–10 mm beyond it with a thin film of adhesive.
- Avoid getting adhesive into the wound.
- Hold the wound edges together for 40–45 seconds to allow the adhesive to set.
- If the edges of the wound are not well aligned, use petroleum jelly to wipe the adhesive off and start again.
- Put three or four coats of adhesive over and around the wound, so that the patch of adhesive extends 10 mm beyond the wound in all directions.
- Wait for each coat to dry before putting on the next: each additional coat takes longer to dry than the previous coat, but do not touch the wound until the final coat is dry.
- Allow the patient to shower but without soaking or scrubbing the wound area, which should be patted dry after the shower.
- Advise the patient to avoid having a bath for seven to 10 days, by which time the adhesive will have peeled off.

Suturing a wound

Note

- The aim of suturing is to keep the edges of the wound together so that healing by primary intention can occur.
- Sutures should not be used:
  - if the edges of the wound cannot be easily brought together; **OR**
  - if the edges of the wound can be securely brought together without sutures; **OR**
  - if healing by primary intention is unlikely to occur.
- If badly performed, suturing will increase the risk of infection and unsightly scarring – more so than skin adhesive or a simple dressing.
- A suture creates another wound and introduces a foreign body into the tissue: it therefore increases the risk of infection in much the same way as any other foreign body does.
- Suture material must be heavy enough and suture needles long enough to ensure a roughly round or squarish suture track in deep wounds.
- In choosing suture material, note:
  - suture thickness is specified by the number on the packet:
    - 1-O: thick; suitable for large scalp wounds;
    - 3-O: suitable for most arm or leg wounds;
    - 5-O: fine; suitable for face wounds in adults;
  - sutures made of braided silk (the traditional "non-absorbable" suture material) are the easiest to use;
  - the thicker the suture material is, the thicker and longer the suture needle must be;
  - most modern suture material comes with a suitable needle permanently attached.
- Suture needles for use in skin are curved, and triangular in cross-section, with one edge sharpened as a cutting edge; the two common types are:

- a "cutting needle" (with the cutting edge on the concave side of the needle), which is best for relatively soft skin);
- a "reverse cutting needle" (with the cutting edge on the convex side of the needle), which is best for thick skin, such on the soles of the feet.

✗ *What not to do*

- Do not use more sutures than are needed to keep the wound edges together.
- Do not put a stitch anywhere unless you are sure there are no important structures under the skin.
- Do not use sutures to drag the edges of a wound into contact: the tension in the sutures can cut off blood supply to the wound, thereby promoting infection and delaying healing.
- Do not suture wounds that are dirty or have foreign bodies in them.
- Do not suture deep penetrating wounds that cannot be washed out thoroughly.
- Do not suture wounds that have crushed or extensively bruised tissues around them.
- Do not suture a wound that is over eight hours old.
- NEVER suture wounds on the fingers: you can easily damage nerves, blood vessels, and tendons. Use a dressing.

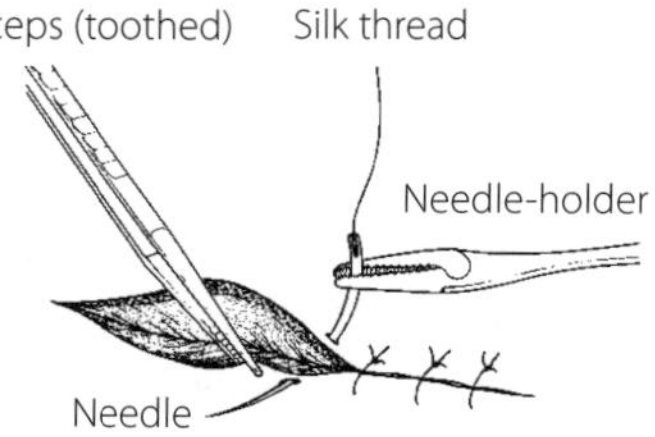

Figure 8.5 Stitching a wound.

✔ *What to do*

- Assemble the following items:
  - one packet of the suture material you have chosen
  - a needle-holder
  - small scissors
  - toothed tissue forceps
  - a kidney dish.
- Sterilize the needle-holder, scissors, forceps, and kidney dish by boiling in water for 20 minutes.
- Place the sterilized needle-holder, forceps, and scissors in the kidney dish.
- Wash your hands.
- Put on clean gloves.
- Open the suture material packet and drop the needle and suture thread into the sterilized kidney dish.
- Use the needle-holder to grasp the needle (hold the needle near its mid-point; if you hold it near to where it joins the thread it will bend when you try to pierce the skin).
- Use the toothed tissue forceps to grasp the edge of the wound nearest to you.
- Holding the needle perpendicular to the skin, drive it with a firm stab through the whole thickness of skin.
- Remember that the needle track should be roughly circular or square, so that the distance from the wound edge to the point where the needle enters the skin should be about half the wound depth (Figure 8.5).
- Rotate the needle-holder, so that the needle point is no longer perpendicular but parallel to the skin.
- Check that the needle emerges from the side and near the base of the wound.

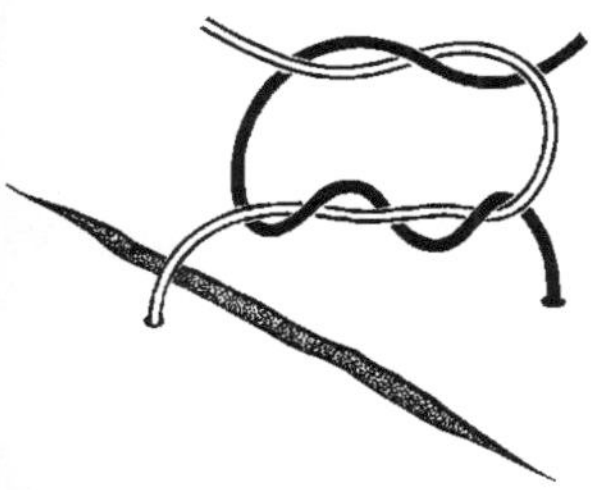

Figure 8.6 How to tie a surgeon's knot.

- Release the needle from the needle-holder, grasp it by the exposed point in the wound, and pull it out of the wound.
- Use the needle-holder again to grasp the needle near its mid-point.
- Use the toothed forceps to grasp the skin on the side of the wound opposite to the first half of the suture.
- Push the needle into the side of the wound directly opposite to where the needle point first emerged.
- Drive the needle upwards through the whole thickness of the skin so that it emerges from the wound edge directly opposite to the point where it first entered, preferably at the same distance from the wound as the first point; note:
  - it is important that the needle comes out opposite to where it went in, otherwise the suture will pull the wound out of shape;
  - it is less important for the needle to emerge the same distance from the wound as it went in.
- Pull the needle and suture thread through the wound with the forceps or needle-holder, and cut the thread so that there is about 4 cm of suture material on either side of the wound.
- To bring the cut edges of the skin together, tie a surgeon's knot (two throws) with just enough tension to keep the skin edges together, but not more (Figure 8.6).
- After tying the knot, cut off the loose ends, leaving about 5–10 mm free to make it easy to remove the stitches later.
- Check that the suture is at right angles to the line of the wound.
- Insert further stitches to prevent the wound from gaping; note:
  - the distance between sutures should be about equal to the distance between the point at which each suture enters the skin and the wound edge, or half the wound depth (Figure 8.7).
- As soon as you have finished suturing, put the needle into a sharps disposal container.
- Consider replacing the sutures if, after wound closure, the cut edges of the skin curve inwards into the wound, making unsightly scarring more likely; note:
  - this problem is especially common with wounds in looser skin, as on the forearms, or if the sutures are too close to the surface.
- If the sutures are not too shallow and if the tissues are elastic, as in a young person, you may be able to pull out the edges of the skin with toothed forceps.
- You may also use a "mattress" suture to keep the skin edges from curving into the wound.
- After suturing, apply a non-adherent gauze dressing on the wound area, followed by a layer of dry gauze:
  - do not dress small scalp wounds or wounds in areas difficult to cover but not likely to become dirty.
- Change the dressing after 24 hours and wash the wound gently with soap and water to remove crusts over the stitches.
- Remove the dressing after 48 hours and leave the wound uncovered.
- Remove sutures after:

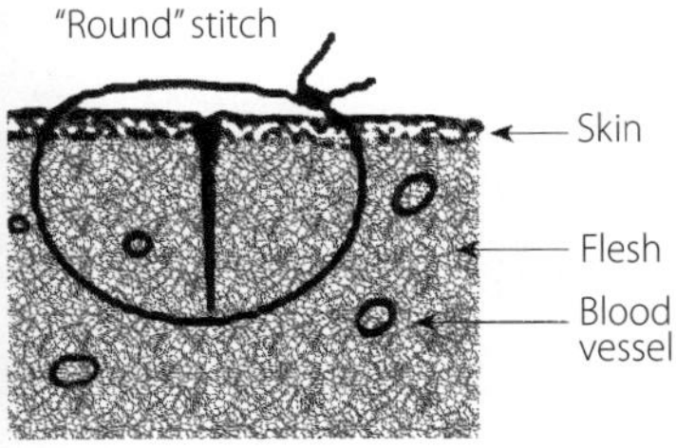

Figure 8.7 Cross section of the stitched wound.

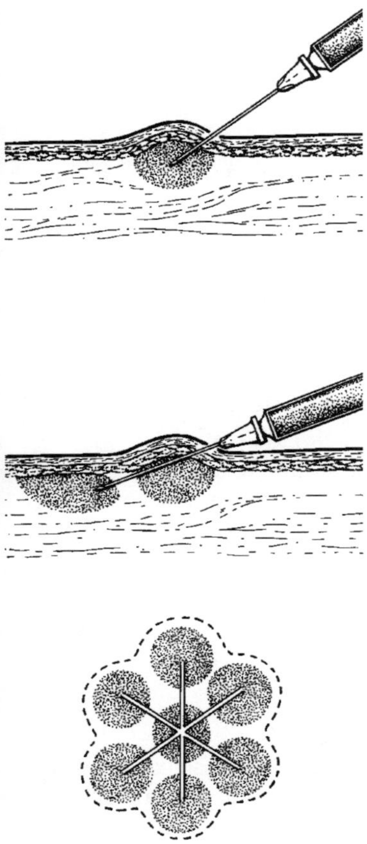

Figure 8.8 Injecting local anaesthetic.

- five days, for wounds on the face;
- seven days, for wounds on the scalp;
- seven to 10 days, for wounds on other sites.

■ To remove sutures:
- assemble toothed forceps, povidone-iodine, gauze swabs, and a stitch-cutter or scalpel blade;
- swab the wound area with povidone-iodine;
- use forceps to grasp one end of the stitch and lift it clear of the skin;
- insert the scalpel blade under the suture and cut it with a movement away from the skin;
- use the forceps to pull the thread out gently.

LOCAL ANAESTHESIA

In a patient who has suffered a painful wound and who anticipates more pain when the wound is being sutured, local anaesthesia can make the task much easier. Local anaesthesia should always be used when sutures are required in parts of the body – the lips, for example – where precision is needed.

✔ *What to do*

- Use lignocaine (lidocaine), 1%, for local anaesthesia, but not more than 20 ml at once; note:
  - lignocaine stings on injection, but only until anaesthesia takes over;
  - lignocaine can cause fits and abnormal heart rhythms if too large a dose is used.
- Inject the anaesthetic directly into the sides of the wound: injecting into intact skin at both sides of the wound is more painful.
- Insert the needle to a depth of about 1 cm into both sides of the wound just below the skin.
- Draw back the plunger to be sure the needle is not in a blood vessel.
- Inject enough anaesthetic to cause visible swelling of the tissues around the wound (Figure 8.8).
- Local anaesthesia lasts about 20 minutes, so if the wound is large and you are inexperienced, and likely to suture slowly, anesthetize only 2 cm or so of the wound at a time.

SPECIAL WOUNDS

Lips

The border between pink-coloured lip and ordinary skin ("the vermilion border") must be matched up precisely: a 1 mm misalignment is noticeable.

✔ *What to do*

- Match the edges of the vermilion border carefully, putting the first stitch exactly through the border on each side of the wound (Figure 8.9).

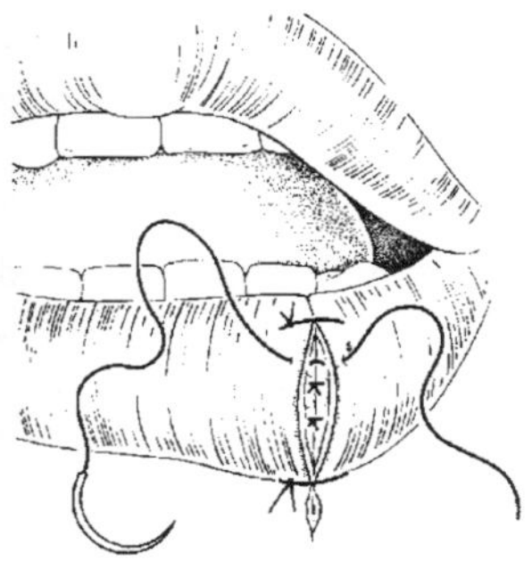

Figure 8.9 Stitching a lip.

- Use only a minimal amount of local anaesthetic and inject it only at the vermilion border, since a large injection into surrounding tissues can distort their shape.
- Whereas the vermilion border nearly always has to be sutured, the inside surface of the lip usually does not, as long as bleeding has stopped and the wound edges have been brought together.

Tongue

Tongue wounds often result from impact injuries to the face and jaw. Because tongue wounds tend to bleed heavily, more serious injuries are likely to be overlooked. Small wounds to the tongue do not need suturing. Large tongue wounds may require suturing, which should be done in a hospital.

✔ *What to do*

- Check for pain and tenderness of the jaws.
- Ask the patient whether some upper teeth feel as if they are out of alignment with lower teeth: this could be due to a fractured jaw.

✘ *What not to do*

- Do not attempt to suture small tongue wounds: you are unlikely to succeed in stopping the bleeding.
- If bleeding of the tongue is slow to stop – and it often is, because of the difficulty of applying pressure to the tongue and of keeping the tongue still:
  - have the patient lie face down, to prevent blood being inhaled;
  - have the patient press ice cubes to the wound, which constricts blood vessels and puts pressure on the wound.

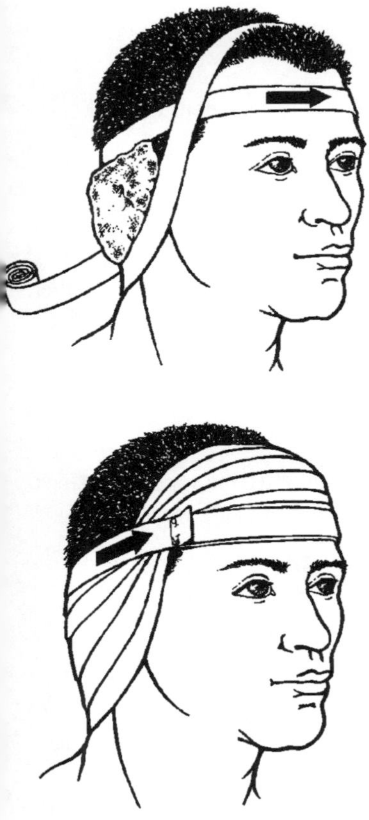

Ears and nose

The ears and the tip of the nose consist of skin over cartilage.

✔ *What to do*

- If the cartilage is not cut or torn, close the skin wound, preferably with butterfly closures or skin adhesive (see above).
- If skin has been lost, so that there will not be enough to cover the cartilage after closure of the wound, do not close the wound.
- Apply a sterile dressing (Figure 8.10) and arrange for the patient to be seen by a medical specialist as soon as possible.

✘ *What not to do*

- DO NOT put sutures into cartilage.

Eyelids

Wounds inflicted on the medial halves of the eyelids (towards the inner corners of the eyes) can damage the tear ducts: patients should be seen by an eye specialist at the next port.

igure 8.10 How to bandage an
njured ear.

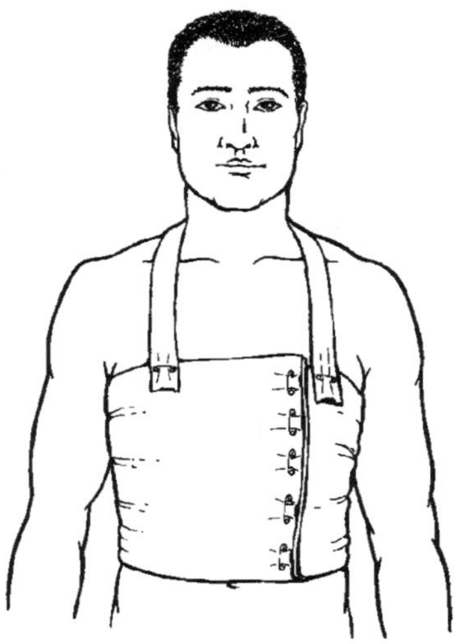

Figure 8.11 How to bandage the chest.

Wounds of the eyelids that are not properly repaired can cause long-term problems: these patients also should see an eye specialist or plastic surgeon at the next port.

Puncture wounds of the soles of the feet

Puncture wounds of the feet can be caused by nails, glass, sewing needles, or wood splinters. Because the object causing the puncture is driven into the foot by the weight of the whole body it often penetrates deeply and the wound may involve bones or joints. The main risk with puncture wounds of the feet is infection, with or without a retained foreign body. In most cases, surgical treatment is needed to detect and remove foreign bodies and ensure proper wound drainage.

✔ *What to do*

- If you are in port, have the patient see a doctor as soon as possible.
- An X-ray is usually needed to locate a foreign body: if this is not possible and walking is painful, have the patient rest until walking is comfortable or until a doctor can be consulted.
- If there are signs of infection – and only then – give amoxycillin/clavulanate, 875/125 mg orally, twice daily and seek medical advice.

✗ *What not to do*

- Do not give antibiotics unless signs of infection appear.
- Do not probe the wound.

WOUND INFECTION

Some bacterial contamination of the wound is inevitable after injury. Infection occurs when the number of bacteria introduced and the conditions in the wound are such that multiplication of bacteria is possible. Dog bites do not usually become infected. Cat and human bites are likely to cause serious infection.

Signs and symptoms

- Redness, heat, swelling, and pain more than 48 hours after the injury or marked worsening of these symptoms earlier.

✔ *What to do*

- Remove clotted blood and debris from the wound.
- If the wound has been stitched, inspect it to see if there is tension on a stitch in any part of the wound which could be caused by swelling of the tissues or pus within the wound.
- If there is tension on a stitch, remove all the stitches that are under tension and allow the wound to drain freely.
- If the redness and swelling are severe or do not improve over 24 hours, give amoxycillin/clavulanate, 875/125 mg orally, twice daily.
- If the infection resolves, leave the wound to heal by secondary intention.

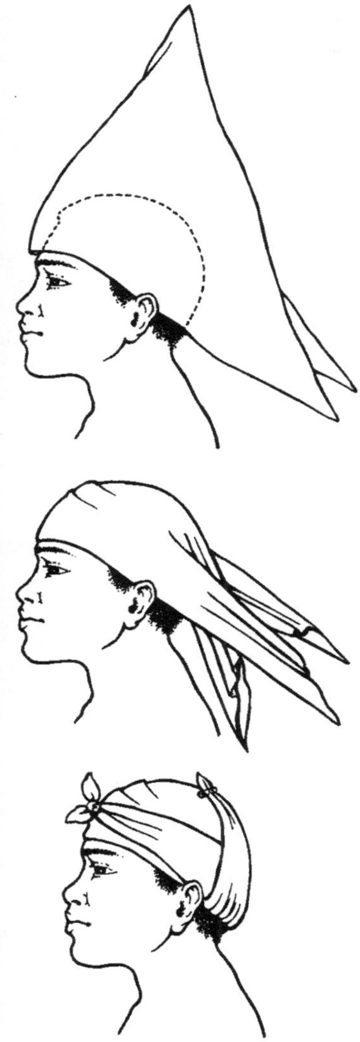

Figure 8.12 How to bandage a scalp wound.

- Dress the wound with a wet-to-dry dressing (see below).
- In the case of an infected cat bite, give ciprofloxacin, 500 mg orally, twice daily.
- In the case of an infected human bite, give amoxycillin/clavulanate, 875/125 mg orally, twice daily.
- In the case of a wound contaminated with seawater or water from a river, lake, or pond, infection can be life-threatening: if redness and swelling spread beyond the immediate wound area or if the patient becomes ill, seek medical advice urgently.

DRESSING WOUNDS THAT CANNOT BE CLOSED

If a wound is allowed to heal by secondary intention, it should be dressed so as to keep it moist and clean. Figures 8.11 and 8.12 show how to bandage wounds on the chest and the scalp.

✔ *What to do*

- Apply a wet-to-dry dressing, as follows:
  - wet a length of surgical gauze with tap water;
  - place it in or over the wound;
  - cover with two or three layers of dry gauze;
  - secure with a bandage or adhesive covering; note:
    - as the gauze dries out it sticks to the wound surface, so that when it is removed bacteria and fluid that has oozed from the wound are removed with it;
  - change the dressing twice daily until the whole base of the wound is pink, without any sign of inflammation or pus formation;
  - apply a non-adherent gauze dressing;
  - change the dressing every second day.

Burns, chemical splashes, smoke inhalation, and electrocution

CLOTHING ON FIRE

✔ *What to do*

- Tell the victim to close the eyes immediately and use a dry-powder fire extinguisher (colour-coded red in many countries) to put out the fire:
  - after the fire is extinguished, have the victim wash out any powder that has entered the eyes.
- If a dry-powder extinguisher is not available, lay the victim down and smother the flames by wrapping the victim in any available material; **OR**
  - throw bucketfuls of water over the victim; **OR**
  - use a hose, if available, to douse the victim.
- Make sure all smouldering clothing is extinguished.

✘ *What not to do*

- **Do not** use a carbon dioxide extinguisher (colour-coded black in many countries), unless nothing else is available: the gas can suffocate the patient:
  - if you must use a carbon dioxide extinguisher, get the victim away from the gas cloud as soon as the fire is out.

HEAT BURNS AND SCALDS

The treatment of burns and scalds is generally the same, whether the cause is dry or wet heat, electricity, or chemicals (for cold burns see Chapter 28, *Medical care for survivors at sea*). With electrical burns, there may be only a small burn on the skin surface but extensive damage to underlying tissue.

Note

- Skin has an outer layer (epidermis) and a deep layer (dermis). The dermis contains sweat glands, hair follicles, and nerves relaying sensation and pain to the skin (Figure 9.1).
- The most important questions to consider in a burn injury are:
  - How deeply does the burn go into the skin?
  - How extensive is the area of skin affected by the burn (Figure 9.2)?
- Burns generally cause loss of fluid from the body:
  - the fluid lost is plasma (the pale-yellow liquid part of blood);
  - generally, the more extensive the burn (as distinct from its depth), the greater the fluid loss and the more severe the degree of shock (see Chapter 2, *Shock*).
- A standard method of estimating the surface area affected by a burn is the "rule of nines" (see section below, *Determining the severity of a burn* and Figure 9.3). For children (not babies), the percentage for the head should be doubled and 1% taken off each of the other areas.

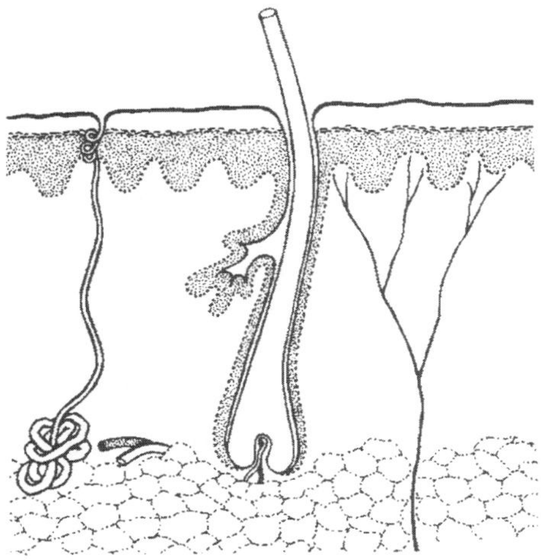

Figure 9.1 The layers of the skin.

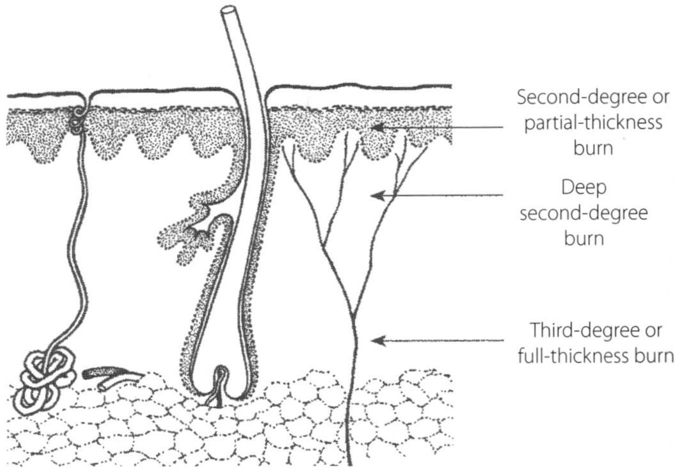

Figure 9.2 The thickness of a burn.

How to determine the severity of a burn

- **First-degree burn:**
  - **skin level:**
    - outer skin layer (epidermis);
  - **signs and symptoms:**
    - redness which turns pale on pressure
    - mild swelling, tenderness, pain;
  - **outcome:**
    - heals in three to seven days without scarring.
- **Second-degree, or partial-thickness, burn:**
  - **skin level:**
    - deep skin layer (dermis).
- **Superficial second-degree burn:**
  - **signs and symptoms:**
    - pain
    - tenderness to pressure and to air blown on the skin
    - redness
    - "weeping" burn area
    - burn area turns pale when pressed
    - blisters;
  - **outcome:**
    - heals in 7–21 days, usually without scarring.
- **Deep second-degree burn:**
  - at first hard to distinguish from third-degree burn (see below);
  - **signs and symptoms:**

Estimating the burned surface area in children

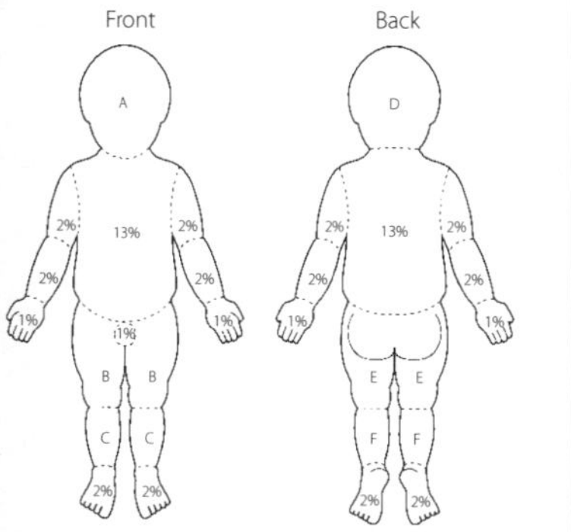

Area	By age in years			
	0	1	5	10
Head (A/D)	10%	9%	7%	6%
Thigh (B/E)	3%	3%	4%	5%
Leg (C/F)	2%	3%	3%	3%

Estimating the burned surface area in adults
The Rule of 9's

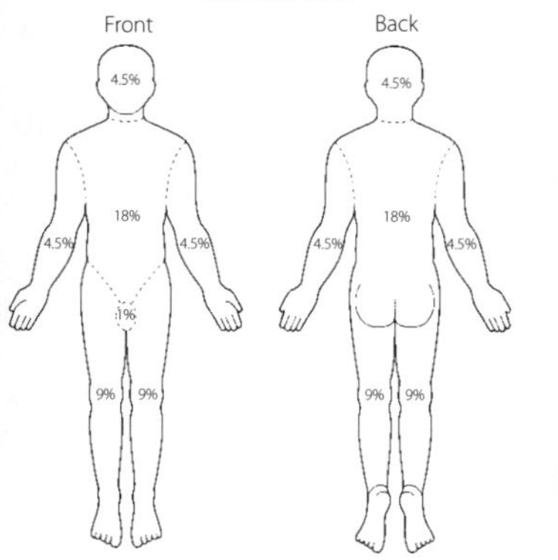

ure 9.3 The rule of nines for children
d adults.

- › pain, possibly severe, from damage to nerve endings
- › tender only to pressure and not to air blown on the skin
- › extensive blisters, which burst readily
- › burn areas weeping or waxy
- › burn areas dry, red or pale
- › red areas do not turn pale when pressed;
- **outcome:**
  - › heals in weeks to months
  - › scarring often severe.

- **Third-degree, or full-thickness, burn:**
  - **skin layer:**
    - › entire thickness of skin
    - › may extend to underlying fat, muscle, and bone;
  - **signs and symptoms:**
    - › skin possibly charred black or dark brown
    - › skin leathery or white
    - › usually no pain (nerve endings destroyed);
  - **outcome:**
    - › untreated, will never heal
    - › treated, usually with skin grafting, will heal within weeks to months
    - › scarring always severe.

✗ *What not to do*

- **Do not treat** a patient with a burn if you have any doubts about whether you can or should:
  - less than perfect care can worsen the outcome;
  - seek medical advice immediately.
- **Do not treat** a burn patient on board who:
  - has any other injury; **OR**
  - is a baby or a child or older than 50; **OR**
  - has a burn on the face, hand, foot, groin, genitals, or anus; **OR**
  - has a burn lying across a large joint; **OR**
  - has a burn going all the way around a limb.

✔ *What to do*

- Seek medical advice in all cases expect for small superficial burns.
- You may be able to treat on board:
  - a partial-thickness burn in:
    - › an adult patient **under 50 years of age**;
    - › whose burn covers less than 15% of the total body surface area;
  - a partial-thickness burn in:
    - › an adult patient **over 50 years of age**;
    - › whose burn covers less than 10% of the total body surface area;

  - a full-thickness burn covering less than 2% of the total body surface area.
- Cool the heat burns as quickly as possible with cold running water (sea or fresh) for at least 10 minutes; **OR**
  - immerse the burned area in basins of cold water.
- If you cannot cool a burn on the spot, take the victim to a place where cooling is possible.
- Try to remove clothing gently but do not tear off any clothing that adheres to skin.
- Cover the burned areas with a dry, non-fluffy dressing larger than the burns, and bandage in place.
- After cooling the burn, remove the patient to a warm cabin with a supply of clean water and dressing material.
- For pain relief in a patient with a small burn give paracetamol or ibuprofen.
- For pain relief in a patient with a large or deep burn give morphine, starting with 15–20 mg intramuscularly, every three to four hours:
  - do not wait for the pain to return before giving the next dose of morphine;
  - increase the dose of morphine by 50% if the patient still has pain one hour after the second dose.
- Encourage the patient to drink oral rehydration solution or hot sweet tea; **OR**
  - insert an intravenous cannula and give 0.9% sodium chloride solution (i.e. normal saline) at a rate of 125 ml/hr.
- If the patient is awaiting evacuation, do nothing further except **keep the patient warm:** take care to prevent blankets from sticking to the burns.
- If the patient is to remain on board, wash the burn gently with soap and potable water:
  - do not use disinfectants such as chlorhexidine because they may delay healing;
  - do not expose several large burn areas at a time;
  - keep the patient warm: loss of skin makes the patient prone to hypothermia;
  - use sterile scissors to cut away loose, dead skin, including broken blisters;
  - leave intact blisters alone, unless:
    - the fluid in the blisters is bloody or cloudy; **OR**
    - the blisters are over a joint; **OR**
    - the patient cannot avoid lying on a blister;
  - for such blisters, use sterile scissors to remove the entire blister roof:
    - do not use a needle to prick blisters;
  - smear the burn with honey and cover it, first with petroleum gauze, then with a sterile non-adherent dressing; note:
    - honey helps prevent infection, and has been shown in scientific studies to be as effective as, but safer than, an antibiotic;
  - cover the dressing with padding to absorb fluid leaking from the burn and hold the dressing in place with a suitable bandage, such as a tubular dressing or crepe bandage for limbs, an elastic net dressing for other body areas;
  - for hand or foot burns, dress fingers or toes separately to prevent them from sticking together;

- leave superficial hand and face burns uncovered or cover only with a non-adherent gauze pad;
- change dressings daily or, over the first day or so, whenever the padding is damp with leaking tissue fluid;
- wash the old honey off with water, put on a new layer, and dress again as before;
- as soon as the burn wound is covered by new pink skin (usually in one to three weeks), stop applying honey and cover the burn with a dry dressing;
- to relieve itching, which often occurs as the burn heals, give cetirizine, 5–10 mg orally, twice daily.

■ For a full-thickness burn greater than 2 cm across, or a large partial-thickness burn, have the patient see a doctor with specialist training in burns at the next port with good medical facilities: a skin graft may be required, but this is best done eight to 10 days after the burn.

Infection of a burn

Because a burn alone causes pain, redness, and swelling, it is difficult to know whether the burn area is infected. Fever or lymph node enlargement or an increase in pain within the first two days of the burn injury suggests infection. Infection in a burn wound is dangerous: it can cause bloodstream infection and can worsen tissue damage in the wound.

✔ *What to do*

■ If you suspect that the burn area has become infected:
- seek medical advice with a view to early evacuation;
- give amoxycillin/clavulanate, 875 mg orally, twice daily.

Respiratory tract burns

A respiratory tract burn should be suspected in any patient with burns around the nose and mouth. The patient must be evacuated urgently. Burns caused by the inhalation of dry gas and smoke do not usually go beyond the throat. Inhalation of superheated steam can cause burns to the lungs as well as to the throat.

✔ *What to do*

■ For a patient with a throat burn and difficulty breathing due to swelling or to blisters in the throat that appeared very soon after the burn injury, arrange for urgent evacuation.

ELECTRICAL BURNS AND ELECTROCUTION

Electrical current causes injury in three main ways:

■ by converting energy into heat within the body, resulting in burns;
■ by direct effects on the heart;
■ by causing falls, which can result in injury.

ELECTRICAL BURNS

There are four types of heat injury associated with electricity:

- **internal burns**: these occur when an electrical current passes through the tissues of the body and heat is generated by tissues that have high resistance to electricity:
  - skin, fat, and bone have high resistance to electricity and are usually severely burned;
  - nerves and blood vessels have lower resistance and are less severely burned;
  - entry and exit wounds are usually present, but can be small even with large internal burns;
- **arc burns**: these occur when an electrical arc strikes the skin but does not enter the body;
- **flame burns:** these occur when clothing is set on fire by an arc or by lightning;
- **lightning burns**: a lightning strike exposes the body to up to 10 million volts for a tenth to a thousandth of a second:
  - the temperature of the air around a lightning bolt is often as high as 30 000°C, and this heat produces an explosive shock wave that causes skin burns;
  - the current in a lightning strike usually travels over the skin surface rather than through the body and so does not usually cause deep tissue burns.

✔ *What to do*

- When approaching a person in contact with electricity, make sure you do not become the next victim.
- If possible, switch off the electrical current.
- If you can not switch off the current, put on rubber gloves and rubber boots, or stand on an insulating rubber mat before approaching and touching the casualty.
- If the victim is entangled in electrical lines, try to remove the lines with a wooden pole, a wooden chair, an insulated cord, or any other suitable non-metal object.
- Check immediately for breathing and heartbeat.
- If the casualty is not breathing, give artificial respiration (see Chapter 1, *First aid*).
- If there is no heartbeat, apply chest compressions (see Chapter 1, *First aid*).
- Send for help.
- When breathing is restored, cool any burned areas with cold water and cover with a clean, dry, non-fluffy dressing.
- Treat as for heat burns (see above) (i.e. relieve pain, prevent or treat shock, and prevent or treat infection).

ELECTROCUTION

Electrocution can stop the heart suddenly or cause it go into an abnormal rhythm, which can cause immediate death. If it does not cause immediate death, an abnormal rhythm can last for several hours, in which case it is usually not dangerous. A patient whose heart has stopped after electrocution may also have enlarged pupils not responsive to light – normally a sign of death, but, in an electrocuted patient, resuscitation efforts can be successful even though the pupils are large and unresponsive. Electrocution causes sudden widespread muscle contraction powerful enough to cause fractures of the vertebrae or falls: always check an electrocuted patient carefully for injuries.

✔ *What to do*

- Serious problems are unlikely if **ALL** the following conditions are present:
  - electrocution has occurred with voltages less than 1000 volts;
  - the patient feels well;
  - pulse rate and blood pressure are normal;
  - pupil size and mental function are normal;
  - speech and walking are normal;
  - there are no skin burns.
- If **ALL** these conditions are **NOT PRESENT**:
  - arrange for evacuation to an onshore hospital;
  - insert an intravenous cannula and administer normal saline (0.9% sodium chloride) at a rate sufficient to produce copious pale urine (start with 150 to 200 ml per hour);
  - treat skin burns in the same way as for other burns (see above).

ELECTRICAL SHOCKS FROM ELECTRONIC WEAPONS

So-called Tasers (electroshock stun guns) and other stun guns are readily available and are used not only by police but also by criminals. They produce electrical shocks that can cause skin burns as well as potentially fatal abnormal heart rhythm. The burns from these weapons should be treated in the same way as other heat burns (see above).

CHEMICAL SPLASHES (see also Chapter 11, *Poisoning*)

✔ *What to do*

- Remove contaminated clothing.
- Drench victim with water to wash the chemical from the eyes and skin.
- **Give priority to washing the eyes**, which are particularly vulnerable to chemical splashes.
- If only one eye is affected, incline the head to the side of the affected eye to prevent the chemical from running across into the other eye.

If the eye is affected, treat as directed in Chapter 5, *Eye injuries and diseases*.

Even small chemical exposures can cause problems, and these may not be apparent until some time after the exposure. A proper medical record entry should be made for all chemical splashes, and the exact chemical involved carefully recorded. Ensure that the crew member is given a copy of this record when he leaves the ship.

Flash burns (arc eye) (see Chapter 5, *Eye injuries and diseases*)

SMOKE INHALATION

Smoke is toxic because it contains carbon monoxide and often hydrogen cyanide, as well as other combustion products that are toxic to the lungs. Because oxygen is consumed in the fire, smoke often contains little oxygen. The carbon monoxide prevents blood picking up oxygen in the lungs and the cyanide prevents oxygen being used in the tissues, so these two toxins and the lack of oxygen in smoke act together. Severe lack of oxygen causes coma and cardiac arrest.

Note

- Haemoglobin is a protein in red blood cells that picks up oxygen in the lungs and carries it to the tissues of the body to keep the cells alive.
- The carbon monoxide in smoke combines with haemoglobin, thus preventing it from picking up oxygen.
- The haemoglobin carrying carbon monoxide is just as red as the haemoglobin that carries oxygen: this means that even patients with severe carbon monoxide poisoning are not blue (cyanotic) but always have a healthy pink skin colour.

Smoke also contains substances which are toxic to the airway lining. Patients who have inhaled these substances in large amounts develop shortness of breath and also coughing that produces large amounts of watery sputum. These symptoms may appear either immediately after inhalation of the smoke or a day or two later.

✔ *What to do*

- Give oxygen, using an oxygen mask rather than tubing in the nostrils, and set the regulator to the highest flow rate.
- Since it takes several hours for carbon monoxide to be removed from the blood, continue oxygen administration for 24 hours or until the oxygen supply runs out.
- Seek medical advice on identifying the nearest port where antidotes to cyanide poisoning are available or, if you are already in port, you should be able to find antidotes in the ambulance station.

Chapter 10

Heat stroke and other heat disorders

HEAT STROKE

Heat stroke is the most severe form of what is called "hyperthermia". Unlike fever, which is due to retention of heat by the body, hyperthermia is due to a failure of the body's temperature regulating systems. Heat stroke results from an overloading of the body's ability to keep a balance between the heat entering the body and the heat leaving the body. Strenuous work in hot conditions or in heavy clothing is a common precipitating factor, but air temperatures do not need to be high. On board ship, seafarers most at risk are those working in the engine room or on deck in the sun or participating in fire-fighting exercises in protective clothing.

Note on natural heat regulation

- A "thermostat" in the brain keeps the body temperature at a setting between 36 °C and 38 °C: it does so by keeping a balance between the amount of heat the body gains and the amount it loses.
- **The body preserves or gains heat** through:
  - **mechanisms**, such as:
    - muscle shivering;
    - muscle contraction during strenuous physical work;
    - the chemical processes of the body's cells (metabolism);
    - narrowing (constriction) of blood vessels in the skin, which reduces loss of blood heat from the body surface;
  - **radiation**, for example, from the sun's rays;
  - **conduction**, when the body is in contact with a hot surface, such as a hot deck;
  - **convection**, when air carries heat from a heat source, such as a ship's engine;
  - **insulation** from thick clothing.
- The body loses heat through:
  - sweating – when sweat evaporates, it takes energy (in the form of heat) from the body:
    - sweating is the main mechanism of heat loss in a hot environment, but is not effective in very humid conditions or when there is so much sweat that it drips off the skin without evaporating;
  - loss of warm faeces, urine and air exhaled from the lung;
  - radiation from the body surface;
  - convection, when air next to the body is heated and then carried away by a breeze:
    - convection is an important mechanism of heat loss, but only if the air is moving and is cooler than skin temperature;
  - conduction, for example, from contact with a cold steel deck.

Signs and symptoms

- Core (internal) body temperature over 40.5 °C as a result of heat load from the environment; note:
  - heat stroke can develop quickly: take action (see below, *What to do*) if there is any rise in body temperature;

    - oral and axillary (armpit) temperatures are slightly lower than the core temperature: if they are elevated, the rectal temperature should be taken in order to determine core temperature.
- Altered mental function, possibly with:
    - aggression
    - confusion
    - delirium
    - fits (convulsions).
- Skin warm and pink, and typically dry, although if heat stroke has developed rapidly the skin may be moist from sweat.
- Rapid pulse rate.
- Rapid respiratory rate.
- Dry cough in some cases.

✔ *What to do*

- Move the patient into a cool environment.
- Remove all the patient's clothing.
- Spray or splash the patient's whole body with cold water and fan him vigorously, or immerse him in a bath of cold water.
- Seek medical advice with a view to evacuation: even if body temperature is brought under control, heat stroke can cause life-threatening damage to internal organs.
- If body temperature does not fall below 39 °C within 30 minutes, place the patient in an ice-water bath. Take the patient out of the bath as soon as rectal temperature has fallen to 39 °C.

✘ *What not to do*

- Do not give anti-pyretic (anti-fever) medicines, such as aspirin or paracetamol: they will not help and may worsen the damage heat stroke can cause to internal organs.
- Do not leave the patient unattended in a bath.

TO PREVENT HEAT STROKE

- Drink plenty of water containing salt before, during, and after exposure to heat – at least 400–500 ml every 20 minutes during exposure.
- Stay as little as possible in a hot, high-risk environment – take a 15-minute break for every hour of exposure.
- Be especially wary when crew are working in warm or hot conditions wearing heavy clothing.

Note on acclimatizing to heat

- A seafarer can become acclimatized to working in hot conditions by gradual exposure to such work.
- Initial acclimatization can take one to two weeks.
- Full acclimatization requires exposure to working in hot conditions three to four times a week for at least four weeks.

Stoker's cramps

Stoker's, or heat, cramps are painful muscular spasms of the large muscles of the arms, legs, and back. They occur following fluid loss caused by heavy sweating during long periods of physical activity.

Signs and symptoms

- Abrupt onset of severe pain in muscles of the limbs and/or back.

What to do

- Give the patient fluid containing salts, ideally oral rehydration solution, or water together with salty food.
- Have the patient sit quietly in a cool, shaded area.
- Allow resumption of physical activity only when the patient has rested for an hour after the cramps have stopped.

Heat exhaustion (or "heat collapse")

Heat exhaustion is a very common heat disorder. It can occur when there is an excessive loss of fluids and salts from the body, from sweating, for example. The result is a reduction in the amount of blood circulating in the body. The symptoms and signs are generally more severe than those of heat cramps.

Signs and symptoms

- Weakness and fatigue
- dizziness
- clammy, ashen skin
- thirst
- heavy sweating
- nausea and vomiting
- **normal** temperature and mental function; note:
  - **any** rise of temperature or abnormal mental function suggests early heat stroke.

What to do

- Have the patient lie down in a cool environment with the feet raised.
- Loosen or remove the patient's clothing.
- Administer fluid, ideally oral rehydration solution, but have the patient drink slowly to avoid nausea and vomiting.
- Check vital signs (temperature, breathing, and heart rate), and mental function.
- Have the patient taken off duty for 24 hours.

Poisoning

Poisoning on board ship may occur after exposure to medical drugs, cargo, or substances used during work. For occupational exposures, this chapter should be used in conjunction with the most recent versions of the International Maritime Organization's *Medical First Aid Guide* and *Emergency Procedures for Ships Carrying Dangerous Goods*. Most cases of poisoning can be dealt with on board ship: only about 5% of serious poisonings require treatment in a hospital and, of these, only 1–2% are fatal. The commonest substances that cause fatal poisoning are carbon monoxide and the simple analgesics paracetamol and acetylsalicylic acid (Aspirin®). The range of potential poisons is very large, whereas the range of body systems that can be affected by poisoning – and thus the range of illnesses that poisons can cause – is small.

The first questions to ask oneself about a case of poisoning or toxic exposure are:

- With what?
- In what quantity?
- When?

POISONING WITH INGESTED DRUGS AND CHEMICALS

Note

- A patient who has deliberately taken an overdose may not say what the drug or chemical was.
- Many patients who poison themselves deliberately take several substances at the same time.
- Poisoning oneself is nearly always done on an impulse, with whatever drug or toxic substance is at hand.
- It is helpful but not essential to know what a patient has taken because, in the treatment of poisoning, it is nearly always enough to provide supportive care while the body excretes the poison.
- There are very few poisons for which a specific antidote exists, and even when there is an antidote, it is needed in only a small minority of poisonings.
- Supportive care in poisoning consists of reducing the absorption of any poison still in the bowel with activated charcoal, maintaining fluid intake so as to favour excretion of the poison from the kidneys, and dealing with the results of impaired consciousness.

✔ What to do

- Search the patient's cabin and belongings for empty medicine containers or a suicide note.
- Check the patient's work environment for opened containers of toxic chemicals, especially insecticide and rat poison.
- Check the medical records to see if the patient has been prescribed any medication, either on board or ashore.
- Remember that tablets and capsules can be identified by their colour, size, shape, and markings: seek medical advice if you find unidentified medicines.

- Examine the patient, paying particular attention to:
  - pupil size;
  - mental state (drowsy/alert) – assess with the Glasgow Coma Scale (see Chapter 26, *Nursing care and medical procedures*) – rational/confused, sad/euphoric;
  - vital signs.
- Decide to which drug type (see Table 11.1, column 1) the patient's condition corresponds:
  - amphetamine-like
  - belladonna-like
  - sedative-hypnotic
  - insecticide-like
  - tricyclic antidepressant.
- For symptoms and signs of intoxication with opioids and hallucinogens, see Chapter 22, *Tobacco, alcohol, and drug use*.
- Seek medical advice at this point.

Table 11.1 Signs and symptoms of poisoning by drug type.

Drug type	Mental state	Pupils	Vital signs	Other symptoms and signs	Drugs
Amphetamine-like	alert, agitated, hallucinating	enlarged	rapid pulse, high BP, fever	sweaty skin, trembling	theophylline, caffeine, "cold" remedies, amphetamine, cocaine
Belladonna-like	alert, agitated, hallucinating	enlarged	rapid pulse, high BP, fever	dry skin, dry mouth	antihistamines, scopolamine, atropine (as tablets or plants, e.g. deadly nightshade, *Datura*), many OTC cold and allergy preparations (eg, Benadryl ®)
Sedative/hypnotic	drowsy, confused, comatose	small or normal	slow pulse, low BP		diazepam, etc., barbiturates, alcohol
Insecticide-like	confused, comatose	small	slow pulse	salivating, tearing (eyes watering), sweating, diarrhoea, frequent urination, excessive lung secretions, wheezing, muscle weakness	organophosphate & carbamate insecticides
Tricyclic anti-depressants	confused, agitated, comatose (in late stage)	enlarged	rapid pulse, fever, high BP at first, low BP later	muscle twitching, seizures	amitryptyline, imipramine, doxepin, etc

BP: blood pressure

- If there is **any** delay in obtaining medical advice, give a single dose of activated charcoal at once, 1 g/kg body weight orally: do not give more than 100 g at a time because vomiting is likely and inhalation of vomit may occur if the patient is drowsy.

✗ *What not to do*

- Although activated charcoal is unpleasant to take, do not try to help the patient by giving small doses repeatedly: they are less effective.
- Do not delay giving activated charcoal: it is half as effective given one hour after a poisoning as it is after 30 minutes.

Red flags

Plan for evacuation of the patient if **ANY** of the following signs, symptoms or conditions are present:

- Glasgow Coma Scale score of 6 or less;
- agitation severe enough to need restraint;
- systolic blood pressure less than 100 mmHg;
- seizures (fits, convulsions);
- pulse rate irregular or less than 50 beats per minute;
- evidence of poisoning with slow-release tablets (often labelled "SR" or "ER" on the packet, after the trade-name);
- chest pain;
- poisoning by a dangerous prescription drug (see below).

COMMON POISONING AGENTS

Paracetamol (acetaminophen)

Paracetamol poisoning is common, largely because the drug is easily available. An overdose can cause liver damage.

Note

- Liver damage is rare in an adult after a single dose of paracetamol up to 7.5 g (15 tablets).
- Liver damage is likely in an adult after a single dose of paracetamol greater than 15 g (30 tablets).
- Severe liver damage is almost certain to occur in an adult after a single dose of paracetamol greater than 20–25 g (40–50 tablets).

► *Signs and symptoms*

- In the first 24 hours:
  - no symptoms, even after a large overdose.
- After 48 hours:
  - pain and tenderness in the right upper abdomen.

- After three to four days:
  - evidence of severe liver damage:
    - jaundice
    - confusion
    - bleeding and bruising.

✔ *What to do*

- If the patient has taken an overdose less than four hours previously, give activated charcoal, 1 g/kg body weight.
- If the patient has taken an overdose more than four hours previously, the drug will have been fully absorbed: consider if the amount taken is dangerous.
- If you suspect that the patient has or is likely to develop liver damage, arrange for evacuation.

Acetylsalicylic acid (Aspirin®)

There are several closely related forms of salicylate (or salicylic acid), which all produce the same signs and symptoms of poisoning:

- acetylsalicylic acid (Aspirin®):
  - tablets used to relieve pain and fever;
- salicylic acid:
  - ointment for warts;
- methyl salicylate (oil of wintergreen):
  - liniment for sore muscles and joints.

Note

- A dose of 10 g (30 tablets) of acetylsalicylic acid or two teaspoons of oil of wintergreen is dangerous in an adult.

► *Signs and symptoms*

- Rapid breathing;
- nausea and vomiting;
- ringing in the ears (tinnitus), which is nearly always present and is typical of salicylate poisoning.

✔ *What to do*

- Give activated charcoal, 1 g/kg body weight.
- Repeated doses may be needed but give them only on medical advice.

Methanol and ethylene glycol

Methanol and ethylene glycol are used in anti-freeze and de-icing liquids, in some cleaners and solvents, and in illicit ("moonshine") alcohol.

Note

- Swallowing more than 150 ml of anti-freeze containing methanol or ethylene glycol is likely to be fatal.

- When first swallowed, methanol and ethylene glycol cause intoxication similar to that caused by alcohol but they are converted by the body to toxic acids that can cause blindness (in the case of methanol) and/or kidney damage (in the case of ethylene glycol) (see Chapter 17, *Kidney and other urinary disorders*).

✔ *What to do*

- Seek medical advice immediately if you believe that early evacuation may be necessary.
- Retrieve the original methanol or ethylene glycol container and have it available when you seek advice.
- Ethanol can slow or prevent the formation of the toxic acids responsible for the poisoning: therefore, if evacuation is not possible immediately:
  - give one standard drink of a concentrated form of ethanol (whisky, vodka, etc.) per 10–15 kg body weight over one hour; **FOLLOWED BY**
  - one to two drinks per hour (adjust the dose to keep the patient obviously drunk but not staggering).

✘ *What not to do*

- **DO NOT** give activated charcoal: it is of little benefit in methanol and ethylene glycol poisoning.

Organophosphate and carbamate insecticides

Poisoning from organophosphate and carbamate insecticides can occur by deliberate self-poisoning, after swallowing contaminated food or inhaling sprays, or through skin exposure, either directly from spraying on the skin or from contaminated clothing. Emergency evacuation is normally required in all cases of organophosphate and carbamate poisoning.

► *Signs and symptoms*

- Within minutes of swallowing or inhaling, or of skin exposure:
  - profuse saliva
  - tears
  - sweating
  - excessive lung secretions
  - diarrhoea
  - frequent urination
  - small pupils
  - slow pulse
  - wheezing
  - in some cases, muscle weakness.
- The most dangerous symptoms are:
  - excessive lung secretions, which can be profuse enough to cause drowning;
  - wheezing;
  - muscle weakness, which can prevent the patient from breathing.

- If you are not sure if the patient has taken an organophosphate, give atropine, 1 mg intramuscularly.
- After 20 minutes, if the pupils have not dilated and the heart rate has not speeded up, you can be sure the patient has organophosphate poisoning.

✔ *What to do*

- Give activated charcoal, 1 g/kg body weight, if the substance has been, or may have been, swallowed, even if symptoms have already appeared.
- Put on rubber gloves.
- Remove all of the patient's clothing likely to have been contaminated by sprayed insecticide and wash contaminated skin with soap and water.
- Give oxygen at the highest possible flow rate via a non-rebreathing mask.
- Give atropine, 2 mg intravenously at once: double the dose every five minutes until the patient stops coughing and wheezing or until you have no more atropine.
- Arrange for emergency evacuation.

Anticoagulants (warfarin, rat poison)

These drugs block blood clotting within two or three days of administration, with the result that minor injuries can cause severe bleeding and there can be internal bleeding.

► *Signs and symptoms*

- Bruising with little or no trauma.
- Stroke (see Chapter 13, *Paralysis, strange behaviour, unconsciousness*).
- Blood in the urine, either obvious or found by dipstick testing.
- Bleeding into the back wall of the abdomen, causing pain in the back and abdomen, with:
  - rapid pulse;
  - falling blood pressure, developing later if bleeding is severe.

✔ *What to do*

- In a case of overdose of rat poison (warfarin), give phytomenadione (phytonadione, vitamin K), 10 mg subcutaneously.
- Seek medical advice: evacuation may be necessary if it is not possible to know what dose of poison was taken or when it was taken.

Petroleum products

Petroleum products are generally not absorbed from the bowel: poisoning results from lung exposure.

Note

- Asphalt, motor oil and axle grease are not toxic.
- Petrol (gasoline), turpentine, kerosene and cigarette lighter fluid cause lung inflammation if they enter the lungs.
- Petrol (gasoline), propane, butane, benzene and toluene form vapours easily, pass through the lungs into the blood, and are then carried to the brain.

Signs and symptoms

- In cases of lung inflammation:
  - breathlessness
  - cough, that may be dry or may produce blood-stained sputum.
- If the brain is affected:
  - drowsiness
  - confusion
  - staggering
  - slurred speech.

What to do

- In cases of exposure to petrol (gasoline), propane, butane, benzene or toluene remove contaminated clothing to prevent further exposure to vapours and have the patient shower with soap for 10 minutes.
- If there is evidence of lung damage, seek medical advice with a view to evacuation.

Caustics

Caustics are strong alkalis, such as sodium or potassium hydroxide (found in drain cleaners), and strong acids, such as sulphuric and phosphoric acid (found in toilet cleaners or battery fluid). Caustics cause burns to the oesophagus and stomach.

Signs and symptoms

- Pain in the chest and upper abdomen;
- vomiting, often of blood.

What to do

- Seek medical advice with a view to urgent evacuation.

What not to do

- **DO NOT** give activated charcoal.
- **DO NOT** provoke vomiting.

Disinfectants and bleach

Disinfectants in the ship's medicine chest are of low toxicity. Liquid bleach (sodium hypochlorite solution) is quite often swallowed but rarely causes serious poisoning.

Dangerous prescription drugs

Most prescription drugs are relatively safe when overdoses are taken. A few cause life-threatening poisoning which requires hospital treatment.

✔ *What to do*

- Seek medical advice urgently and give a single dose of activated charcoal, 1 g/kg body weight orally, if you suspect poisoning with any of the following drugs, even if they were taken in small doses:
  - chloroquine (but ***not*** other antimalarial drugs);
  - verapamil, diltiazem, nifedipine, and other drugs with names ending in "-dipine";
  - metoprolol and other drugs with names ending in "-olol";
  - colchicine (used for gout);
  - theophylline (used for lung disease).

POISONING FROM EXPOSURE TO COMMON GASES OR VAPOURS

✔ *What to do*

- Leave the danger zone at once and get into the open.
- While escaping, cover your nose and mouth with a wet cloth, if possible.
- If you feel irritation in your eyes or throat, hold your breath and keep your eyes closed as much as possible while escaping.
- If a crew member has been exposed to a toxic gas or vapour, put on rubber gloves and remove the crew member's clothing and seal it in a plastic bag.
- Have the crew member shower, washing all over with soap for 15 minutes, then rinse the eyes with water for 10 minutes.

Carbon monoxide

Carbon monoxide prevents haemoglobin, the oxygen carrying pigment of red blood cells, from releasing its oxygen to the tissues. Carbon monoxide poisoning, which is often mild but may be chronic or frequently recurring, can occur when a person inhales smoke from a large fire or from poorly ventilated internal combustion engines, fuel stoves and heaters.

► *Signs and symptoms*

- Onset within minutes of exposure to the gas; disappearance over several hours after the patient has left the area.
- Normal pink skin colour (**not** blue) even in very severe cases, because oxygen is trapped in the blood.
- In mild cases, in which the following symptoms are often interpreted as cold- or flu-like symptoms:
  - headache
  - feeling unwell
  - nausea
  - dizziness.

- In more severe cases:
  - confusion
  - drowsiness
  - loss of consciousness.

✔ What to do

- See Chapter 9, *Burns, chemical splashes, smoke inhalation, and electrocution.*

Cyanide

Cyanide is used to fumigate ships. Exposure can occur if fumigation is carried out carelessly or by untrained workers. Sodium and potassium cyanide are solids, which on contact with acids produce hydrogen cyanide, which is a gas. Hydrogen cyanide is lighter than air, accumulates at the top of enclosed spaces, and is rapidly dispersed by adequate ventilation.

Signs and symptoms

- Irritation of the eyes and nose
- soon after, difficulty breathing and headache
- vomiting
- confusion
- weakness
- seizures
- coma
- death after 5–10 minutes of exposure.

Irritant gases – phosgene, chlorine, ammonia

These gases are heavier than air and accumulate at the bottom of enclosed spaces.

Signs and symptoms

- Irritation of the eyes, skin, lungs and airways;
- severe burns;
- irritation of the nose and throat;
- cough and breathlessness, suggestive of lung injury:
  - in mild cases, these symptoms may appear only 24 hours or so after exposure;
  - the heavier the exposure, the sooner these symptoms develop;
- burning of the eyes, especially with ammonia exposure.

✔ What to do

- Seek medical advice with a view to evacuation of the patient.
- Meanwhile, give oxygen by a non-rebreathing mask at the highest possible flow rate.
- Treat eye burns as directed in Chapter 5, *Eye injuries and diseases.*

Carbon dioxide

Carbon dioxide is one of the most abundant gases in the atmosphere. It is formed during respiration, combustion and organic decomposition, and is used in food refrigeration, carbonated drinks, fire extinguishers and aerosols. It is not toxic but displaces breathable air from enclosed spaces. It is heavier than air and accumulates at the bottom of enclosed spaces.

Signs and symptoms

- Breathlessness
- headache
- a feeling of warmth and sweatiness.

What to do

- Remove the patient from the area of exposure: symptoms should disappear within minutes.

Flammable liquid vapours

Most flammable liquids, including liquified petroleum gas (LPG and Calor gas, propane and butane), and most solvents, form vapours that are heavier than air. These tend to accumulate at the bottom of holds and storage lockers, and although not directly toxic displace breathable air and can asphyxiate crew who enter these areas.

Freons

Freons are a group of hydrocarbon compounds containing fluorine ("fluorocarbons"). They are widely used as refrigerants. If a freon is inhaled, it can cause severe cold injury (frostbite) of the respiratory tract. Heavy exposure can damage the heart, causing abnormal heart rhythm and sudden death.

Hydrogen sulphide ("Rotten egg gas", "Sewer gas")

Hydrogen sulphide is produced in oil refining, and from decomposition of organic matter, especially manure. It is heavier than air and accumulates at the bottom of holds.

- Hydrogen sulphide is explosive and toxic.
- The smell is obvious at first, but the gas poisons the sense of smell so that after a few minutes the smell appears to have gone away even if concentrations are rising.
- Low concentrations irritate the nose, mouth and eyes.
- Higher concentrations cause poisoning identical to that of hydrogen cyanide.

Note

- People working with dangerous goods should adhere strictly to basic safety precautions and be familiar with the conventional labelling of these goods.
- A poison should never be stored in anything other than its original container.
- **Special measures to prevent poisoning are described in the sections pertaining to each individual group of substances in** *Medical first aid guide for use in accidents involving dangerous goods*, London, International Maritime Organization, 2004.

- Protective clothing (e.g. rubber or plastic gloves, aprons, boots) and breathing apparatus (compressed air systems, smoke helmets) for the handling of dangerous goods must be readily available on board ship and regularly inspected and cleaned or replaced.
- Adequate washing and showering facilities should be available close to the workplace.
- In the event of a leakage or spillage involving dangerous gases or fumes, a gas detector should be used before declaring a space safe.
- Gas masks should be available: they will not provide complete protection but may help during an escape from a contaminated site.
- An appropriate neutralizing substance should be applied to the site of a leakage or spillage: the area should be covered with sand or vermiculite, which should afterwards be removed to a safe place in a special container.
- Holds and enclosed spaces in which toxic vapours and gases might accumulate should be properly ventilated and checked with a gas detector (not an explosimeter) before anyone is allowed to enter these places and also during cargo-handling operations.
- Places used for the storage of dangerous goods should be decontaminated after use and/or before reuse.
- Dangerous goods should not be stored or carried close to foodstuffs.

BITES AND STINGS

Human and animal bites (for cat and dog bites, see Chapter 8, *Wounds*, and for tetanus and rabies, Chapter 23, *Infectious diseases*).

Rat bites

Rat bites are rare on board ship. In most cases, disease is transmitted by rats through contact with the animals' urine or faeces or with fleas living on them, rather than by bites. Antibiotics are not required for rat bites unless symptoms, such as pain, redness, warmth and swelling, last more than three days after the bite.

Snake bites

Unless provoked or accidentally trodden on or handled, snakes seldom bite humans. Most snakes are not dangerous and many bites, even by dangerous species, do not cause serious poisoning.

✔ *What to do*

- Take the patient away from the snake.
- Lay the patient down and keep the patient warm and at rest.
- Wash the wound.
- If the snake is dead, pick it up with a stick and place it in a bag for later identification but **DO NOT** handle its head: it may be capable of biting for two hours after death.
- If you are at sea and the snake is dead, take digital photographs of the whole snake and a close-up of the top and side of its head.
- If the snake is not dead and is no longer in sight, **DO NOT** attempt to look for it.

- Take the patient to the nearest hospital or seek medical advice with a view to evacuation.
- Apply a compression bandage to the bitten limb:
  - use a wide crepe bandage, if available, but any fabric torn or cut into strips about 5–10 cm wide will do;
  - start at the fingers or toes and bandage upwards as far as possible;
  - wrap the bandage no tighter than you would for a sprained ankle;
  - the bandage should be comfortable enough to be kept in place for several hours;
  - once the bandage is in place, apply a splint to a bitten leg and place a bitten arm in a sling.
- Do not remove clothing before applying the bandage: the movement will increase absorption of the venom.

✗ *What not to do*

- **DO NOT** give the patient alcohol or any medicine.
- **DO NOT** cut or suck the wound.
- **DO NOT** apply an arterial tourniquet.
- **DO NOT** remove a pressure bandage before the patient sees a doctor or before you receive medical approval to do so.

Jellyfish stings

Jellyfish live in salt water. There are many species. The Portuguese-man-of-war is not a jellyfish but it causes a similar sting.

Jellyfish venom is contained in stinging capsules (nematocysts) attached to the tentacles. A jellyfish fires its poison whenever its tentacles brush against an object. The capsules can continue to fire after being detached from the body of the jellyfish.

► *Signs and symptoms*

- Immediate pain at the site of the sting; then
- redness, itchiness, and an intense burning sensation at the site of the sting.

✔ *What to do*

- Apply shaving cream to the stung area to trap any undischarged nematocysts.
- Use a spoon or similar object to scrape off the shaving cream, together with the tentacle and nematocysts.
- To relieve pain, immerse the stung area in water at a temperature of 40°C.

✗ *What not to do*

- **DO NOT** rub the stung area.
- **DO NOT** apply vinegar, ethanol (alcohol), or urine.

Venomous fish

Venomous fish are present in most tropical waters, especially around the islands of the Indian Ocean and Pacific Ocean. Stonefish and lionfish are the most likely species to affect humans. Both species have long dorsal spines with venom.

Signs and symptoms

- Intense, often agonizing pain, at the spot where fish spines have pierced the skin.

What to do

- To reduce pain, have the patient immerse the affected part in water as hot as can be comfortably tolerated.
- If pain continues or infection occurs, arrange for the patient to have the affected part X-rayed at the next port to check if spine fragments have broken off inside the wound: surgery will be required to remove them.

Sea urchins

Sea urchin spines are coated with toxin. They cause deep wounds and the tips may break off and remain deeply embedded in the wound.

Signs and symptoms

- Severe pain
- redness
- swelling.

What to do

- Note that if symptoms resolve over a day or two, it is unlikely that a spine fragment has been left in the wound.
- Immerse the wounded part in water as hot as the patient can comfortably tolerate.
- Remove any spines that are accessible from the surface; **BUT**:
    - **DO NOT** attempt to remove spine fragments lodged deeply under the skin: have a surgeon remove them at the next port.
- If redness, swelling, and pain arise or worsen more than three days after the wound was inflicted, give amoxycillin/clavulanate, 875/125 mg orally, twice daily.

Scorpions and spiders

All spiders and scorpions are venomous but very few are dangerous to humans. Only large spiders, which have fangs strong enough to penetrate the skin, cause significant human bites. Scorpions inhabit desert areas and are very unlikely to be found on board ship.

- Spider bites are most likely to occur when animals are accidentally brought on board in cargo.
- *Phoneutria* (see below) have been found on board ships in cargoes of bananas from South America.
- Most spider bites cause only:
    - redness and swelling at the site of the bite, with mild soreness; and
    - in some cases, a firm red nodule that lasts a few days.

- Brown recluse (*Loxosceles)* spiders of North and South America can cause:
  - a spreading area of redness 5–20 cm across; followed by
  - formation of a 1–2 cm blister over the next 24 hours or so; then
  - bursting of the blister, leaving an ulcer that may take months to heal.
- A few spiders can cause severe poisoning from venom absorbed into the bloodstream. These are:
  - brown recluse (*Loxosceles*) spiders; poisoning causes
    - fever, vomiting, and blood in the urine;
    - deaths have not been reported.
- Widow (*Latrodectus*) spiders, which are present in most warm areas of the world, Wandering (*Phoneutria*) spiders of South America and Funnel-Web (*Atrax* and *Hadronyche*) spiders of Australia have venom which affects the nervous system; they cause:
  - severe pain at the site of the bite;
  - sweating, high blood pressure, agitation and vomiting;
  - painful muscle spasms, usually near the bite or in the legs and abdomen;
  - deaths have occurred in healthy adults.

Examination of the patient

Note

- This chapter outlines the general principles which the shipboard caregiver – the captain, master, or other crew member assigned to this role – should consider when called upon to examine a patient on board.
- The examination of patients with specific health problems is dealt with in the chapters of this guide dealing with these problems and listed in the Contents page.

INTRODUCTION

The severity of an injury or an illness cannot be properly assessed without a careful, systematic examination of the patient. The examination is performed in two stages. The first stage involves taking the patient's history, which traces the sequence of events related to the injury or illness from the time of the injury or the onset of the symptoms to the present examination. The second stage consists of the physical examination of the patient, in which signs are looked for that might indicate the severity and/or cause of the patient's health problem.

The history and the findings of the physical examination must be recorded concisely, accurately and completely, since this information may have to be communicated by radio or provided to a shore-based physician taking over the case.

The length of time and depth of detail required for an examination will clearly depend on the complexity of the health problem.

CONSENT

In general, no one, medically qualified or not, can conduct a physical examination of another person, or give them any form of treatment, without their consent. Failing to obtain a patient's consent to examination or treatment may result in civil liability and can constitute a criminal offence.

You must always (with the exceptions noted below) have the patient's consent to examination and treatment **before** you begin any examination or give any treatment.

Each crew member should be informed of his or her right to give or refuse consent to examination and treatment, and of the other rights listed here, when arriving in the sickbay, if his or her condition makes it possible. Giving the crew member a copy of these pages is suggested as a convenient way to do this.

It is not necessary for the patient to sign a document to indicate consent, or for his consent to be witnessed, unless there may be disputes later over whether consent was given. If you think that for this reason you should have another person present when the patient consents, note that the witness must observe not only the patient's agreement but also the information he is given about the examination and treatment.

When you ask a patient for their consent to examination or treatment you must:

- inform them of what you propose to do; the information you give must cover everything you would want to know if you were in the patient's position **and** you must answer truthfully any question the patient asks;

- make sure the patient understands the information you have given him (for example, if you tell a patient you need to perform a rectal examination, you are responsible for checking that the patient understands what that involves);
- not use coercion or threats, actual or implied (except a "threat" to impose or maintain medically necessary isolation);
- be sure that the patient has expressed his consent explicitly (it is **NEVER** the case that silence implies consent);
- consent is **not** valid, and may not protect you legally, if it is:
  - too general (agreement to phrases such as "any treatment deemed necessary by the master" does **not** constitute consent); or
  - too old; consent to examination and treatment should be sought for each new illness.

A patient is **NEVER** under any obligation to explain or justify a decision not to consent to examination or treatment. He can make his decision for good reasons, bad reasons, or no reason at all, and his decision must be respected just the same. A patient's reasons may be so bizarre as to suggest mental illness, but refusing consent to a treatment that other people think would be a good idea is not, in itself, an indication of mental illness.

A patient can withdraw his consent to treatment or examination at any time, and he does not have to give any reason or explanation for this decision.

You can give treatment without consent:

- in an emergency, when taking the time to seek consent might endanger the patient;
- to an unconscious patient – **BUT** if a patient refuses treatment when conscious and then becomes unconscious the treatment cannot be given;
- to a mentally ill patient endangering others;
- in some countries, **but not in others**, to a mentally ill patient endangering themselves, and to some patients with infectious diseases.

Seek medical advice whenever:

- a patient asks a question which they consider relevant to their consent but which you cannot answer confidently;
- a patient refuses treatment of a serious illness or injury;
- a patient refuses treatment for an infectious disease or one likely to impede the safe operation of the ship;
- a mentally ill patient is endangering himself.

Patients also have the right to:

- read all notes and records made in connection with their treatment;
- be given a copy of their medical records when leaving the ship or going to see a doctor;
- see a doctor of their choice at the next port.

PRIVACY AND CONFIDENTIALITY

Everything you learn about a patient while caring for them is confidential, or secret. This applies both to things the patient tells you and things you learn by examining them or from their medical records. Even if a patient tells his shipmates some of these things, it is better if you avoid all discussion of them.

Information about a patient should not be given to others not involved in the patient's care unless it is absolutely necessary. For example, the master may need to make a decision to divert the vessel to a nearby port. However, you should give only as much information as is necessary for this decision to be made. Be careful that any discussion involving confidential information is held out of hearing of those who do not need to be involved.

Charts and medical records should be kept where visitors cannot read them.

Many people may be eager to find out the details of a patient's illness. These include family members, ship owners, representatives of insurance companies, police and so on. Although these people may have legitimate reasons to want this information, and may claim that they have a right to be informed, **do not** provide any information until you have asked the patient. **Always ask the patient before you give any information to anyone, even family members.**

If the patient is too sick to be asked, seek medical advice before giving any information to anyone.

If the patient refuses to allow you to give out information you must not do so unless:

- you are legally obliged to, by a subpoena or search warrant, for example; or
- because the patient's illness is one which you are required to notify to police or port authorities; or
- the patient's condition requires that for the safety of others the master be informed.

In these cases you should provide no more information that you are obliged to and you should inform the patient of the disclosure before you make it.

How to take a patient's history

- Write down the time, date and your name on the case record.
- Record that the patient has consented to the examination.
- Begin by asking general questions (let the patient respond without interrupting), such as:
  - When were you last perfectly well?
  - What was the first thing that made you think you were not well?
  - What happened then? And then?
- Ask specifically about each symptom the patient reports:
  - What were the first symptoms?
  - Exactly how, where and when did the symptom start?
  - Has the symptom changed over time? If so, how?
- Ask about other symptoms that the patient may not have reported:
  - Have you noticed any changes in other parts of your body or in any bodily functions, since this problem appeared?

- Ask if there has been even slight:
  - breathlessness
  - change in bowel habit
  - change in the amount, colour, or consistency of urine passed
  - headache
  - rash
  - fever.
- Ask the patient to clarify or expand on vague complaints like tiredness (ask: "Do you mean you needed to sleep more, or didn't feel like doing anything, or something else again?"), weakness (ask: "What everyday things could you still do and which could you not do?"), and loss of appetite (ask: "Did you not feel hungry, or did food taste bad when you ate it, or did eating cause pain or nausea?"), which occur with almost any illness.
- Pay careful attention to the **exact** sequence of events at the beginning of the illness.
- Avoid leading questions (questions that suggest an answer), such as: "The pain is worse when you breathe in, isn't it?". Instead ask "When you breathe in, does it make the pain better or worse?"
- Avoid ambiguous questions, such as: "Do you have any pain or numbness in your feet?"
- Ask if the patient:
  - has consulted other physicians or caregivers about the problem and, if so, what they said or did;
  - if any treatment has been taken for the problem and if so:
    - what treatment;
    - how regularly taken;
    - for how long;
    - prescribed by whom;
    - if this treatment is still being taken and if not, why it was stopped;
    - what effect the treatment had.
- Ask what other illnesses and surgical procedures the patient has had in the past:
  - do not accept either the patient's or another caregiver's diagnosis uncritically: ask the patient what symptoms appeared with each past illness;
  - ask what medications, including herbal and folk remedies, the patient takes routinely.
- Ask about smoking habits:
  - How many cigarettes a day?
  - For how many years?
  - Does the patient smoke commercially made or own-rolled cigarettes?
  - Note that a 30-gram packet of tobacco consumed in a week corresponds roughly to 20 commercially made cigarettes per day.
- Ask about alcohol consumption:
  - On how many days per week is alcohol consumed?
  - How many drinks are consumed on an average "drinking day"?

- Ask about recreational drug use.
- Ask about sexual activity.
- Ask about previous occupations – the kind of work done not just the position occupied.
- Ask about illnesses of parents and siblings or illness known to run in the family.
- Ask about allergies to anything or any bad reaction experienced to any medication.
- If the diagnosis is not obvious, question the patient using a checklist of symptoms organized, from head to toe, by organ or organ system (see Table 12.1)
- Remember, however, that leading questions of this type provide less reliable information than spontaneous complaints.

THE PHYSICAL EXAMINATION

Unlike the first stage of the basic medical examination, which focuses on subjective symptoms experienced and described by the patient, the physical examination looks for objective signs of abnormal functioning of the body. Again, a systematic head-to-toe approach should be adopted (Table 12.2).

Table 12.1 Checklist of common symptoms by organ or organ system.

Organ or system	Ask the patient about past or present occurrences of:
Head	■ wounds (injuries or trauma), headache;
Eyes	■ blurred vision, double vision, pain, yellow colour of the sclera (the white of the eye), pain or discomfort on looking at a light source;
Ears	■ loss of hearing, dizziness, pain, or drainage of fluid;
Nose	■ bleeding, runny, or stuffy;
Mouth and throat	■ sores, pain, difficulty swallowing;
Neck	■ stiffness, enlarged lymph glands, pain;
Respiratory system	■ coughing, sputum production, coughing up of blood, chest pain when breathing, shortness of breath;
Cardiovascular system	■ chest pain, swelling of one or both legs, shortness of breath on exercising, breathlessness when sleeping flat in bed, strong or rapid heart beat, high blood pressure, heart attack, rheumatic fever;
Gastrointestinal system	■ poor appetite, indigestion, nausea, vomiting, diarrhoea, constipation, jaundice (yellowish skin), stomach pain, blood in stool or in vomit;
Genitourinary system	■ pain when urinating, pain in middle of the back, frequent urination, straining to urinate, blood or pus in urine, discharge from penis;
Nervous system	■ paralysis or weakness of a part of the body (arms or legs), convulsions (fits or seizures), pain in the feet, numbness or abnormal sensation anywhere, difficulty keeping balance in the dark.

Table 12.2 Checklist for physical examination.

General appearance	■ Is there anything unusual or noteworthy about the patient's posture? ■ Is there anything unusual or noteworthy about the patient's facial appearance, expression, or movements? ■ Is the body tense, restless, or lethargic? ■ Is there anything abnormal or noteworthy about the patient's manner, speech, or behaviour? ■ Is the patient feverish and/or sweating?
Vital signs	■ Take the patient's blood pressure 3 times at 5-minute intervals, ideally with the patient sitting and the arm resting on the table. See Chapter 26, *Nursing care and medical procedures*, for illustrations of measuring blood pressure. ■ Note down if the blood pressure is taken with the patient lying down. ■ What is the pulse rate at the wrist or neck (carotid)? ■ Is the pulse strong or weak, regular, or irregular? ■ What is the body temperature?
Skin	■ Are there rashes or sores on the skin? ■ If there is a rash, where is it? Is it elevated (slightly above the level of the skin surface) or flat? What colour is it? Does it consist of small or large spots? Are the spots separate or do they run together? Do the spots itch? Are there scratches? If possible, photograph the rash, preferably in daylight. ■ Is the skin hot and dry or cold and damp? ■ What is the colour of the skin: pale, bluish, yellowish? Is there evidence of jaundice? ■ What colour are the lips?
Head	■ Is there evidence of trauma, such as a cut, bruise, or swelling? ■ Is there blood in the ear canal (a sign of head injury)? ■ Is there bleeding or an abnormal discharge from the nose?
Eyes	■ What size are the pupils? Are they round or irregular? Are both pupils the same size? Do the pupils become smaller or stay the same size when a light (a penlight, for example) is shone into the eyes? ■ What colour is the sclera (white of the eye)? Is it yellowish or reddish when examined in natural daylight? ■ Ask the patient to look left, right, up and down: do both eyes move in all directions? Does this exercise cause double vision?
Mouth and throat	■ Using a tongue depressor or teaspoon to push the tongue down, is there swelling, unusual redness, white spots, or ulcers on the back of the throat? ■ Is there swelling, unusual redness, white spots, or ulcers on the gums or under the tongue (ask the patient to open his mouth and touch the roof of his mouth with the tip of his tongue)? ■ Are the colour and movement of the tongue unusual? ■ Are the teeth in good condition? ■ Give the patient a sip of water: is there difficulty swallowing? Does the patient cough immediately after attempting to swallow?

(Continued)

Table 12.2 (continued)

	■ Does the patient's breath have an unusual or unpleasant smell?
	■ Does the patient's mouth seem to be unusually dry?
	■ Ask the patient to lie down, extend the knees, and relax. Put your hands behind the patient's head and lift the head gently, bending the neck forward. Can the patient bend the neck so that the chin touches the chest?
	■ Are the neck lymph glands (lymph nodes) swollen, painful, movable or fixed, soft or hard?
Chest	■ How many breaths a minute does the patient take? Is the breathing superficial, noisy, or deep? Is it regular or irregular?
	■ Can the patient breathe without difficulty or pain? If there is pain, is touching the spot painful?
	■ If the patient has suffered an injury, are the ribs damaged? Holding the patient's chest on either side, squeeze gently. Is there pain and if so where? Is there swelling at this spot?
	■ Using a stethoscope, listen to the breath sounds on the front and back and on each side. Are the sounds the same comparing one side to the other and comparing top to bottom?
	■ Listen to the heart sounds: are there added sounds or murmurs?
Abdomen	■ With the patient lying comfortably in a warm, well-lit environment, does the contour of the abdomen appear symmetrical? Is it flat, drawn in, distended?
	■ Are there any abnormal-looking swellings on the abdomen?
	■ Does the abdomen feel soft or rigid on palpation? Is there guarding (tensing of the muscles), in one area or over the whole abdomen?
	■ Does the patient's facial expression show grimacing or other indications of pain when your hand or finger touches a particular spot on the abdomen?
	■ Are there scars on the abdomen? What is the origin of each scar? Has the gallbladder or appendix been removed?
	■ Using a stethoscope, can you hear bowel sounds?
Genitalia, inguinal (groin) area, anal area	■ Can you see any rashes, swelling, skin ulcers? Are any lymph glands swollen or painful, particularly in the groin? Is there any sign of hernia?
	■ Is there a discharge from the penis? Is the tip or opening of the penis red or abnormally moist?
	■ Is there swelling or tenderness in the scrotum?
	■ Is there swelling or skin redness or are there nodules around the anus?
Limbs	■ Is there weakness or paralysis in the patient's arms or hands? Ask the patient to squeeze your hands forcefully and then to push you away: is there any difference in strength between the right and left arm or hand? If there is a difference, is it because of pain?
	■ If there is pain does the patient feel it when moving the hand or arm himself or when you move it while he is relaxed?
	■ Is there weakness or paralysis in the patient's legs? Ask the patient to bend his knees and push both feet forcefully toward the foot of the bed against your hands, and to straighten his legs and then raise them off the bed while you push down: is there a difference in strength between the right and left leg? If there is a difference, is it because of pain?

(Continued)

Table 12.2 (continued)

	■ If there is pain does the patient feel it when moving the leg himself or when you move it while he is relaxed? ■ Is there a change in skin colouring or swelling or deformity around the joints? Do the joints feel unusually warm? ■ Are there varicose (swollen) veins or red or swollen areas on the legs? Does gentle palpation of the legs reveal painful areas?
Back	■ Is there tenderness or deformity of the back? Assess tenderness of the spine by hitting the vertebrae gently with a closed fist, starting at the top and going down to the bottom. ■ Does bending forward, backwards, or to the side cause the patient pain? ■ Does the patient feel pain in the kidney area when you hit firmly with your fist over the lower two ribs 5 cm or so on either side of the midline?
Nervous system	■ Does the patient show unusual concern or unconcern about this episode of illness? ■ Is the patient's emotional state or behaviour unusual in any way? Does he or she have delusions (false beliefs) or hallucinations (abnormal sensory experiences)? ■ Is the patient's memory and orientation normal? Ask specific questions: Where are we? What is the date? Who am I? What was the last port we visited? Who is the President of the United States (or another appropriate country)? ■ Is the patient's gait normal? Ask the patient to walk a few steps and to pick up an object from a table or a chair with each hand. ■ Ask the patient to walk around a chair in a clockwise and then in an anti-clockwise direction. ■ Ask the patient to stand with his feet together. Does he sway or fall? ■ Ask the patient to stand with his feet together and then to close his eyes. Does he become more unstable? ■ Ask the patient to squat and stand up without holding on to anything.

Paralysis, strange behaviour, unconsciousness

STROKE

Stroke is a loss of brain function caused by failure of blood supply to the brain. The loss of function can be temporary, when it is called a transient ischaemic attack (or a "ministroke"), or permanent.

Common causes of stroke are:

- blockage of an artery supplying blood to the brain (ischaemic stroke), which is caused in turn by:
  - a plaque or clot (thrombus) that has formed inside the artery from accumulated fats and other substances (atherosclerosis); this causes 65–75% of strokes; **OR**
  - a clot formed in a blood vessel elsewhere in the body that has travelled to the brain (embolism); this causes 5–10% of strokes;
- bleeding into the brain (haemorrhagic stroke) from a ruptured artery supplying blood to the brain; this is the cause of about 20% of strokes and is more often fatal than other forms of stroke; there are two types of haemorrhagic stroke:
  - intracerebral haemorrhage, caused by rupture of a vessel inside the brain;
  - subarachnoid haemorrhage, caused by rupture of a vessel on the surface of the brain.

Signs and symptoms

Typical patterns of signs and symptoms in stroke:

- symptoms gradually progress over hours or days;
- in many cases, periods of stability or improvement of the patient's condition, followed by further worsening;
- in a few cases, particularly of embolism or haemorrhage, onset of symptoms over minutes with no further worsening.

The commonest pattern of symptoms in stroke is:

- weakness of the face, arm and hand, and leg on one side of the body; note:
  - the patient may complain not of weakness but of "clumsiness" or "heaviness" or even "numbness", but you will find weakness when you examine him;
  - weakness of the face is shown by drooping of the corner of the mouth;
  - in stroke, the patient can still wrinkle the forehead;
  - if the mouth droops **and** the forehead on the side of the droop is smooth, the diagnosis is probably Bell's palsy (see below);
- abnormal speech (especially if the right side of the body is affected) with thick, slurred speech, difficulty finding words, or complete inability to speak or understand.

When you examine the patient you will find:

- the arm and leg weak and floppy on examination; note:
  - if you are not sure if an arm is weak, ask the patient to hold both arms straight out in front of him: a weak arm will drift down and away from the body over the next 10 to 15 seconds.

Less common symptoms in stroke are:

- dizziness and staggering;
- blurred or double vision, often with weakness of one side of the face and the opposite side of the body;
- loss of vision in one eye lasting a minute or two.

Note

- Loss or impairment of consciousness can occur in stroke but it is not common and is rarely the only symptom.
- Weakness of both legs is **not** likely to indicate a stroke.
- Headache with no other symptoms is **not** likely to indicate a stroke.

✔ *What to do immediately*

- Seek medical advice: evacuation may or may not be needed, and, if needed, may or may not be urgent, depending on the circumstances.
- If there is any reason to suspect head injury, seek medical advice immediately.
- Otherwise, before calling for medical advice, do the following:
  - have the patient lie flat in bed with the body, shoulders, and head at the same level: allow a single pillow if the patient is uncomfortable lying flat;
  - check the blood pressure, pulse rate and level of consciousness.
- **Blood pressure**:
  - blood pressure is usually increased soon after a stroke;
  - systolic blood pressure above 170 mmHg or below 120 mmHg suggests a poor outcome: these patients should normally be evacuated as soon as possible;
  - blood pressure that is very high in a young patient suggests cerebral haemorrhage, and these patients also should be evacuated urgently.
- **Pulse rate**:
  - a rapid, irregular pulse suggests that an embolism has caused the stroke: this requires medical treatment in hospital.
- **Consciousness**:
  - assess the Glasgow Coma Scale score (see Table 26.3 in Chapter 26, *Nursing care and medical procedures*);
  - if consciousness is impaired, have the patient evacuated urgently.
- Give the patient a sip of water: if there is any difficulty swallowing, or if the patient coughs or splutters, you will have great difficulty caring for the patient on board.
- Have this additional information ready when you speak to the doctor:
  - the patient's age and detailed past medical history;
  - any evidence of treatment (medication in the patient's locker, entries in the medical record, etc.) for:
    - high blood pressure;
    - diabetes – if the patient is on treatment for diabetes and is drowsy or confused blood sugar levels may be low (hypoglycaemia): give sugar, by mouth if the patient can swallow or glucagon, 1 mg intramuscularly, if the patient cannot swallow.

- › epilepsy – occasionally, repeated fits can cause weakness of one side of the body resembling stroke (for advice on treatment, see under *Epilepsy*, below);
- › any evidence of cocaine or amphetamine use.

✗ *What not to do immediately*

- **DO NOT** give supplementary oxygen.
- **DO NOT** give anything by mouth to any patient with impaired consciousness.
- **DO NOT** give anything by mouth to any patient until you are sure that they can swallow water normally.

✔ *What to do while awaiting evacuation*

- Have the patient lie as flat as possible for the first 24 hours, but then the patient can sit up.
- If there is impaired consciousness, put the patient in the recovery, or coma, position (see Chapter 1, *First aid*).
- To avoid bedsores or pressure sores turn the patient as recommended in Chapter 26, *Nursing care and medical procedures*.
- If swallowing is difficult or impossible, insert an intravenous cannula, and give normal saline (0.9% sodium chloride), one litre every eight hours.
- If the patient can swallow normally encourage him to drink (aim for three litres daily), but only clear fluids (problems with swallowing causing food to enter the lungs are still possible).
- Set up a condom catheter device (see Chapter 26, *Nursing care and medical procedures)*.
- Nursing patients with stroke is demanding: try to arrange for crew caring for a stroke patient to have frequent breaks.
- If evacuation is likely to be delayed for more than 24 hours give:
  - docusate with senna, two tablets every evening; **AND**
  - acetylsalicylic acid (Aspirin®), 150 mg orally, daily; **UNLESS**:
    - › the patient cannot swallow;
    - › the patient is known to have an active peptic ulcer or has had major surgery or a trauma within the past two weeks.
- If signs and symptoms of loss of brain function disappear after a few minutes, suspect a transient ischaemic attack, which is followed in many cases by a major stroke.

Transient ischaemic attack (TIA)

A TIA is defined as symptoms of stroke that go away in less than 24 hours. In most cases they go away much faster, usually in a few minutes.

A TIA often means that the patient will have a major stroke in the near future.

✔ *What to do*

- Measure the pulse and blood pressure; if the blood pressure is high or low, or the pulse is very fast or irregular, seek medical advice immediately.

- Give acetylsalicylic acid (Aspirin®), 150 mg orally at once, and then daily.
- Have the patient seen by a doctor at the next port.
- Seek medical advice about the need for evacuation if a second TIA occurs which lasts longer than the first or affects more of the body.

HEADACHE

COMMON CAUSES OF HEADACHE

- **Acute infection**:
  - headache with fever and malaise: the diagnosis is usually apparent.
- **Tension headache**:
  - the commonest type of headache, affecting about a third of adults over a 12-month period;
  - a diffuse, usually mild-to-moderate pain, often described as a tight band, on both sides of the head;
  - no other symptoms;
  - may last for hours or days;
  - most patients are able to continue normal activities despite the headache.
- **Migraine**:
  - the second-commonest type of headache, affecting about 15% of adults;
  - the commonest headache for which medical attention is sought;
  - usually begins in early adult life, so most patients will have had repeated episodes;
  - pain is felt most often in the forehead, on one side in about two thirds of cases, on both sides in the rest;
  - pain comes on gradually, steadily worsening over an hour or two;
  - severe pain lasts a few hours in most cases, but a mild pain then often hangs around for 48–72 hours;
  - touching the patient's skin over the scalp or face during a migraine attack generally worsens the pain, sometimes making it hard to distinguish from local tenderness;
  - the patient is distressed by the pain and is unable to carry on with everyday activities;
  - ordinary physical activity and bright light worsen the pain, forcing the patient to rest in a dark room;
  - nausea and vomiting are common a few hours after onset of pain;
  - some patients experience warning of an impending migraine attack as an "aura", which:
    - lasts about an hour;
    - consists of bright but uncoloured zigzag lines in the centre of vision;
    - is sometimes accompanied by numbness or tingling of the face and hands; OR
  - some patients experience changes in mood and appetite 24–48 hours before an attack;
  - a stuffy, runny nose, and warmth of the skin over the forehead on the painful side is common in migraine and may lead to a mistaken diagnosis of sinusitis (see next section).

UNCOMMON CAUSES OR FORMS OF HEADACHE

- **Sinusitis** (see Chapter 15, *Respiratory diseases*):
  - headache is felt only in the face or forehead;
  - headache is made worse by leaning forward;
  - there is a purulent nasal discharge in all cases;
  - chronic sinusitis is over-diagnosed as a cause of headache: most patients who have been given this diagnosis have migraine.
- **Cluster headache**:
  - pain is very severe on one side of the head, usually around the eye or temple, and is associated with tearing and redness of the eye on the painful side;
  - clusters of one or two attacks occur each day over a few weeks, after which the headaches stop for months or years;
  - onset is sudden, peaking in severity within a few minutes;
  - pain lasts from 30 minutes to an hour or two.
- **Temporo-mandibular joint disorders**:
  - the headache is described as a deep aching pain mainly around one ear but spreading to the jaw or temple;
  - the pain is often worse in the morning.

Red flags

Seek medical advice before giving treatment to a patient who has **any** of these conditions:

- a headache occurring for the first time that peaks in severity within a few seconds (thunderclap headache);
- a headache occurring for the first time with weakness or numbness of the face or limbs;
- a new headache that steadily worsens, becoming severe over two to six weeks;
- headache with drowsiness or confusion;
- a new headache during pregnancy;
- headache with neck stiffness (inability to put the chin on the chest when lying flat).

✔ *What to do in a case of migraine or tension headache*

- Give paracetamol, 1000 mg orally; **OR**:
  - acetylsalicylic acid (Aspirin®), 600 mg to 1000 mg orally; **OR**
  - ibuprofen, 800–1200 mg orally; note
  - you should give the higher doses for migraine, since it often responds better to a large dose given early than to smaller repeated doses.
- If the patient has a history of vomiting early in a migraine attack, give ondansetron, 4 mg orally, together with one of the above analgesics.
- If migraines are occurring more than once a week, have the patient see a doctor to consider using migraine-specific drugs and drugs to reduce the frequency of attacks; **note**:
  - frequent use of analgesics, such as acetylsalicylic acid (Aspirin®) and paracetamol, can worsen headaches.

✔ *What to do in a case of cluster headache*

- As soon as the headache starts, give oxygen, 6 litres per minute, by non-rebreathing mask, for 20 minutes.
- If the patient has not had a previous diagnosis of cluster headache, seek medical advice about whether to give prednisone, 50 mg orally, daily to reduce attacks until the patient can see a doctor at the next port of call for more specific treatment.

SEIZURES AND EPILEPSY

There are several types of seizure, or fit. The most common are epileptic seizures, which are caused by characteristic abnormal electrical activity in part or throughout the brain. Seizures can also be caused by kidney failure or severe shortage of oxygen or of glucose in the brain: these patients do not show the abnormal electrical activity characteristic of epilepsy. Epilepsy can begin at any age. In about half of patients, a cause can be identified, such as stroke, brain injury, or a birth defect. Many patients who have a seizure never have another one, and if further seizures do occur, they may not do so for months or years. Seizures, whether in patients known to have epilepsy or in patients who have never had seizures before, can be triggered by fever, alcohol, sleep deprivation, and certain drugs (see list below).

Types of epileptic seizure

There are two main types of epileptic seizure: a **partial seizure**, in which only part of the brain is affected, and a **generalized seizure**, in which most or all of the brain is affected. Partial seizures are further divided into **simple partial seizures** and **complex partial seizures**. Generalized seizures are divided into **non-convulsive (or absence) seizures** and **convulsive seizures**.

PARTIAL SEIZURES

- **Simple partial seizures**:
  - do not impair consciousness;
  - last seconds to a few minutes;
  - may precede, as an aura or as a warning seizure, a complex partial or generalized seizure;
  - consist of:
    - seeing flashing lights;
    - jerking of a hand or foot;
    - perception of unusual smells or sounds;
    - in a small number of cases, fear or rage, or unusual behaviour such as undressing in public.
- **Complex partial seizures** (or temporal lobe epilepsy):
  - the commonest form of epileptic seizures in adults;
  - do not cause falling or jerking;
  - last a minute or two;

- consist of:
  - unresponsiveness to the environment and other people;
  - a vacant stare;
  - repetitive gestures, typically chewing or smacking the lips;
  - repeating words or phrases;
  - walking about without purpose;
  - in many cases, for a few hours after the seizure, headache, sleepiness, and confusion.

GENERALIZED SEIZURES

- **Absence seizures** (or non-convulsive seizures, or petit mal epilepsy):
  - occur mainly in children;
  - last only a few seconds;
  - may occur several or many times a day;
  - cause sudden loss of consciousness but not falling;
  - all an observer sees is the patient standing still and staring blankly.
- **Generalized convulsive seizures** (or grand mal epilepsy or tonic-clonic epilepsy):
  - the classical form of epilepsy;
  - cause sudden loss of consciousness, sometimes preceded by a simple partial seizure (an aura) and often associated with a loud cry;
  - there is then a tonic phase, in which all the muscles of the body contract, so that the patient becomes rigid and stops breathing; this phase lasts 15 seconds or so;
  - a clonic phase starts after the tonic phase and lasts a minute or so, during which:
    - the patient's limbs jerk;
    - in many cases, the patient becomes cyanotic (blue), incontinent of urine or faeces, and may bite his tongue;
  - after the end of the clonic phase the patient goes into a deep sleep, and then gradually wakes up, often still confused and with a headache.

✔ *What to do in a case of non-convulsive seizures*

- Wait for the seizure to end: no immediate action is required.
- Do not try to restrain the patient: patients with complex partial seizures may become violent if restrained during a seizure.
- Arrange for the patient not to work in conditions likely to make a seizure dangerous, such as at a height, in the galley, or in the engine room.

✔ *What to do in a case of convulsive seizures*

- To reduce the risk of injury to the patient, remove sharp objects, electrical cables, etc.
- Wait for the seizure to end, then place the patient in the coma, or recovery, position (see Chapter 1, *First aid*) until speaking and standing are possible.

- If the seizure does not stop within five minutes or recurs before the patient recovers consciousness, see below, under *Status epilepticus*.
- Allow the patient to rest for a few hours.
- After the patient's recovery, if there are no ***Red flags*** (see below), wait until the patient can answer questions before calling for medical advice.
- When the patient can answer questions, ask:
  - what medication, if any, the patient is taking;
  - whether the patient takes illicit or recreational drugs or alcohol and to what extent (how often? how much?);
  - whether the patient has been deprived of sleep for any reason;
  - whether the patient has suffered a stroke or head injury in the past;
  - whether any member of the patient's family has suffered or is suffering from epilepsy.
- If the patient is known to have epilepsy and is on drug treatment, record:
  - the doses being taken;
  - whether all prescribed doses have been taken;
  - whether there has been any diarrhoea or vomiting that could have prevented absorption of the drugs.
- If this is the patient's first seizure, there is no need for urgent treatment or evaluation: drugs taken for epilepsy are rarely started after the first seizure.
- Have the patient see a doctor at the next port.
- Meanwhile, arrange for the patient not to work in conditions likely to make a seizure dangerous, such as at a height, in the galley, or in the engine room.
- Because of the possible long-term implications of epilepsy with regard to work at sea, advise the patient to see a specialist on returning home to form a plan for future care.

✗ *What not to do*

- **DO NOT** attempt to open the patient's mouth by force or to place anything in the mouth to prevent tongue biting.

Red flags

If any one of these conditions is present, seek medical advice urgently:

- seizures with fever;
- new seizures less than a week after a head injury;
- status epilepticus (see next section);
- a second seizure during a single voyage in a patient not known to have epilepsy.

STATUS EPILEPTICUS

- This is a seizure, of any type, that continues for longer than five minutes or when repeated seizures occur without the patient recovering consciousness between seizures;
- usually occurs in patients with known epilepsy, often when they stop taking or cannot absorb their usual drugs;

- can also occur during withdrawal from alcohol or benzodiazepine drugs (drugs with names ending in - azepam) and in some brain infections;
- can occur with any type of epilepsy, and:
  - is easy to diagnose in generalized tonic-clonic epilepsy;
  - is difficult to distinguish from psychiatric illness or other causes of confusion in complex partial epilepsy.

✔ ***What to do***

- Give midazolam, 0.1–0.2 mg per kg body weight, intramuscularly, or 10 mg intranasally (open two ampoules and give one drop at a time into alternate nostrils until the ampoules are empty).
- As soon as you have administered this treatment, seek medical advice with a view to evacuation.
- Midazolam is short-acting, and, under medical advice, the dose may be repeated if further seizures occur.

Drugs that can precipitate seizures

- Drugs in the ship's medicine chest (see Chapter 33):
  - ciprofloxacin
  - metronidazole
  - lignocaine (lidocaine)
  - metoprolol.
- Other common drugs:
  - penicillin G
  - caffeine
  - theophylline
  - amphetamine.

LOSS OF CONSCIOUSNESS

There are three situations that may pose a problem for a medical officer, or crew member acting as such, in relation to loss of consciousness: a patient with sudden loss of consciousness; finding a person who is unconscious; and a patient with diabetic coma (diabetic ketoacidosis).

Sudden loss of consciousness (syncope)

Sudden loss of consciousness is usually caused by a sudden drop in blood pressure: this is called syncope. Syncope is often described by patients "as if the lights went out". Once the patient has fallen, recovery is rapid and complete because blood flow to the brain is restored. This distinguishes syncope from conditions such as hypoglycaemia (low blood sugar), in which consciousness is lost slowly. Syncope can be due to:

- a very slow heart rate;
- an abnormal heart rhythm;
- loss of small blood vessel tone, causing pooling of blood in the legs.

There are three common forms of syncope likely to be seen on board ship: postural syncope, micturition syncope, and vaso-vagal syncope.

POSTURAL SYNCOPE

- The patient becomes dizzy and pale, then loses consciousness after standing up.
- Postural syncope often occurs after a period of bed rest lasting more than a few days, such as during an illness.
- Medicines, especially those used for treating high blood pressure, are a common cause of postural syncope.
- Postural syncope can be the first symptom of blood loss, as from a bleeding peptic ulcer.

MICTURITION SYNCOPE

- An attack usually occurs immediately after urination, often during the night.

VASO-VAGAL SYNCOPE (FAINTING)

- A fainting episode can occur after a few seconds or minutes of nausea, skin pallor, sweating, and light-headedness.
- The episode may be precipitated by a strong emotion or fear.

Note

- In most cases, syncope is not a sign of serious illness.
- Syncope can be the first or only indication of serious heart disease, especially if:
  - an attack occurs while the patient is lying or sitting;
  - the patient has a history of heart disease.
- In a few cases, generalized epilepsy can occur without tonic-clonic movements (see above) and can mimic syncope:
  - epilepsy is likely to be the correct diagnosis if the patient:
    - is dusky blue (cyanosed) rather than pale;
    - recovers slowly and is confused for a period after the episode.

✔ *What to do*

- Lay the patient flat.
- Check for injuries (one third of patients with syncope injure themselves falling).
- If you think that medications may have caused postural syncope, seek medical advice about stopping these medications.
- If there are indications of a serious cardiac cause seek medical advice with a view to evacuation.
- If no cause can be found, keep the patient lying down and check frequently for evidence of bleeding, such as blood in the stools.

Finding an unconscious person

Common causes of unconsciousness include:

- alcohol intoxication: remember that alcohol and trauma often go together, so be wary of singling out alcohol as the only cause of unconsciousness;
- epileptic seizures;

- hypoglycaemia (low level of sugar in the blood), usually caused by insulin treatment;
- overdose of a narcotic drug, usually heroin, or a benzodiazepine (drugs with names ending in - azepam);
- compression of the brainstem by high pressure in the skull forcing part of the brain through the hole at the base of the skull through which the spinal cord leaves the skull:
  - a common cause of this compression is bleeding in the skull caused by trauma or intracerebral haemorrhage (see Chapter 4, *Head injuries*).

✔ *What to do on finding an unconscious patient*

- If there is no evidence of major head injury, immediately give:
  - glucagon at once, 1 mg intramuscularly; **AND**
  - naloxone, 0.8 mg intramuscularly or intravenously, repeated twice if there is no response.
- If the patient remains unconscious, seek medical advice.

Diabetes mellitus and coma

There are two forms of diabetes: Type 1 diabetes and Type 2 diabetes:

- **Type 1 diabetes** (juvenile-onset diabetes or insulin-dependent diabetes) is caused by insufficient production by the pancreas of insulin, a hormone that regulates the use of sugar by the body.
- **Type 2 diabetes** *(*adult-onset diabetes or non-insulin dependent diabetes mellitus*)* is much more common than Type 1 diabetes and is due partly to deficiency of insulin secretion but mainly to resistance of the body's tissues to the action of insulin. This resistance is related to obesity, lack of exercise, and inherited factors. Most problems with Type 2 diabetes are due to the long-term complications of the disease, which take 10 to 20 years to develop.

  There are two ways in which diabetes mellitus can cause coma: under-treated diabetes can cause diabetic ketoacidosis (see below) and over-treated diabetes can cause lack of glucose in the blood (hypoglycaemia) (see below).

Signs and symptoms of Type 1 diabetes

- Frequent urination with large volumes of urine
- thirst
- hunger or increased appetite
- in some cases, weight loss despite increased intake of food.

Signs and symptoms of Type 2 diabetes

- Blindness
- kidney failure
- neurological problems.

Note

- You do not need to provide a diabetic with special food but in insulin-using diabetics ensure that meals are given at regular and predictable times to keep the correct balance between insulin injections and food intake.
- An insulin-using diabetic who cannot eat because of severe vomiting, for example, still needs some insulin: seek medical advice about the correct dose.

Diabetic ketoacidosis

Diabetic ketoacidosis occurs only in Type I diabetes: the deficiency of insulin causes the body to produce large amounts of glucose and the fat cells to pump out large amounts of fat, which are converted in the liver to substances called "ketoacids". The result is a dangerous chemical imbalance in the body.

Diabetic ketoacidosis develops over days. The symptoms of Type I diabetes (see above) will have been present for at least this long before consciousness becomes impaired.

Signs and symptoms

- Flushed, dry skin
- a distinctly fruity breath odour (similar to nail polish remover or acetone)
- large amounts of urine
- drowsiness or confusion
- rapid, deep, sighing breathing
- sometimes abdominal pain and vomiting
- in severe cases, confusion, followed by coma and death.

✔ *What to do*

- Remember that in a patient from a less developed country diabetes may be present but may not have been diagnosed.
- Test the urine for sugar (see Chapter 26, *Nursing care and medical procedures*): for practical purposes on board ship, the presence of glucose in the urine strongly suggests that the patient has diabetes and the absence of glucose in the urine suggests that the patient, if not under treatment, does not have diabetes.
- If, in addition to a strongly positive glucose finding, the urine also tests strongly positive for ketones, arrange for urgent evacuation; note:
  - the finding of ketones in the absence of glucose is not an indication of disease, especially when there has been limited food intake over 24 hours.
- If the glucose test is positive but the ketone test negative and if the patient is well, medical care will depend on the patient's age and body weight:
  - most of these patients will be older and overweight: advise them to see their usual doctor after the voyage;
  - in a patient under 25 years, consider Type I diabetes as a likely diagnosis and arrange for a medical consultation as soon as possible: diabetic ketoacidosis can develop quickly.

Hypoglycaemia

Treatment for diabetes aims at lowering the level of sugar (glucose) in the blood. If the treatment is too strong or given too often, or if sugar in the blood is already low because of exercise or because no food has been eaten, low blood sugar (hypoglycaemia) can occur.

Signs and symptoms

- Hunger
- sweating
- rapid pulse
- rumbling stomach
- "silly" or inattentive behaviour
- in severe cases, confusion or loss of consciousness.

✔ *What to do*

- Suspect low blood sugar if a patient under treatment for diabetes exhibits silliness, bizarre or irrational behaviour, followed by confusion and eventually unconsciousness: in this case:
  - give sugar, preferably in an easily absorbed form, such as a sugary drink or candy;
  - if the patient is unconscious, give glucagon, 1 mg intramuscularly;
  - give sugar as soon as the patient wakes up, since glucagon is short-acting and hypoglycemia may recur.
- Remember that a diabetic is far more likely to have hypoglycaemia than diabetic ketoacidosis: always give sugar or glucagon to a diabetic displaying abnormal behaviour or impaired consciousness.
- Note that many patients with Type 2 diabetes are treated with drugs rather than insulin: some of these drugs can also cause dangerous hypoglycaemia.

BELL'S PALSY

Bell's palsy is a relatively sudden weakness or paralysis of the muscles on one side of the face, which is often mistaken for stroke (see above). It is caused by a virus infecting the facial nerve, usually herpes simplex virus (the same virus that causes cold sores). The facial nerve supplies the muscles of the face, the taste buds at the front of the tongue, the tear glands, and some salivary glands.

Bell's palsy is common and causes a great deal of distress because of the unsightliness that accompanies it. The condition usually improves within three weeks and resolves completely within five to six weeks.

Signs and symptoms

- Onset over a few hours of weakness or complete paralysis of the muscles on one side of the face.
- The weakness is often first noticed on waking in the morning.
- The most obvious indication of face weakness is drooping of the mouth on the affected side.

- The patient cannot close the eye or raise the eyebrow on the affected side, or wrinkle the forehead (ask the patient to frown) on the affected side (this is important, since weakness of the face with the ability to frown preserved suggests a stroke).
- There are no tears in the eye on the affected side.

✔ ***What to do***

- If the patient cannot shut the affected eye properly, damage to the eye can occur: tape a gauze pad over the eye to keep it closed;
  - **DO NOT** put the tape directly on the eyelid;
  - have the patient keep the gauze pad on all the time at first, then only at night as recovery occurs.
- Give Aciclovir, 400 mg orally, five times daily, for one week; **AND**:
  - prednisone, 50 mg orally, every day for a week.
- Have the patient see a doctor at the next port.

MENTAL ILLNESS

Psychosis

Psychosis is a term used to denote a group of mental disorders in which the patient loses contact with reality. It involves delusions, hallucinations, and thought disorder.

SYMPTOMS OF PSYCHOSIS

- Delusions:
  - are patently false beliefs, not related to a patient's religion or culture, which the patient insists are true despite overwhelming evidence to the contrary;
  - include:
    - **delusions of persecution**, in which the patient believes he is the victim of a plot;
    - **delusions of grandeur,** in which the patient believes he is extremely important or can do things beyond his normal capacities (like flying or being a king);
    - **delusions of reference**, in which the patient believes that his environment – television or radio broadcasts or signs in the ship or the behaviour of other people – contains messages directed to him;
    - **delusions of thought control,** in which the patient believes that his thoughts are under outside control or have been inserted into his mind or are being broadcast so that others can read his mind.

Delusions are not always obviously ridiculous (e.g. "The cook is trying to poison me"). If you are patient, and ask the patient to explain his belief in detail ("Why do you think he is doing that?"), its delusional nature will eventually come out.

- Hallucinations:
  - are false sensory perceptions, such as seeing or hearing or smelling things that are not perceived by others;

- in most cases of psychosis, hallucinations are of hearing (auditory hallucinations), such as hearing voices, especially voices that are abusive and threatening.
- Thought disorder:
  - is characterized by disorganized thinking;
  - causes a patient to jump from one idea to another that is not linked logically to the first other than by involving a similar sounding word or similar memory;
  - is manifested in illogical, incoherent, even nonsensical speech, with words "tumbling out" in a chaotic fashion.

Forms of psychosis

SCHIZOPHRENIA

- Is the most common form of psychosis;
- is a chronic, disabling condition in which episodes of psychotic symptoms occur repeatedly, with progressive impairment of social and occupational functioning;
- most often begins in late adolescence or early adult life and lasts for years;
- involves positive symptoms, negative symptoms, and cognitive symptoms;
- **positive symptoms**:
  - delusions, hallucinations, and thought disorder;
  - occur not continuously but periodically;
  - are those that most often prompt hospitalization of the patient;
  - are those most readily treated by medication;
- **negative symptoms**:
  - a diminished range of emotions;
  - loss of interest in normally pleasurable activities and in social interaction;
  - often cause long-term problems with work and relationships;
- **cognitive symptoms**:
  - defects in memory and reasoning;
  - disabling and not readily treated by medication.

BIPOLAR AFFECTIVE DISORDER (or manic depressive psychosis)

- Characterized by manic phases dominated by extreme elation (euphoria) or excitement, alternating with depressive phases, in which the patient is irritable and severely depressed;
- usually, between these two phases, there are periods when the patient is well and is able to lead a productive life;
- usually comes to medical attention in the manic phase, which can involve:
  - irritability
  - increased activity
  - reduced sleep
  - rapid speech, that can become overtly irrational
  - grandiose ideas, that can become delusional, with hallucinations
  - impulsiveness and poor judgement.

BRIEF REACTIVE PSYCHOSIS

- Produces typical symptoms of psychosis following a significant or stressful life event, such as:
  - a birth
  - a bereavement
  - a marriage break-up
  - the start of a new job
  - falling in, or out of, love;
- resolves when the stress is no longer felt by the patient.

DRUG-INDUCED PSYCHOSIS

- In which psychotic symptoms are triggered by taking drugs such as amphetamine or cocaine.

ORGANIC PSYCHOSIS

- Results from brain damage due to:
  - a head injury
  - meningitis
  - epilepsy
  - physical illnesses involving the liver, kidney, or endocrine glands.

✔ *What to do in a case of psychosis*

- Assess the patient for risk of suicide and for risk of violence or aggression (see below).
- If you can talk to and examine the patient, look for evidence of a medical illness, such as alcohol withdrawal.
- Consider the possibility of intoxication with a drug such as amphetamine, cocaine, or phencyclidine: in such cases, the psychotic symptoms will resolve as the effects of the drug wear off.
- If the patient is relatively calm and does not appear to pose a risk to himself or others, have him kept under continuous observation and seek medical advice.
- If the patient is very agitated or there is an immediate risk of suicide or violence give haloperidol, 2.5–5 mg intramuscularly or intravenously, repeated every two to six hours as needed, up to a maximum dose of 15 mg per day (up to 30 mg per day if, despite 24 hours' treatment, the patient's condition is still dangerous); **AND**:
  - diazepam, 5 mg orally, four times daily, if the patient remains agitated after receiving haloperidol and can take oral medication;
  - if haloperidol cannot be used or if dangerous violence is taking place, give midazolam, 10–15 mg intramuscularly:
    - give the higher dose to control dangerous violence quickly and to patients who drink alcohol regularly;
    - midazolam acts quickly but wears off quickly: give haloperidol as soon as possible;
    - in rare cases, midazolam can precipitate violent behaviour (especially if haloperidol has not been given).
- Seek medical advice once the patient is under control.

Depression

Sadness becomes pathological depression when it interferes with the activities of everyday life: work, relationships, and self-care. About 10% of men and 20% of women suffer depression at some time in their lives and 2–3% of men and 5–10% of women suffer depression at any given time.

Note

- Depression has a complex relationship to alcohol abuse: a patient with depressive symptoms and a problem of alcohol abuse should consult an expert.
- The relationship between depression and grief or bereavement is complex:
  - depressive symptoms occurring within two months of bereavement are normal;
  - beyond two months, the likelihood increases of true depression developing;
  - depressive symptoms that persist for one year after bereavement are definitely abnormal.

Signs and symptoms

- A feeling of "rotting inside" or of " being unattractive";
- fatigue;
- difficulty sleeping;
- appearing sad most of the time: note that patients with depression do not often complain spontaneously of excessive or abnormal sadness.

What to do

- Diagnose depression if the patient:
  - appears depressed; **AND**
  - has problems of work, relationships, or self-care; **AND**
  - most of the time over a two-week period, experiences five or more of the following symptoms or signs:
    - loss of interest in or pleasure from normally pleasurable activities
    - weight gain or weight loss
    - poor sleep
    - fatigue and loss of energy
    - slow movements and responses
    - agitation
    - feelings of worthlessness or guilt
    - poor concentration
    - thoughts of death or suicide.
- If you suspect depression, check for the risk of suicide (see below, under *Suicide*).
- If suicide does not seem to be a risk, have the patient see a doctor at the next port.

Violent or threatening behaviour

A person who is aggressive, violent, or otherwise threatening may:

- have taken drugs, particularly amphetamine;
- be drunk;
- be suffering from schizophrenia.

SIGNS OF POTENTIAL DANGER TO OTHERS

- A history of previous physical violence against a person or object in the past few weeks – the more recent and the more serious the past violence, the greater the risk of present violence.
- An expressed desire to harm a named person or hallucinations of being ordered to harm a named person.
- Threatening, yelling or swearing at others in the immediate vicinity.
- Signs of alcohol or amphetamine intoxication (see Chapter 22, *Tobacco, alcohol, and drug use*).
- Extreme restlessness, pacing, "nervous" smoking, or fidgeting.

✔ *What to do when faced with a violent or threatening patient*

- Confront the patient quickly with overwhelming force.
- If it is necessary to overpower the patient, assemble several crew members; give each a thick mattress; and have them together rush the patient, holding the mattresses out in front, so as to bundle the patient to the ground.
- Give haloperidol, 5–10 mg intramuscularly, **AND** midazolam, 5–10 mg intramuscularly.

✘ *What not to do*

- **DO NOT** attempt to talk to the patient alone.
- **DO NOT** ask directly if the patient has a weapon or demand that the patient surrender a suspected weapon.

Suicide

Suicide is a common cause of death in most communities. Men are at greater risk than women; adolescents and the elderly are at greater risk than people in middle-age.

Overall, there are at least 10 unsuccessful suicide attempts for every death from suicide. However, the proportion of successful suicide attempts is higher in men and is particularly high when guns or other lethal means of suicide are available. Few illnesses occurring on board ship are more likely to kill the patient than depression associated with a high risk of attempted suicide.

Nearly everyone who commits suicide is suffering at the time from some form of mental illness: the more severe the illness, the higher the risk of suicide. Depression or alcohol abuse is frequently associated with suicide (about 25% of people who commit suicide are drunk at the time), as are schizophrenia and mania (see above).

✔ *What to do*

- Ask these questions (they will **NOT** "suggest" suicide to a patient who has not already thought about it):
  - Have you ever had thoughts of harming yourself?
  - Do you intend to harm yourself?
  - Have you made a specific plan to harm yourself?
  - Have you started making preparations to carry out the plan (such as obtaining a gun and ammunition)?
  - Have you practised carrying out the suicide (e.g. loading a gun and holding it to different parts of the head)?
- If the patient has a plan, consider:
  - whether the patient could carry it out (if the plan involves a gun, does the patient have access to one?);
  - how likely it is that the plan would result in a fatal outcome if it was carried out as described;
  - whether the plan includes steps to reduce the chance of rescue (e.g. choosing a time when the patient is on watch alone in a remote part of the ship).
- There is a **high** risk of a successful suicide attempt **in the next 48 hours** in any patient who:
  - intends to commit suicide; **AND**
  - has a clear and effective plan for doing so; **AND**
  - has the capacity to carry out the plan.
- If these risk factors for a successful suicide attempt are present:
  - make sure the patient is not left alone;
  - remove anything from the patient's surroundings and clothing that could be used to commit suicide;
  - seek medical advice urgently with a view to evacuation.
- If the patient has thought about suicide but has no plan, the risk of suicide is lower but still significant; in this case:
  - ensure that the patient has no access to a weapon or other means of suicide likely to be lethal;
  - make sure support is available from crew members trusted by the patient;
  - emphasize your commitment to helping the patient through his difficulties;
  - provide increased contact with the patient's family, if he desires it;
  - ask the patient to promise not to commit suicide (for many people a promise they have given to someone they respect can restrain impulsive behaviour).
- Arrange for the patient to see a doctor at the next port.

After an unsuccessful suicide attempt

- Seek medical advice.
- Treat injuries or poisonings as required.
- Assess suicide risk as above.

- Whatever you assess the suicide risk to be, keep the patient under observation – one suicide attempt always means there is a risk of a further suicide attempt.

✗ What not to do

- **DO NOT** give diazepam: it may cause disinhibition and precipitate violence.
- **DO NOT** allow the patient to drink alcohol.
- **DO NOT** be critical or judgemental.

Post-traumatic stress disorder

Post-traumatic stress disorder (PTSD) occurs after a stressful event, such as experiencing a physical assault, including rape, or being in a motor vehicle accident or a natural disaster, or witnessing the death of a loved one. Most people experience a reaction following a stressful event: bad dreams, for example, or difficulty getting the event out of their minds. In PTSD these symptoms are more severe and prolonged, and interfere with everyday work and social activities. The frequency of PTSD varies with the type of triggering event: over 50% after rape, about 15% after witnessing the death of a loved one, and 5% after an accident or natural disaster.

Signs and symptoms

- Intrusive thoughts about the traumatic event;
- "flashbacks", i.e. vivid and intensely distressing "re-experiencing" of the event;
- intense reactions to reminders of the trauma, which may be only remotely associated with it;
- avoidance of reminders to an extent which may be socially and occupationally disabling;
- edginess and irritability;
- insomnia.

✔ What to do

- Remember that PTSD is a long-term problem: the patient will not "get over it" without professional help.
- Although controlled exposure to traumatic memories is part of the psychological treatment of PTSD, on board ship you should help the patient to avoid reminders of the trauma.
- Ask the patient about over-use of alcohol or drugs, which the patient may be resorting to in an attempt to control the symptoms.
- Ask the patient whether he or she has thoughts of self-harm (see above, *Suicide*).
- If the patient can continue to function with support, arrange for a consultation with a doctor either at the next port or at the patient's home port.

Chest pain and other disorders of the heart and circulation

Blood is supplied to the heart by two coronary arteries (see Chapter 31, *Anatomy and physiology*). These arteries can be narrowed by a fatty deposit (atheroma) that accumulates on their inner walls. A blood clot can form in the section of a coronary artery narrowed by atheroma (coronary thrombosis), blocking the artery and causing myocardial infarction, in which an area of heart muscle dies. When the coronary arteries are narrowed but not altogether blocked and when the workload on the heart is increased by exercise, the heart can become short of blood: the result is angina (angina pectoris).

All these conditions come under the term "coronary artery disease", which mostly occurs in people over 50 years of age but can also occur in younger people. The term "heart attack" is usually used to mean myocardial infarction but some people use it to mean angina or attacks of severe breathlessness caused by heart disease: it is important, therefore, to be clear about what a patient means by "heart attack".

ANGINA PECTORIS

Angina pectoris is pain or discomfort in the chest caused by inadequate blood supply to the heart. There are two main forms of angina pectoris: stable angina and unstable angina.

Stable angina is angina pectoris that has been occurring in episodes for weeks or months, each time after about the same amount of exercise but rarely when the patient is at rest. With stable angina, there is only a low risk of a heart attack occurring in the near future.

Unstable angina is angina pectoris that began only recently or occurs at rest or occurs following much less exercise than the patient was in the habit of doing previously: with unstable angina there is a high risk of a heart attack occurring in the near future.

Note

- Angina and the pain of myocardial infarction are similar in location and character but the pain of myocardial infarction is usually more severe and longer-lasting.
- Some patients with myocardial infarction have only mild pain, and some will be reluctant to call it "pain" at all, preferring "weight" or "heaviness".
- Angina comes on after a few minutes' exercise and forces the patient to stop or slow down, then goes away after a few minutes' rest.
- The amount of exercise needed to bring on angina is often less in the morning than in the evening, less after than before meals, and less when exercising in the cold than in warmer temperatures.
- It is not very important whether a patient has unstable angina or a myocardial infarction. The important thing is to recognise that the pain is coming from the heart and that it is getting worse.

Chest pain is probably coming from the heart if:

- **it is felt**:
  - in the middle of the chest under the breast bone (sternum); **AND/OR**
  - in the left arm or in the neck and lower jaw;
- **it is described by the patient as**:
  - "heavy" or "like a heavy weight on the chest";
  - "a tightness";
  - "a pressing";
  - "a squeezing"; and
  - the patient clenches one fist over the centre of his chest when trying to say what he feels;
- **it**:
  - is consistent over different episodes in the same patient (patients can reliably recognize pain as myocardial infarction if they have had one before);
  - is like pain previously happening on exercise but more severe;
  - comes on gradually;
  - lasts from 30 minutes to one to two hours;
  - is accompanied by breathlessness, nausea, and sweating.

Pain is probably not coming from the heart if it is:

- felt in the lower abdomen or upper jaw;
- described as "sharp" or "stabbing";
- pain that starts suddenly;
- pain that the patient can point to with one finger;
- a stab that lasts a few seconds and is felt in a small area near the left nipple;
- pain felt on one side of the chest that gets worse with deep breathing;
- likely to be associated with tenderness at the rib extremities near the breastbone;
- pain:
  - with a "burning" rather than a "heavy" or "pressing" character;
  - associated with an acid taste in the mouth;
  - coming on after meals and not exercise;
  - lasting for many hours and not just for 30 minutes to one or two hours;
  - this pain is more likely to be due to gastro-oesophageal reflux disease (see Chapter 16, *Gastrointestinal and liver diseases*).

✔ *What to do in a case of myocardial infarction or unstable angina*

- Seek medical advice with a view to evacuation: act promptly, because the benefit of treatment for myocardial infarction is reduced after only a few hours' delay and is largely lost after 24 hours.
- Before seeking medical advice, collect the following information:
  - age
  - smoking habits
  - presence of diabetes mellitus

- history of heart disease in mother, father, brothers, or sisters
- duration of pain
- pulse rate and rhythm
- blood pressure
- ability of patient to breathe comfortably lying flat.

- While awaiting evacuation or if evacuation is impossible, have the patient stay in bed except to go to the toilet.
- Restrict the patient to a light diet with fluids as desired.
- Give acetylsalicylic acid (Aspirin®), 150 mg (half a tablet) orally, at once and then daily.
- Give metoprolol, 50 mg orally, twice daily; **UNLESS**:
  - the blood pressure is less than 120 mmHg systolic; **OR**
  - the pulse rate is less than 65 beats per minute; **OR**
  - the patient has asthma.

✔ *What to do in a patient with stable angina*

- Give acetylsalicylic acid (Aspirin®), 150 mg (half a tablet) orally, daily.
- Give metoprolol, 50 mg orally, twice daily; **UNLESS**:
  - the blood pressure is less than 120 mmHg systolic; **OR**
  - the pulse rate is less than 65 beats per minute; **OR**
  - the patient has asthma.
- Restrict the patient to activities that do not cause pain.
- Advise the patient strongly not to smoke.

Complications of myocardial infarction

CONGESTIVE HEART FAILURE

- If the area of heart affected by myocardial infarction is extensive, there may not be enough heart muscle to pump blood effectively; this causes:
  - **in severe cases**:
    - extreme difficulty breathing, made worse when the patient lies flat;
    - low blood pressure;
    - cool, blue or grey, sweaty face, hands and feet;
    - if the blood pressure is less than 90mmHg systolic, cardiogenic shock is present; (see Chapter 2, *Shock*); this is nearly always fatal;
  - **in moderate cases**:
    - the above signs and symptoms, except that blood pressure remains normal;
  - **in mild cases**:
    - breathlessness made worse by lying flat and, after one or two days, swelling (oedema) of the ankles.

ABNORMAL HEART RHYTHM (CARDIAC ARRHYTHMIA)

- The dead (infarcted) area of heart muscle can give rise to abnormal heart rhythms, most often during the first 24 hours after the myocardial infarction.

- In most cases, the abnormal rhythm consists of fast heart beats that may become chaotic: this can cause sudden death.
- The dead area of heart muscle can block the normal pathways through which the heart is triggered to contract, causing it to beat at a very slow rate – usually 30–40 beats per minute: the result is a fall in blood pressure, faintness and, in some cases, breathlessness.

✔ *What to do in a case of congestive heart failure*

- **In severe cases**:
  - give frusemide, 40 mg intravenously (preferably) or intramuscularly; **AND**
  - morphine, 5–10 mg intravenously (preferably) or intramuscularly;
  - if there is no improvement in 30 minutes, give frusemide, 80 mg intravenously (preferably) or intramuscularly.
- **In moderate cases**:
  - give frusemide, 40 mg intravenously (preferably) or intramuscularly, and repeat if there is no improvement in 30 minutes.
- **In mild cases**:
  - give frusemide, 20 mg intramuscularly.

✔ *What to do in a case of abnormal heart rhythm*

- If you cannot feel a pulse, begin cardiopulmonary resuscitation (see Chapter 1, *First aid*).
- Seek medical advice.
- If the pulse is slow, give atropine, 0.6 mg intravenously (preferably) or intramuscularly: repeat twice if there is no response in 10 minutes or if there is an initial effect but the pulse slows again later.

Palpitations

The term "palpitations" refers to a feeling or awareness by the patient that the heart is beating abnormally fast or abnormally forcefully. Common patterns of palpitation are:

- **a feeling that the heart has stopped**, followed by one or two forceful, pounding beats, sometimes described as "the heart turning over":
  - this feeling is due to extra beats inserted into to the normal heart rhythm, causing a pause in the beating of the heart followed by a strong beat;
  - this palpitation is often associated with excessive consumption of caffeine and with anxiety;
- **regular palpitations** (i.e. the interval between one heart beat and the next is always the same) that occur:
  - in episodes that start and end gradually and last less than five minutes;
  - at a pulse rate of about 120 beats per minute;
  - with a dry mouth and light-headedness but not loss of consciousness;
  - these palpitations are usually due to anxiety;

- **rapid, regular palpitations** that occur:
  - in episodes that start and end suddenly and last more than five minutes;
  - at a pulse rate of more than 150 beats per minute;
  - in young people, who often describe repeated episodes that began in childhood;
  - these are rarely dangerous in young people; but
  - can be dangerous in patients over 50, who usually have a known heart disease;
- **irregular palpitations** that:
  - start suddenly;
  - often last for hours or days at a pulse rate of 150 to 180 beats per minute;
  - are often associated with an alcoholic binge or (less often) heart disease in patients under 50;
  - are usually due to heart disease in patients over 50 years of age.

✔ *What to do in the case of palpitations*

- Ask the patient these questions:
  - Did the palpitations begin suddenly or gradually?
  - Are they, or were they, regular or irregular in rhythm?
  - Do you still have palpitations? **IF NOT**:
    - Did they stop suddenly or gradually?
    - Is there, or was there, chest pain or heaviness or tightness when you felt the palpitations?
    - Do you, or did you, feel dizziness or light-headedness during the palpitations?
    - How long did/do the episodes of palpitation last?
- Note that episodes lasting more than five minutes are more likely to be due to heart disease than episodes lasting less than five minutes.
- What do the palpitations feel like in your chest?
- Have the patient tap out the rhythm of the palpitations on a table or on your hand.
- If the palpitations are still present, feel and count the pulse and take the blood pressure.
- If the pulse rhythm is irregular when you feel the pulse, give acetylsalicylic acid (Aspirin®), 150 mg (half a tablet) orally, daily and have the patient see a doctor at the next port.
- Seek medical advice with a view to evacuation, if:
  - there is a very rapid or irregular pulse rhythm when you feel the pulse; **AND**
  - the patient feels heaviness, tightness, or pain in the chest; **OR IF**:
    - the patient has lost consciousness completely (i.e. has not just felt light-headedness) during an episode of palpitations.
- If you cannot obtain medical advice, give metoprolol, 50 mg orally, twice daily, **unless** the patient has asthma.

Blocked arteries in the legs

The leg arteries can be blocked by atheroma. The patient is nearly always a smoker and over 50 years of age. Occasionally, in patients of any age, a leg artery can be blocked by a clot that formed elsewhere, such as in the heart or in a large artery, and then travelled to the leg artery.

Signs and symptoms

- In most cases, a long history of pain in the calf muscles when walking that disappears on rest.
- In cases in which a leg artery is completely blocked:
  - severe pain in the leg
  - the leg is cold and pale
  - pulses in the feet are absent
  - after a few days, the toes die (necrosis) and turn black.

✔ What to do

- Seek medical advice.
- Give acetylsalicylic acid (Aspirin®), 150 mg (half a tablet) orally, daily.
- For pain relief, give morphine, 5–10 mg intramuscularly or 10–20 mg orally, every three to four hours.

Deep vein thrombosis

In deep vein thrombosis, clots form in the large veins that run deep inside the leg. The clots can become dislodged from the leg and travel to the heart and lungs, where they can block blood flow to the lungs and cause death.

Deep vein thrombosis usually occurs in patients who:

- have had surgery or suffered a major injury during the previous four weeks; **OR**
- have been immobile for more than 10 hours, such as during a long plane flight; **OR**
- have an inherited tendency to form blood clots easily and to suffer repeated episodes of deep vein thrombosis.

Signs and symptoms

- Pain in one leg, with swelling.
- In severe cases, purplish skin over the affected leg, which is very painful.

✔ What to do

- Measure the circumference of the thickest part of the two calves with a tape measure at the same height: a difference of more than 2 cm is abnormal.
- Confine the patient to complete bed rest.
- Give acetylsalicylic acid (Aspirin®), 150 mg (half a tablet) orally, daily.
- Seek medical advice.

Respiratory diseases

BRONCHITIS

Bronchitis is an inflammation of the bronchi, the branches of the windpipe inside the lungs. There are many causes of bronchitis, but the commonest are infections, asthma, and cigarette smoking. The main symptom of bronchitis is a cough that produces sputum.

Bronchitis due to infection

Most cases of bronchitis in otherwise healthy people are caused by viruses. The only common bacterial infection causing bronchitis is whooping cough (pertussis) (see Chapter 23, *Infectious diseases*).

Signs and symptoms

- Sore throat;
- feeling unwell;
- cough producing small amounts of usually clear, colourless sputum;
- no fever, unless influenza virus is the cause (see Chapter 23, *Infectious diseases*);
- respiratory rate and pulse rate normal;
- **treat as pneumonia** if:
  - pulse rate is over 100 beats per minute; **OR**
  - respiratory rate is over 24 breaths per minute; **OR**
  - body temperature is over 38°C;
- if symptoms arise following contact with a person with a long-lasting cough occurring in paroxysms, suspect whooping cough.

✔ *What to do*

- No treatment is required.
- If whooping cough is suspected, give antibiotics as recommended for pertussis (see Chapter 23, *Infectious diseases*).

Bronchitis due to cigarette smoking

Bronchitis is the cause of "smoker's cough" and is an early indication of lung damage due to cigarette smoking.

Signs and symptoms

- Coughing every day, producing small amounts of clear, colourless or pale-yellow sputum;
- if a common cold or other minor viral infection is present:
  - worsening of cough
  - increased amount of sputum
  - sputum thicker, opaque, and yellow or green;
- no fever;
- shortness of breath on exertion of a degree that posed no problem previously – often the first sign of serious lung damage.

✔ What to do

- If a patient who smokes cigarettes has symptoms of a viral infection and has developed a new or worse cough which produces opaque, coloured sputum, and if the patient also has shortness of breath on exercise:
  - give amoxycillin/clavulanate, 875/125 mg orally, twice daily for five days.
- Otherwise no treatment is needed: bronchitis due to cigarette smoking disappears a few weeks after the patient has stopped smoking.

BRONCHIECTASIS

Bronchiectasis is a condition in which the bronchi are abnormally dilated, do not clear mucus normally, and are prone to repeated infection. Bronchiectasis in adults often results from an episode of severe pneumonia in childhood and can also be due to the inherited disorder cystic fibrosis.

► Signs and symptoms

- A chronic cough producing large amounts of white or pale-yellow sputum (usually more than half a teacup a day).
- If infection is present:
  - sputum quantity is increased
  - sputum changes in colour to dark yellow or green
  - in some cases, blood is mixed with the sputum
  - fever may be present, but if the temperature is higher than 38°C, assess and treat as pneumonia.

✔ What to do

- Give amoxycillin/clavulanate, 875/125 mg orally, twice daily.
- Have the patient see a doctor in his home port: bronchiectasis causes gradual deterioration in lung function.

COMMON COLD

Colds are spread mainly by direct hand-to-hand contact or by indirect contact via objects or surfaces touched by the hands of a person with a cold.

► Signs and symptoms

- Blocked, runny nose
- feeling unwell
- a sore or "scratchy" throat
- no fever or chills
- cough, usually three to four days after the cold starts:
  - cough at onset of the illness is a sign of influenza or asthma, or bronchitis due to cigarette smoking.

✔ What to do

- No treatment is needed.
- If a blocked nose interferes with sleep or work, give drops (e.g. oxymetazoline 0.5 mg/ml or an equivalent medication) that constrict the blood vessels in the nose.
- To limit spread of the infection to other crew members:
  - have the patient wash the hands frequently;
  - have other crew members wash their hands after contact with the patient or with objects touched by the patient.

PLEURISY

Pleurisy is inflammation of the pleurae, the two membranes that, respectively, line the chest cavity and surround the lungs. The space between the two pleurae can fill with fluid (pleural effusion), or with pus (empyema, see section below, under *Pneumonia*) or with air (pneumothorax, see Chapter 7, *Abdominal and chest injuries*). Pleurisy is most often part of another illness. The commonest cause of pleurisy is pneumonia (see below).

► Signs and symptoms

- A sharp stabbing pain on one side of the chest, made worse by breathing movements or coughing:
  - the patient can point with one finger to the spot where the pain is worst;
  - resembles pain from a fractured rib, in which case the patient has a history of injury and marked tenderness over the fracture.

✔ What to do

- Treat with a nonsteroidal anti-inflammatory drug, such as ibuprofen, 400 mg orally, every six hours:
  - if pain is not controlled **ADD** tramadol, 50–100 mg orally, every six to eight hours;
  - if pain is still not controlled after two doses of tramadol, **GIVE**:
    - morphine, 10–20 mg orally, every four hours; OR
    - morphine, 5–10 mg intramuscularly, every three to four hours.
- If there is no clear evidence of pneumonia causing the pleurisy, have the patient see a doctor at the next port to investigate the possible cause.

Pneumothorax (see Chapter 7, *Abdominal and chest injuries*)

PNEUMONIA

Lobar pneumonia

Lobar pneumonia is an inflammation of one lobe or, occasionally, two lobes of the lung. It is usually caused by the bacterium *Streptococcus pneumoniae*, also called the *pneumococcus*.

Signs and symptoms

- Abrupt onset;
- fever, usually over 38° C;
- shaking chills;
- cough, producing thick, yellow or blood-tinged ("rusty") sputum;
- in about half of cases, a stabbing, often severe, pain on one side of the chest, made worse by breathing movements or coughing;
- breathing often rapid and shallow because of pain, with increased respiration rate (often to 30 breaths per minute and sometimes higher) in about half the cases.

What to do – generally

- Put the patient to bed.
- To alleviate fever, and if you are not giving ibuprofen (see next point), give paracetamol, 1 g orally, every six hours.
- To relieve chest pain, give ibuprofen, 400–800 mg orally, every six hours:
  - if the pain is still troublesome after two doses:
    - continue the ibuprofen; and ADD
    - tramadol, 50–100 mg orally, every six to eight hours; **OR**
    - morphine, preferably 10–20 mg orally, every four hours; **OR**
    - morphine, 5–10 mg intramuscularly, every three to four hours.
- Encourage the patient to drink (water, tea, fruit juice), to compensate for the loss of fluid from rapid breathing and sweating.

What to do – specifically

- Determine the severity of the illness.
- Mild pneumonia:
  - pulse rate less than 100 beats per minute
  - respiratory rate less than 25 breaths per minute
  - blood pressure normal
  - urine output normal
  - mental function normal.
- Moderate pneumonia:
  - any two of the following three signs:
    - pulse rate more than 100 beats per minute
    - respiratory rate more than 24 breaths per minute;
    - body temperature over 38.5°C; **BUT** blood pressure, urine output and mental function normal.
- Severe pneumonia:
  - any one of the following:
    - low or falling blood pressure (100 mm Hg systolic or less)
    - reduced urine output (i.e. has not passed urine for six hours)

- mental confusion
- respiratory rate more than 40 breaths per minute.

- For mild pneumonia, give amoxycillin/clavulanate, 875/125 mg orally, twice daily.
- For moderate or severe pneumonia, seek medical advice, and meanwhile, give:
  - ceftriaxone, 1 g intramuscularly or intravenously, twice daily AND azithromycin, 500 mg orally, twice daily.
- Once the patient has had no fever for 24 hours, replace ceftriaxone with amoxycillin/clavulanate, 875/125 mg orally, twice daily.
- For patients allergic to penicillin, give **only** azithromycin, 500 mg orally, twice daily, throughout.
- Since most patients will improve quickly, if your patient still has fever after three days, seek medical advice.
- Continue antibiotics for five days or until the patient has had no fever for three days.
- Note that most patients do not feel entirely well for several weeks.
- Do not authorize a patient who has had pneumonia to return to duty before seeing a doctor and obtaining chest X-ray confirmation that the pneumonia has cleared.

Empyema

Empyema is an accumulation of infected fluid (pus) that has spread from the lungs into the pleural space. The infected fluid can build up to more than a litre, putting pressure on the lungs and causing shortness of breath and pain. Empyema is the most serious complication of pneumonia. It usually occurs a few days after the onset of pneumonia, often when the patient's condition has begun to improve. The patient feels unwell again and the fever returns.

✔ *What to do*

- Since empyema cannot be diagnosed with confidence on board ship and requires a surgical operation to drain the infected fluid, seek medical advice with a view to early evacuation.
- Meanwhile, continue antibiotic treatment (which alone will not cure the infection).

Aspiration pneumonia and lung abscess

Aspiration pneumonia is an inflammation of the lungs and bronchi caused by vomit or other fluid entering the lungs. It can arise, for example, when a person's mental state is abnormal, as in drunkenness or during an epileptic fit. In some patients, bacterial infection leads to the formation of a collection of pus in the lungs (lung abscess). Aspiration pneumonia or lung abscess should be suspected if fever and cough develop in a patient after an alcoholic debauch or an epileptic fit. Distinguishing between simple aspiration pneumonia and lung abscess requires a chest X-ray, but the initial treatment is the same.

► *Signs and symptoms*

- Gradual onset, so that the patient often has difficulty knowing exactly when the illness started.
- Fever, often mild and never accompanied by shaking chills.

- Cough producing foul-smelling sputum, gradually worsening over days or weeks.
- In some cases, weight loss despite a good appetite.

✔ *What to do*

- Give amoxycillin/clavulanate, 875/125 mg orally, twice daily; note:
  - you may have to continue this treatment for several weeks.
- In some cases, a lung abscess must be drained surgically, so the patient should see a doctor at the next port.

SINUSITIS

Sinusitis is an inflammation of the so-called "accessory sinuses" (air cells or hollow air spaces) of the skull (Figure 15.1). The larger sinuses in each cheek bone (maxillary sinuses) and in the forehead just over the eyes (frontal sinuses) are most commonly affected. Sinusitis can be due to viruses or bacteria but most cases with severe symptoms are due to bacteria. A diagnosis of sinusitis is highly likely in a patient with typical cold symptoms who continues to have nasal blockage and pain over a sinus seven to 10 days after the onset of the cold.

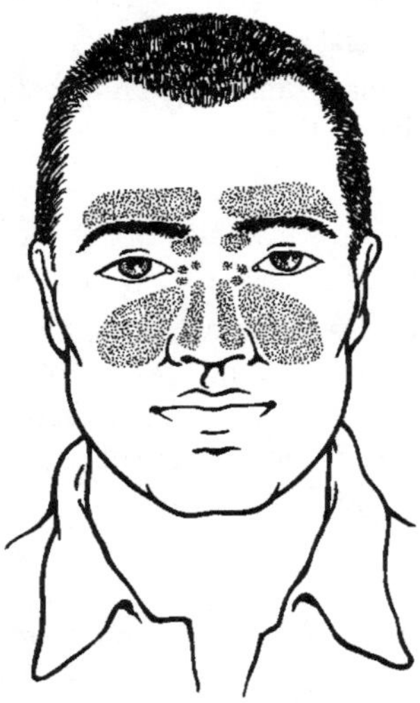

Figure 15.1 Sinuses.

► *Signs and symptoms*

- Onset usually following a cold;
- blocked nose;
- pain and tenderness over the affected sinus;
- pain made worse by leaning forward;
- thick yellow discharge from the nose;
- fever;
- mainly headache, if the frontal sinus is affected;
- pain in the upper teeth, if the maxillary sinus is affected.

✔ *What to do*

- In mild cases, have the patient use a vasoconstrictor spray or drops (oxymetazoline, 0.5 mg/ml) to encourage drainage of the sinus.
- If there is fever or severe pain, add amoxycillin/clavulanate, 875/125 mg orally, twice daily.
- If the patient develops double vision or blindness, confusion or drowsiness, or swelling around the eye, arrange for urgent evacuation: the infection has probably spread to the skull bones.

HAY FEVER

Hay fever is an immune response that affects the upper respiratory tract and is triggered by an allergy-causing substance (allergen) in the environment (see Chapter 31, *Anatomy and physiology*, under *Allergy*). In cooler climates the allergen is generally pollen, so symptoms are most troublesome in the spring. In warmer climates, moulds and perennial grasses are usually responsible, so symptoms can occur throughout most of the year. Some patients with hay fever also have asthma. Attempting to avoid the allergen responsible for hay fever is usually impractical. Nasal congestion, the main symptom of hay fever, can lead to obstruction of the sinuses and bacterial or viral sinusitis (see above).

Signs and symptoms

- Congested, runny nose
- itchy, tearing eyes
- sneezing.

What to do

- If the symptoms are interfering with the patient's work give cetirizine, 5–10 mg orally, once or twice daily.
- Note that cetirizine may cause drowsiness, especially in higher doses, and you should exercise caution in allowing the patient to take watch or perform hazardous work when he has taken cetirizine.
- In the long term the patient should obtain a corticosteroid drug for nasal use (e.g. budesonide, fluticasone, or many others).

ASTHMA

Asthma is a chronic disease that affects the airways (the tubes that carry air in and out of the lungs). In asthma, the inner walls of the airways are inflamed, making the airways very sensitive, so that they tend to react strongly to things to which the patient is allergic, to viral infections, or to certain drugs. When the airways react, they become narrower and less air flows through them to the lung tissue. This causes symptoms like wheezing (a whistling sound with each breath), cough, chest tightness, and difficulty in breathing. All of these symptoms are worse at night and in the early morning.

Signs and symptoms

- Coughing attacks, worse at night and after exercise, sometimes the only symptom;
- a feeling of tightness in the chest;
- wheezing;
- in severe cases, shortness of breath.

What to do – generally

- Determine how severe the asthma attack is:
  - since severe asthma attacks nearly always occur in patients who have had previous severe attacks, note the circumstances of the patient's previous asthma attacks, including previous response to treatment;
  - treat for severe asthma any patient who:

    - › has been hospitalized for asthma many times in the past or within the last six months;
    - › is not responding to his or her usual asthma medication.

- If the patient talks:
  - in full sentences, this suggests mild asthma;
  - in short phrases, this suggests likelihood of speedy recovery with treatment; **BUT**:
    - › if speech is still in phrases after four hours' treatment, treat for severe asthma;
  - in single words, this suggests severe asthma.
- Suspect life-threatening asthma if:
  - the patient is initially breathless, coughing, and wheezing but does not respond to treatment and becomes drowsy or confused; note:
    - › a drowsy patient may appear less breathless and less distressed, and wheezing may become less pronounced or disappear altogether;
    - › if you suspect severe or life-threatening asthma, obtain medical advice with a view to evacuation.
- Once the patient's lips and tongue take on a bluish tinge, death is likely to occur in a few minutes.

✔ *What to do – specifically*

- If the patient uses frequent doses of bronchodilator drugs, make sure that "preventer" (or long-term "control") medication is also taken (this is usually a steroid, either inhaled or taken by mouth).
- To prevent dehydration, encourage the patient to drink plenty of fluids.
- For mild asthma:
  - give salbutamol, two to four puffs via a plastic spacer: repeat every 10 minutes for three doses, then every 30 minutes for two hours, then hourly;
  - if the patient has not recovered after four to six hours, treat for severe asthma (below);
  - if the patient does not have an inhaled steroid preventer, give prednisone, 25 mg orally, every day for one week.
- For severe asthma:
  - give salbutamol, four puffs via a plastic spacer every 10 minutes for three doses then every 30 minutes for two hours, then hourly; **PLUS**
  - prednisone, 50 mg orally at once, then 25 mg orally morning and night;
  - after one week, reduce the dose to 25 mg each morning for one week, then to 12.5 mg (half a tablet) each morning for one week.
- For life-threatening asthma:
  - give 0.5 ml adrenaline (epinephrine) 1:1000 by subcutaneous injection and repeat as necessary;
  - once the patient has improved, give salbutamol and prednisone as for severe asthma.
- Note that neither bronchodilator syrups and tablets (e.g. of salbutamol) nor theophylline and aminophylline are effective.

✗ *What not to do*

- Do not **under any circumstances** give any form of sedative.
- If the patient has his own supplies of syrups or tablets for asthma **do not** allow him to take them in addition to the treatment above.

Gastrointestinal and liver diseases

ABDOMINAL PAIN – GENERAL POINTS

There are many conditions that can cause abdominal pain and not all of them arise from processes inside the abdomen. For this reason, identifying the cause of abdominal pain can be difficult. Useful diagnostic information, however, can be obtained from the patient's description of the pain.

Questions to ask the patient:

- How intense is the pain: slight, mild, moderate, or severe?
- Does the pain prevent normal activity?
- Does the pain prevent sleep?
- What is the pain like: aching, burning, scalding, cramping, gnawing, stabbing, nagging, stinging, throbbing, tingling, sharp, or dull?
- When did the pain begin?
- Did the pain reach its greatest severity straight away or did it get gradually worse?
- Does the pain come and go or is it constant?
- Where do you feel the pain? Can you point with one finger to where it hurts?
- Does the pain travel to other parts of the body? If so, where?
- What makes the pain worse?
- What makes the pain less intense?
- What other symptoms began at around the same time? For example:
  - nausea and vomiting (note that vomiting can occur without nausea, especially if there is bowel obstruction);
  - constipation or diarrhoea;
  - passing wind (farting) even if there is constipation;
  - any change in the stools: colour, odour, ease with which they are flushed away in the toilet, and presence of blood or slime;
  - change in appetite;
  - change in colour of urine?
- What medication, if any, are you taking?
- Have you ever had this pain before? If so, what happened then?
- What disorders or diseases have you had in the past?

How to examine the abdomen

- Have the patient lie flat, face upwards, with only a single pillow under the head and the arms at the side of the body:
  - **NEVER** attempt to examine the abdomen with the patient propped up.
- Sit down, or if necessary squat or kneel, next to the patient's bunk, so that your back is straight and your hand and forearm are parallel to the floor when you examine the abdomen.
- If you are right-handed, place yourself on the right side of the bunk:
  - **NEVER** examine the abdomen leaning over the patient.
- Observe if the patient is lying still, or restless and constantly moving around:
  - a patient lying still to avoid worsening the pain may have peritonitis;
  - a patient may be restless because of colicky pain.

- Note whether the whites of the patient's eyes are yellowish (jaundice).
- Note whether the tongue is dry, suggesting dehydration.
- Note whether the abdomen is swollen (distended).
- Look for the position of the belly button in relation to the lower end of the sternum:
  - even in obese patients, the belly button is in about the same horizontal plane as the sternum when the patient lies flat;
  - if the belly button is higher than the sternum, suspect abdominal swelling (distension).
- Look for localized swelling, bruising, or one or more scars on the abdomen that could suggest injury or previous surgery.
- Look for swellings in the groin or the scrotum that might indicate hernia.
- Listen for bowel sounds, placing your stethoscope on the skin at a point two to three centimetres below and to the side of the navel (belly button) and listen for one full minute (see also Chapter 12, *Examination of the patient*).
- Palpate the abdomen (see below, *How to palpate the abdomen*).
- Examine the rectum (see below, *How to do a rectal examination*).

How to do a rectal examination

- Put a glove on your right hand and smear petroleum jelly on the index finger.
- Have the patient lie on his side facing away from you with his knees drawn up.
- Part the buttocks and examine the anus for fissures, abscesses, and haemorrhoids.
- With your right index finger pointing forwards (not upwards), press on the anus with the pulp of your finger: after a second or two you will feel the anal sphincter (the muscle that keeps the anus closed) relax.
- Flex your finger so that it enters the rectum.
- Sweep your finger around the rectum, feeling for faeces and lumps in the wall of the rectum.
- Press gently in all directions, noting masses and tenderness.
- Withdraw your finger, note the colour of the faeces on the glove and look carefully for blood.

How to palpate the abdomen

- **Warm your hands.**
- **Watch the patient's face, not the abdomen.**
- **The harder you press, the less you will feel.**
- Place your right hand flat on the abdomen with your forearm and hand in alignment and parallel to the floor.
- Keep the palm of your right hand in contact with the abdomen throughout the examination.
- Place your left hand loosely over your right hand and use the fingers of your left hand to press the fingers of your right hand down onto the abdomen: keep your right hand relaxed.

- Beginning in an area some distance from where the worst pain is felt, move your hands systematically over the abdomen, a hand's width at a time, pressing lightly in each place (the fingers of your right hand should depress the skin to a depth of one centimetre or so).
- Talk to the patient as you do this, to distract attention.
- As you press in each place, watch the patient's face for evidence of tenderness and feel for firmness due to muscle spasm (guarding).
- Go back to the place where you started and repeat the process, pressing more firmly, so that your right-hand fingers depress the skin to a depth of two to four centimetres (remember to use your left hand to press and keep your right hand relaxed).
- **Watch the patient's face, not the abdomen, for evidence of tenderness**.
- To feel for the liver:
  - place your right hand flat on the right side of the abdomen with your fingers pointing towards the patient's head;
  - ask the patient to take slow, deep breaths;
  - with every inspiration, push your fingers gently inwards and upwards, beginning below the belly button and moving upwards, two centimetres or so with each breath, until you reach the ribs;
  - you will feel the liver as a firm edge that comes down and meets your fingertips as the patient breathes in;
  - if you feel the liver more than two or three centimetres below the lower edge of the rib cage, it is almost certainly enlarged;
  - note whether the edge of the liver is tender and whether it is smooth or knobbly.

Red flags in abdominal pain

On board ship, the main aim in examining a patient is to determine whether or not the patient is seriously ill and needs evacuation. Red flags are clues to a seriously ill patient: seek medical advice quickly if any of these are present:

- constant severe pain;
- abdominal tenderness and muscle spasm, localized or generalized;
- absence of bowel sounds;
- marked vomiting;
- no bowel movement or passage of air (farting) for 24 hours;
- tarry or blood-stained stools and/or passage of pure blood;
- signs of shock: giddiness on standing upright, rapid pulse, low blood pressure, clammy skin, low urine output;
- dark or bloodstained urine;
- jaundice (yellowish skin around the eyes and yellowish whites of the eye);
- a patient who looks sick or very apprehensive.

✔ *What to do if there is a red flag*

- Seek medical advice and anticipate evacuation.
- Have the patient rest in bed.

- Give nothing by mouth if you can insert an intravenous cannula; if you cannot, give only oral rehydration solution and water.
- If you have inserted an intravenous cannula and the patient is not drinking, give 0.9% sodium chloride solution, one litre every six hours:
  - give additional sodium chloride to an amount equal to loss of fluid from vomiting or diarrhoea;
  - if the urine is scanty and concentrated (specific gravity > 1.010) and the patient is thirsty, give additional sodium chloride, up to two litres every six hours, until the urine is plentiful and pale.
- To relieve pain, give morphine, 10–15 mg intramuscularly, every three to four hours (but first see *Bowel obstruction* and *Inflammatory bowel disease*, below).
- Give antibiotics as advised by the medical consultant.

✔ What to do if there are no red flags

- Have the patient stay in bed.
- Put the patient on a light, low-fat diet, with liquids to drink as desired (water, lemon juice, fat-free milk, or tea).
- If the pain is in the upper abdomen, give omeprazole, 20 mg orally, twice daily.
- If the pain is colicky **AND** you can feel hard faeces in the rectum, give a laxative.
- Otherwise, wait and see.
- Repeat the examination of the abdomen twice daily.
- If the patient is not better in 24 hours, seek medical advice.

✘ What not to do

- Do not give acetylsalicylic acid (Aspirin®) or ibuprofen.

SEVERE ABDOMINAL PAIN

Appendicitis

The appendix is a small, finger-shaped pouch that projects out of the large intestine (colon) at the lower right side of the abdomen. If it becomes blocked, the appendix can become inflamed and filled with pus. This condition is called appendicitis. The swelling can block off the blood supply to the appendix, which dies (becomes necrotic) and bursts, leading to a life-threatening infection and inflammation of the peritoneum (peritonitis), the membrane that lines the wall of the abdomen.

► Signs and symptoms

- At first:
  - indigestion

- passing wind (farting)
- mild diarrhoea
- vague malaise.

- After a few hours:
  - pain in the centre of the abdomen, usually constant and mild or moderate.
- After a few more hours:
  - pain in the right lower abdomen, becoming sharper and more severe;
  - tenderness and muscle firmness (guarding) in the painful area.
- There is little nausea or vomiting; if there is any vomiting it occurs only **after** the pain is well established.
- Loss of appetite in most cases: if the patient is hungry, the diagnosis is not likely to be appendicitis.
- Mild fever (not over 38 °C) in some cases: a high fever in a patient with symptoms of appendicitis suggests a ruptured appendix.

Note

- In a young man with the above symptoms, appendicitis is by far the most likely diagnosis.
- In a woman, pelvic inflammatory disease (see Chapter 19, *Sexually transmitted infections)* is an alternative diagnosis.
- In older patients, several conditions can produce the symptoms of appendicitis: establishing the diagnosis will not generally be possible on board ship.

✔ What to do

- Seek medical advice with a view to evacuating the patient.
- If pain is severe, give morphine, 10–15 mg intramuscularly.
- Insert an intravenous cannula and give normal saline (0.9% sodium chloride), one litre every six hours.
- Give ceftriaxone, 2 g intravenously or intramuscularly, daily.

✘ What not to do

- DO NOT give the patient any food, unless evacuation is going to be delayed for more than 72 hours and the medical consultant suggests doing so.

Pancreatitis

Pancreatitis is an inflammation of the pancreas, an organ situated just behind the stomach. Most cases are mild and resolve in 7–10 days. Some cases are life-threatening. It is difficult to predict which cases will become severe. Pancreatitis can be acute (a single severe episode) or chronic (sustained but less intense inflammation); in chronic pancreatitis episodes of severe pain, similar to those of acute pancreatitis, occur as well.

Common causes of pancreatitis include:

- gallstones (in 35–40% of cases);
- alcohol abuse (in 35–40% of cases).

Uncommon causes of pancreatitis include:

- high triglyceride (fat) levels in the blood, often associated with diabetes mellitus;
- high calcium levels in the blood;
- certain medicines, notably:
  - nonsteroidal anti-inflammatory drugs, including acetylsalicylic acid (Aspirin®)
  - diuretics (e.g. frusemide)
  - antibiotics (metronidazole and sulfonamides)
  - viral infections (especially mumps and HIV/AIDS).

Signs and symptoms

- **Acute pancreatitis**:
  - severe pain, that is constant, felt most often at the centre of the upper abdomen, and continuing for days;
  - in about half of cases, pain is also felt in the back;
  - relief of pain by bending forwards can occur, and is characteristic of pain from the pancreas;
  - in nearly all cases, nausea and vomiting;
  - in many cases, vomiting constant and continuing for days;
  - tenderness in the upper abdomen, but surprisingly mild given the severity of the pain.
- **Chronic pancreatitis**:
  - pain, often severe, which is:
    - mostly felt in the upper abdomen but often radiating to the back;
    - often relieved by bending forward;
    - constant in some patients, intermittent with long pain-free intervals in other patients;
  - nausea and vomiting;
  - signs of failure of pancreatic function, such as:
    - weight loss, despite normal appetite and eating habits;
    - oily, foul-smelling stools that are difficult to flush away;
    - diabetes mellitus.

✔ *What to do in a case of acute pancreatitis*

- Seek medical advice with a view to evacuation.
- Insert an intravenous cannula and give 0.9% sodium chloride at a rate of 250 ml/hr for the first 48 hours, then at half this rate: the aim is to keep urine output above 50 ml/hr.
- Increase the rate of fluid infusion if the urine is scanty and dark.
- Give morphine, 10–15 mg intravenously, every three to four hours.
- Give nothing by mouth for five days.
- If pain is subsiding after five days, have the patient take clear fluids and then food if there is no recurrence of pain over the next 48 hours.

✘ *What not to do in a case of acute pancreatitis*

- DO NOT give any fat (oil, butter or margarine), fatty foods (fried food, cheese, mayonnaise) or fat-containing fluids (milk, ice cream, etc.) even after the attack resolves.

✔ *What to do in a case of chronic pancreatitis*

- Insist that the patient stop drinking alcohol.
- Give small, frequent meals with minimal fat.
- To relieve pain give:
  - ibuprofen, 400 mg orally, every six hours;
  - if this is inadequate after a trial of several days, try tramadol, 100 mg orally, two or three times daily;
  - if this is inadequate after a trial of several days, give morphine, 20 mg orally, every four hours.
- If episodes of severe pain are accompanied by vomiting, treat as for acute pancreatitis (above).

Bowel obstruction

Bowel obstruction is a blockage in the gut that prevents food, fluid, digestive secretions, and gas from passing through the digestive tract. About 75% of cases are caused by adhesions – scar tissue in the abdomen caused by surgery performed in the past. In the remaining 25% of cases, hernias are the cause of bowel obstruction. Bowel obstruction is dangerous because the gut swells and can become strangulated and then rupture, causing life-threatening infection of the abdominal cavity.

► *Signs and symptoms*

- Abdominal pain (usually the first symptom) that:
  - is crampy;
  - is felt around the navel (belly button);
  - comes and goes frequently, with spasms lasting a minute or so and occurring every few minutes.
- In some cases, constant pain, which suggests strangulation.
- Vomiting – early and copious with an obstruction high in the bowel but late and less marked if the colon is obstructed.
- Abdominal swelling (distension), which is less marked with an obstruction high in the bowel and more marked if the colon is obstructed.
- Constipation and inability to pass wind (fart), arising early with an obstruction in the colon but only after several days with an obstruction high in the bowel.
- Indications of strangulation:
  - fever
  - rapid pulse
  - marked or local tenderness.

✔ *What to do*

- Seek immediate medical advice and plan to evacuate the patient.
- Insert an intravenous cannula and give 0.9% sodium chloride (normal saline) in sufficient quantities to produce a urine output of 50 ml/hr: large amounts may be needed (six litres a day or more).

✗ *What not to do*

- DO NOT give anything by mouth.
- DO NOT give morphine.

DIARRHOEA

Foodborne illness

There are three main patterns of illness caused by foodborne infections: vomiting with little or no diarrhoea, watery diarrhoea with little or no vomiting, and blood-stained diarrhoea.

VOMITING AS THE MAIN SYMPTOM

The main causes are gastrointestinal poisons (enterotoxins) released by bacteria, most commonly *Staphylococcus aureus* and *Bacillus cereus*, and infection with a virus called norovirus (also called Norwalk virus).

- The bacteria *Staphylococcus aureus* and *Bacillus cereus* multiply and produce a toxin in food that has been contaminated, usually by a food handler, and then left for a few hours at room temperature. The toxin causes nausea and vomiting within six hours of ingestion of the contaminated food. The bacteria are killed by cooking but the toxin is resistant to heat, so the contamination can occur either before or after cooking.
- Norovirus (Norwalk virus) causes sudden onset of vomiting, sometimes accompanied by mild, watery diarrhoea. Infection occurs when cooked food is contaminated by a food handler. Large amounts of food can be contaminated, and many people can be affected at once in enclosed communities, such as passengers and crew on a cruise ship who eat food served in a buffet. The illness lasts two to three days and resolves without treatment. It does not produce immunity to subsequent infection.

WATERY DIARRHOEA AS THE MAIN SYMPTOM

- The bacterium, enterotoxigenic *Escherichia coli* (ETEC), is the commonest cause of watery diarrhoea in the less developed countries ("traveller's diarrhoea", see below) but other bacteria and occasionally viruses can be responsible.
- *Clostridium perfringens* is an important cause of diarrhoea in developed countries. This bacterium produces a toxin that causes diarrhoea, but only after a large number of the bacteria have been ingested. Infection is, therefore, mainly associated with food kept at room temperature for a long time after cooking.

DIARRHOEA WITH BLOOD IN THE STOOLS AS THE MAIN SYMPTOM

- Blood in diarrhoea is due to damage to the bowel wall by an infectious organism.
- Without laboratory tests it can be difficult to know whether or not there is blood in the faeces: a patient with diarrhoea containing obvious blood or mucus, **or** with

severe abdominal pain or fever should be treated as having damage to the bowel wall from an infectious organism.

- In most cases the patient passes a few large volume stools a day, which are loose or watery and have varying degrees of blood-staining. This syndrome must be distinguished from dysentery (see below), in which the patient passes many small stools mixed with blood.
- The common causes of profuse diarrhoea with blood are the bacteria *Salmonella* and *Campylobacter*, which are found in poultry and eggs contaminated by poultry faeces. People acquire infection by eating the food uncooked (including foods, such as mayonnaise, prepared with uncooked eggs) or under-cooked, **or** left to stand at room temperature after cooked food has been contaminated through contact with raw food residue.

✔ *What to do in a case of foodborne illness*

- If **vomiting** is the only or main symptom:
  - you do not usually need to treat the patient: the illness disappears in a few hours without treatment;
  - encourage the patient to drink large quantities of clear fluids.
- If **diarrhoea** (watery or containing blood) is the only or the main symptom:
  - give ciprofloxacin, 500 mg orally, twice daily for three days (but not to a woman who is or may be pregnant);
  - if it is essential for a crew member with diarrhoea to return to duty, give **ALSO** loperamide, 4 mg (two tablets) initially, then 2 mg (one tablet) after each subsequent diarrhoeal motion, up to a maximum of eight tablets in 24 hours;
  - do not give loperamide without giving cirpofloxacin.

✔ *What to do to prevent foodborne illness*

Note that:

- nearly all raw food has some microorganisms on or in it: in many cases these are disease-causing organisms;
- adequate cooking destroys all disease-causing organisms;
- foodborne illness is, therefore, associated with:
  - contamination by a food handler, usually after cooking;
  - uncooked or under-cooked food (such as, raw or under-cooked oysters, or salads washed in contaminated water);
  - food contaminated after cooking by contact with raw food (for example, by slicing a cooked chicken on a cutting board used to prepare raw chicken).

To avoid foodborne illness on board:

- make sure all crew members, but especially food handlers, wash their hands often and meticulously;
- discourage consumption of raw or under-cooked food;
- insist that:
  - food be purchased from suppliers with high standards of hygiene;
  - raw food be kept separate from cooked food;

- perishable raw food be refrigerated until cooking;
- cooked food not intended for immediate consumption, and left-overs, be promptly refrigerated;
- food handlers with diarrhoeal disease be transferred to other duties until certified not to be excreting *Shigella*, *Salmonella*, or *Campylobacter* organisms.

Dysentery

Dysentery is an illness usually caused by bacteria of the *Shigella* group, although other bacteria can cause a similar illness and *Shigella* can cause an illness producing watery diarrhoea. Dysentery is spread by food or water contaminated with human faeces containing the *Shigella* organism. Only a few individual bacterial organisms are needed to cause disease, so that, unlike *Salmonella*, multiplication of the organism in food is not a causative factor and infection can be acquired from freshly prepared food.

Signs and symptoms

- In most cases, about 10 (but sometimes many more) low-volume motions a day.
- Only minor fluid loss, because of the small volume of the motions.
- Initially, faeces with only slime or mucus.
- Later, blood-stained faeces: in about half of the cases the blood is not obvious, although it can be detected by laboratory tests.
- In otherwise healthy adults, disappearance of diarrhoea in a few days, even without treatment; note:
  - organisms may be excreted in the stools for some time after symptoms have disappeared, so that disease transmission remains a risk.

Traveller's diarrhoea

Traveller's diarrhoea generally occurs in travellers to areas of the world where hygiene is poor. In the less developed countries, 90% of cases are due to bacteria, the commonest being enterotoxigenic *Escherichia coli* (ETEC). *Escherichia coli* are the commonest bacterium found in the human colon and make up a substantial part of the weight of normal faeces, but not all *Escherichia coli* produce entero-toxin. Infection is acquired by inadvertently ingesting human faeces containing ETEC, usually in contaminated water or food. Most cases are mild and symptoms disappear without treatment in three to five days. In a small proportion of cases, loss of fluid may be severe enough to cause dehydration, especially if there is vomiting as well.

Traveller's diarrhoea occurs in nearly all cases within a few days of ingestion of the organisms. Diarrhoea that begins more than a week after leaving a port is probably due to infection on board.

Signs and symptoms

- Diarrhoea, with usually large, watery motions, but rarely more than six per day;
- loss of appetite;

- nausea;
- vomiting in moderate and severe cases;
- abdominal cramps in moderate and severe cases;
- fever only in severe cases.

✔ What to do to avoid traveller's diarrhoea

- Eat only food that is – and, if possible, that you have seen being – thoroughly cooked and eaten immediately after it is cooked.
- Do not eat any uncooked food, including salads and ice cream.
- Plates and cutlery are often washed in contaminated water: if you eat at street stalls bring your own plate and fork or choose food served directly from the cooking surface.
- Eat fruit only if you peel it yourself.
- You can drink a bottled drink safely if the bottle has an intact plastic cap seal: otherwise choose a carbonated beverage and drink it only if it is fizzy when first opened.
- Do not use ice with drinks: it is not safe.
- Tea and coffee made with coffee beans or tea leaves are usually safe but it is better if you use your own cup.
- Instant coffee is not reliably safe: it is often made with water from the hot tap.

Food poisoning from marine toxins

CIGUATERA FISH POISONING

Ciguatera is the commonest cause of seafood toxin poisoning. The toxin is produced by single-celled organisms that grow on coral reefs. The organisms are eaten by small fish that are unaffected by the toxin but that are eaten in turn by larger predatory fish. When humans eat these predatory fish, the toxin can make them ill. A predatory fish carrying ciguatera looks, smells, and tastes normal. The toxin is not destroyed by cooking.

► Signs and symptoms

- Onset a few hours after eating an affected fish;
- initially, vomiting and diarrhoea;
- soon afterwards, abnormal sensation (burning, "pins-and-needles") in the limbs and blurred vision lasting for a few weeks or, in a few cases, for months.

✔ What to do

- There is no treatment for the immediate symptoms.
- After recovery, warn the patient to avoid all fish, caffeine (coffee, tea, Cola-type fizzy drinks) and alcohol, which may cause relapse of the nervous system symptoms.

✔ What to do to prevent ciguatera

- When travelling in tropical areas avoid large predatory fish, particularly reef fish such as barracuda.

SCOMBROID FISH POISONING

Scombroid fish poisoning is common and occurs in all regions of the world. It is caused by bacterial contamination of dark-fleshed fish, typically tuna or mackerel (which belong to the *Scombridae* family of fish). If the fish is not properly refrigerated, the bacteria multiply and generate histamine in the flesh of the fish. The histamine, which is not destroyed by cooking, may cause symptoms that can be mistaken for a "fish allergy".

► Signs and symptoms

- Onset within an hour of eating the fish;
- sudden flushing of the face, a feeling of warmth, and a blotchy rash on the chest and face;
- disappearance of symptoms within a few hours.

✔ What to do

- If symptoms are troublesome, give cetirizine, 10 mg orally.

✔ What to do to prevent scombroid poisoning

- Refrigerate fish carefully: scombroid can be caused by canned tuna not refrigerated after opening.
- Avoid dark-fleshed fish caught from boats lacking efficient facilities for onboard refrigeration.

Inflammatory bowel disease (colitis)

There are two main inflammatory bowel diseases: ulcerative colitis and Crohn's disease. A third form of infectious colitis can follow a course of antibiotics, whatever the reason for the antibiotic use. A fourth illness, ischaemic colitis, is caused by lack of blood flow to the bowel. It usually occurs in elderly individuals suffering from extensive coronary artery and cerebrovascular disease and will not be considered here.

Ulcerative colitis

The cause of ulcerative inflammation of the colon is not known. Most patients have a history of symptoms going back months or a few years, with one or more similar episodes that have come and gone without treatment. This history distinguishes ulcerative colitis from infectious diarrhoea. In a few patients ulcerative colitis begins as a sudden severe illness and these cases can easily be confused with infectious diarrhoea.

► Signs and symptoms

- Onset gradual in most patients.
- In patients with mild disease:

- two or three small, semi-formed motions per day, usually with mucus or slime and blood mixed into the stool;
- mild abdominal pain;
- no fever.

- In patients with severe disease:
  - frequent diarrhoea (10–20 motions per day) with obvious blood;
  - more marked abdominal pain, sometimes severe;
  - fever;
  - weight loss in some cases.

Note

- Patients with severe disease are at risk of perforation of the colon and a life-threatening peritonitis.
- This usually occurs after seven to10 days of severe disease, so it is not likely to be a problem on board ship.
- If the colon perforates:
  - pain becomes more severe and is felt over the whole abdomen;
  - shock soon follows, with rapid pulse, falling blood pressure, and tenderness and distension of the abdomen.

✔ *What to do*

- Seek medical advice.
- If the patient has more than 10 bowel motions per day or has fever or marked abdominal pain, arrange for evacuation.
- It is safe to keep a patient with mild disease on board but consider evacuation now if a future evacuation, needed because of deterioration in the patient's condition, might prove difficult.
- **For a patient with mild-to-moderate disease**, allow a normal diet.
- **For a patient with moderate-to-severe disease**, give prednisone, 50 mg orally, daily, while waiting for evacuation.
- **For a patient with severe disease**:
  - allow only clear fluids by mouth;
  - insert an intravenous cannula and give normal saline (0.9% sodium chloride), one litre every eight hours;
  - give ceftriaxone, 1 g intravenously or intramuscularly, twice daily, and metronidazole, 500 mg orally, three times daily.

✘ *What not to do*

- DO NOT give loperamide, morphine or tramadol.

Crohn's disease

Crohn's disease is a chronic inflammatory disease that can affect any part of the gastrointestinal tract. Unlike appendicitis, most patients have had symptoms for years before the condition is diagnosed. Unlike ulcerative colitis, Crohn's disease rarely causes severe acute illness.

Signs and symptoms

- Mild diarrhoea;
- pain in the abdomen, often in the right lower quadrant, where there may be tenderness or a mass;
- colicky pain and vomiting, suggestive of bowel obstruction;
- weight loss;
- low fever.

✔ What to do

- If the patient can eat a normal diet without pain, vomiting, or abdominal distension, plan for a consultation with a doctor at the next port.
- If the patient cannot eat, seek medical advice with a view to evacuation.

✘ What not to do

- DO NOT give loperamide, morphine, or tramadol.

Antibiotic-associated colitis

Antibiotic-associated colitis is caused by the bacterium *Clostridium difficile*, which infects the bowel once the bacteria that ordinarily live in the bowel have been killed by antibiotics that the patient has taken to treat an infection. In most cases the illness is mild but some patients develop a severe colitis called pseudomembranous colitis.

Signs and symptoms

- Onset after a few days of antibiotic treatment.
- In mild cases:
  - a few episodes of watery diarrhoea daily;
  - crampy abdominal pain;
  - no fever.
- In patients with pseudomembranous colitis:
  - diarrhoea more frequent (10–15 motions per day);
  - pain more severe;
  - fever, which may be high in some cases.

✔ What to do

- Take the patient off the antibiotic:
  - note that antibiotic-associated colitis usually begins after several days of treatment, by which time the antibiotic treatment should be almost completed;
  - seek medical advice if you think that stopping the antibiotic might be dangerous.
- Give metronidazole, 500 mg orally, three times daily for 10 days; **IF**
  - medical advice confirms that you should not stop the patient's original antibiotic treatment; **OR IF**
  - the patient has severe diarrhoea or fever; **OR IF**
  - diarrhoea continues for more than one or two days after stopping the antibiotic treatment.

- Have the patient stay in a single-berth cabin with only one attendant.
- Have the attendant wear gloves whenever coming into contact with the patient and wash the hands **with soap and water** after removing the gloves: note that *Clostridium difficile* is resistant to alcohol gels.

INDIGESTION AND PAIN RELATED TO MEALS

The main conditions that cause indigestion and pain after meals are gastro-oesophageal reflux, peptic ulcer, and gallstones (see *Gallstones*, below, under *Liver and biliary disease*).

Gastro-oesophageal reflux disease

Gastro-oesophageal reflux disease (GERD) is a common condition caused by acid from the stomach splashing back into the oesophagus and causing inflammation of the oesophageal lining. Normally, this reflux is prevented by contraction of a muscle (lower oesophageal sphincter) at the lower end of the oesophagus: the main problem in cases of GERD is failure of the sphincter to prevent reflux.

► *Signs and symptoms*

- Heartburn, usually after meals or after drinking alcohol or coffee.
- Regurgitation of swallowed food back into the mouth, without nausea or retching.
- In some cases, particularly of severe or long-standing GERD, difficulty in swallowing.

✔ *What to do*

- Advise the patient to avoid alcohol and caffeine.
- Advise the patient to sleep with the head higher than the chest.
- Give omeprazole, 20 mg orally, once every night or, if symptoms are severe, 20 mg twice daily.
- In cases where there is difficulty swallowing or where symptoms do not resolve promptly with omeprazole, have the patient see a doctor at the next port.

Peptic ulcer

Peptic ulcers are ulcers of the lining of the stomach or, more commonly, the duodenum. There are two main causes: infection with the bacterium *Helicobacter pylori* and use of acetylsalicylic acid (Aspirin®) or any other non-steroidal anti-inflammatory drug (NSAID). Either factor alone can lead to peptic ulcer but the two combined cause more damage.

The bacterial infection is acquired in childhood but the route of infection is not known. Infection is commoner in poorer than in more developed communities: improved living standards in a community can produce a rapid fall in the frequency of *H. pylori* infection. In the more developed countries, about 50% of adults older than 60 are infected, while in the less developed countries 80% of people between 40 and 50 years of age are infected.

Signs and symptoms

- In about half of patients, a burning pain in the centre of the upper abdomen starting three to four hours after a meal and relieved by additional food or by antacid drugs.
- In about a third of patients, "indigestion", with:
    - a feeling of fullness and bloating after meals
    - belching
    - nausea
    - in some cases, vomiting.
- In about a third of patients, GERD-like symptoms (see above, under *Gastro-oesophageal reflex disease*).
- The symptoms of peptic ulcer usually last a few weeks or months, disappear for weeks or months, and then return.
- Many patients have a mixture of the three patterns of symptoms described above.

COMPLICATIONS

- Penetration by the ulcer of the whole thickness of the back wall of the gastrointestinal tract, reaching into the organs behind the bowel, especially the pancreas, and causing:
    - severe pain in the centre of upper abdomen that goes through to the back and is not relieved by food or omeprazole.
- Perforation of the gastrointestinal tract as a result of the ulcer eating through the anterior bowel wall, forming a communication between the gastrointestinal tract and the peritoneal cavity, causing:
    - dramatically sudden, severe pain over the whole abdomen.
- Scarring around the ulcer, causing:
    - obstruction of the passage from the stomach to the duodenum;
    - vomiting one or two hours after a meal.
- Bleeding from the ulcer, causing:
    - potentially life-threatening loss of blood (see below, *Heavy bleeding from the gastrointestinal tract*).

✔ *What to do*

- Have all patients with pain or indigestion after meals see a doctor: in most cases an endoscopic examination will be required, since a definite diagnosis can rarely be made from the symptoms alone.
- Meanwhile, to relieve the pain or indigestion after meals, give omeprazole, 20 mg orally, once a day, until the patient can be seen by a doctor.

Red flags

Patients with pain or indigestion after meals **and** any of these symptoms should see a doctor as soon as possible because they have an increased risk of cancer of the stomach or oesophagus:

- weight loss
- difficulty swallowing or pain on swallowing
- vomiting

- jaundice
- a family history of stomach cancer
- a history of surgery of the stomach.

✗ *What not to do*

- DO NOT give acetylsalicylic acid (Aspirin®), ibuprofen, or any other non-steroidal anti-inflammatory drug.

HEAVY BLEEDING FROM THE GASTROINTESTINAL TRACT *(gastrointestinal haemorrhage)*

- About half of all cases of gastrointestinal haemorrhage are caused by a bleeding peptic ulcer.
- The second commonest cause of gastrointestinal haemorrhage is bleeding from oesophageal varices (dilated veins beneath the lining of the oesophagus that tend to develop in patients with cirrhosis of the liver).
- Bleeding from peptic ulcers usually stops after hours or days.
- Bleeding from oesophageal varices usually does not stop without treatment.
- It is not possible to tell where a patient is bleeding from without direct inspection of the bowel by endoscopy.
- Gastrointestinal haemorrhage carries a significant mortality rate even in well-equipped hospitals in the more developed countries:
  - the risk of death is much higher:
    - in patients with gastrointestinal haemorrhage due to oesophageal varices than in those with peptic ulcer;
    - in older patients;
    - in patients with other serious illnesses.

Heavy upper gastrointestinal bleeding

Upper gastrointestinal haemorrhage usually originates in the stomach, oesophagus, or duodenum.

► *Signs and symptoms*

- Vomiting of blood (haematemesis).
- Passage of black, tarry, foul-smelling faeces containing partially digested blood (melena).

✔ *What to do*

- Take the pulse and the blood pressure with the patient lying flat and then standing up (if the patient is able to stand).

- There has been significant blood loss if:
  - systolic blood pressure is below 100 mmHg;
  - systolic blood pressure drops by more than 20 mmHg when the patient stands up;
  - the pulse rate is greater than 100 beats per minute.
- Insert an intravenous cannula into both of the patient's hands or arms, using the largest size cannula available, and start an infusion of normal saline (0.9% sodium chloride).

Table 16.1 Clues to diagnosis of gastrointestinal disease in vomit, stools, and urine.

Vomit	Suggested diagnosis
▪ Contains partly digested food. ▪ If the vomited food is undigested and tastes normal to the patient (i.e. contains no acid or bile), the obstruction is probably above the stomach, i.e. in the oesophagus. ▪ Generally, the shorter the time between eating and vomiting the higher the site of obstruction in the gut.	▪ One of several diseases or disorders of the upper gastrointestinal tract (oesophagus, stomach, duodenum), of which the commonest are: oesophageal scarring from an ulcer, cancer, and gastric outlet obstruction due to scarring from an ulcer or from past surgery.
▪ Contains bile (a yellow-green liquid); the obstruction must be below the mid-duodenum, where the bile duct enters the bowel.	▪ One of several gastrointestinal diseases or disorders, of which the commonest are obstructed hernia and "adhesions" from previous surgery.
▪ Shows bright-red blood or dark "coffee-grounds" blood.	▪ Bleeding from the oesophagus, stomach, or duodenum.
▪ Contains or smells like faeces.	▪ Colon obstruction.
Stools (faeces)	**Suggested diagnosis**
▪ Contain bright-red blood.	▪ Bleeding from large intestine, rectum, or anus.
▪ Are a black and tarry with a very foul smell.	▪ Bleeding from upper gastrointestinal tract.
▪ Contain pus.	▪ Ulcer or abscess of gastrointestinal tract or inflammatory bowel disease.
▪ Are slimy.	▪ Inflammatory bowel disease.
▪ Are pale, voluminous and hard to flush away.	▪ Failure to absorb fat (steatorrhoea), due to: • reduced bile production due to disease of liver or gall-bladder; • pancreatic disease.
▪ Contain threadworm, tapeworm, or roundworm.	▪ Worm infestation (threadworms, tapeworms, roundworms).
Urine	**Suggested diagnosis**
▪ Is dark-brown or greenish.	▪ Obstructive jaundice (i.e. blockage of the bile duct in the liver), with accumulation of bilirubin (a yellowish-green pigment present in bile).
▪ Is cloudy, with sandy deposits.	▪ Urinary infection or urinary stones.
▪ Is reddish or smoky, or with blood clots.	▪ Bleeding from genitourinary tract (due to stones, infection, cancer, medicines).

- Obtain medical advice urgently about the amount of fluid needed: this will depend on the blood pressure and pulse but could be a substantial amount.
- If you have to decide yourself how much fluid to administer, start with one litre every four hours and adjust the amount to keep urine flow above 50 ml/hr.
- Arrange for evacuation.
- Meanwhile, give omeprazole, 40 mg (double the usual dose) orally, at once and then twice daily.
- Give ciprofloxacin, 500 mg orally, twice daily.
- Ensure that vomited blood is cleaned up using universal precautions.

✗ *What not to do*

- DO NOT give the patient anything to eat.
- DO NOT give:
  - acetylsalicylic acid (Aspirin®), ibuprofen, or any other nonsteroidal anti-inflammatory drug;
  - paracetamol.

Heavy lower gastrointestinal bleeding

Heavy bleeding from the lower bowel causes the passage of maroon or bright red blood, often unmixed with faeces, but not black or tarry or foul-smelling like melena. As with upper gastrointestinal bleeding, there are a number of causes which cannot be distinguished on board ship. However, lower bowel haemorrhage is less likely than upper gastrointestinal haemorrhage to be life-threatening and not all patients need to be evacuated.

► *Signs and symptoms*

- Passage of maroon or red blood, often un-mixed with faeces.

✔ *What to do*

- Take the pulse and blood pressure with the patient lying flat and then standing up.
- Insert an intravenous cannula and give normal saline (0.9% sodium chloride), one litre every eight hours.
- Seek medical advice; you can probably keep the patient on board safely if he:
  - is under 40;
  - is otherwise healthy;
  - has had only a single episode of bleeding;
  - has a pulse rate less than 100 beats per minute;
  - has a systolic blood pressure of over 110 mmHg;
  - on standing up shows a drop in systolic pressure of less than 20 mmHg;
  - if the doctor agrees, put him to bed and wait to see if there is any further bleeding.
- If further bleeding occurs, increase the rate of fluid infusion to match the blood loss and seek medical advice with a view to evacuation of the patient.

Anal fissure

An anal fissure is a tear in the lining (mucosa) of the anus caused by trauma to the anal canal, as may occur with a large, hard stool. Once the mucosa is torn the injury tends to become chronic.

Signs and symptoms

- Pain, usually described as sharp and tearing, as faeces are passed.
- A small amount of bright blood on toilet paper or on the surface of faeces.
- In some cases, itching or irritation of the skin around the anus.
- Presence of a visible fissure, most often at the back of the anus, resembling a fresh cut if the fissure occurred recently, or pale with raised edges if the fissure is of long standing.

✔ What to do

- To keep the stool soft, have the patient increase the fibre content of the diet by eating plentiful fresh fruit and vegetables, and bran.
- If constipation is a problem, give docusate with senna, 1–2 tablets orally, each day at bedtime.
- Have the patient sit in a bath in five to eight centimetres of warm water for 10–15 minutes twice a day (without using soap or bubble-bath preparations).
- If the fissure has not healed when you reach port, have the patient see a doctor.

✗ What not to do

- DO NOT attempt to perform a digital rectal examination: it will cause severe pain.

Haemorrhoids (piles)

Haemorrhoids are enlarged veins in the lower rectum. They can be inside the rectum (internal haemorrhoids) or under the anal skin (external haemorrhoids), or in both places at once. Haemorrhoids are usually due to straining when passing stools, as may occur in chronic constipation.

Hemorrhoids are the commonest cause of loss of small amounts of blood from the rectum.

Signs and symptoms

- Bright red blood, seen:
  - on the surface of the stool; **OR**
  - as a smear on toilet paper; **OR**
  - as a few drops in the toilet bowl;
- anal itch (see below);
- pain if the haemorrhoid clots;
- in cases of external haemorrhoids, smooth purplish swellings visible under the anal skin;

- in some cases of internal haemorrhoids, protrusion of the swollen veins through the anus.

✔ *What to do*

- To keep the stool soft, have the patient increase the fibre content of the diet by eating plentiful fresh fruit and vegetables, and bran.
- Have the patient sit in a bath in five to eight centimetres of warm water for 10–15 minutes twice a day (without using soap or bubble-bath preparations).
- If constipation is a problem, give docusate with senna, 1–2 tablets orally, each day at bedtime.
- Push internal haemorrhoids back into the rectum: if this is not possible:
  - have the patient lie in bed face downwards with an ice-pack on the protruding haemorrhoids;
  - after 30–60 minutes, the protruding haemorrhoids should have shrunk and you will be able to push them back inside the rectum.
- In a patient with thrombosed (clotted) haemorrhoids:
  - give tramadol, 100 mg orally, twice daily;
  - have the patient sit frequently in warm baths, as described above;
  - if you are in port, have the patient undergo immediate surgical treatment.
- If you are at sea, have the patient see a doctor at the next port of call.

Anal pruritis (anal itch)

Patients with pinworms (see Chapter 23, *Infectious diseases*) often have itching around the anus at night, when the worms emerge from the bowel.

Anal pruritis is usually caused by soiling of the skin around the anus by faeces. This can be due to:

- haemorrhoids
- diarrhoea (of any cause)
- in some patients by an abnormality of the muscles of the anus; in these cases the problem is long-standing.

✔ *What to do*

- Have the patient clean the anus after each bowel motion with water, without rubbing or scratching.
- Have the patient apply 1% hydrocortisone cream to the anus twice daily, but not for more than one week.
- If the itch is still troublesome, have the patient apply zinc oxide paste to the anus after each bowel motion.

HERNIA

Hernia occurs when there is a defect in the wall of the abdomen through which some of the

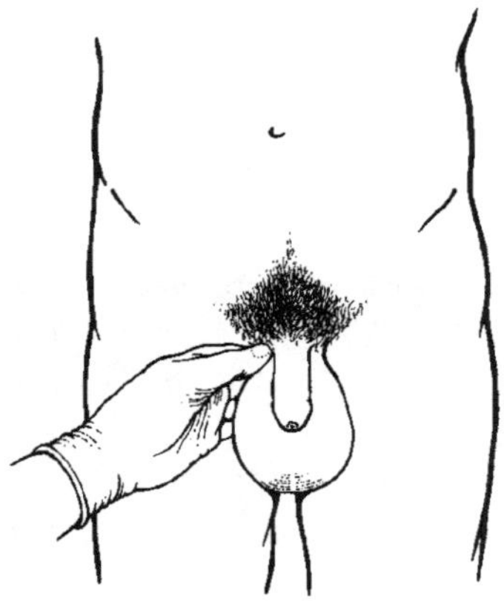

Figure 16.1 How to examine the scrotum for a hernia.

contents of the abdomen can protrude. This can occur in several places around the abdomen but the groin is the commonest site for hernia and the one where hernia is most likely to cause problems on board ship.

Inguinal (groin) hernia

An inguinal hernia occurs when there is a weak spot or a tear in the muscular wall of the abdomen around the groin, through which, in some cases, a segment of bowel (intestine) may protrude and be trapped (see below *Incarceration*, under *Complications*). Men are more often affected than women.

There are two common types of inguinal hernia: indirect inguinal hernia and direct inguinal hernia. Both occur just above the inner half of the crease that separates the abdomen from the upper thigh.

- **In an indirect hernia**, the defect is present from birth, because the passage (inguinal canal) by which the testes pass from the abdomen to the scrotum before birth does not close after the testes have passed through: a detectable hernia may appear in children, adolescents, or adults.
- **In a direct hernia**, there is a defect in the muscle wall of the abdomen through which a segment of intestine may or may not have protruded.

Signs and symptoms

- In most patients, discomfort (not usually pain) in the lower abdomen made worse by lifting or straining and relieved by lying down.
- A bulge in the groin, easily seen with the patient standing but not usually visible when the patient lies down.
- Enlargement of the hernia when the patient coughs.

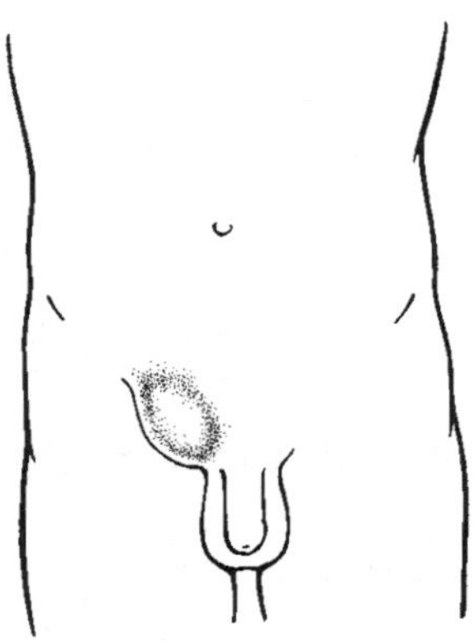

Figure 16.2 A bulge in the groin may be a sign of a hernia.

COMPLICATIONS

- Incarceration of the bowel (trapping of the bowel within the hernia, so that it cannot be pushed back into the abdomen);
  - incarceration can result in bowel obstruction (see below); **OR IN**
  - strangulation, with severe pain and tenderness at the site of the hernia, and swelling and blockage of blood supply to the bowel, which dies (necrosis);
  - incarceration is most likely to occur soon after a hernia first appears;
  - incarceration is commoner with small hernias than with large ones.

✔ *What to do*

- If there are no symptoms of incarceration or strangulation, advise the patient to see a doctor when convenient.
- Note that hernia can only be cured by surgery but the risk of complications is low if there are no symptoms other than a lump.
- If a formerly reducible hernia (i.e. a hernia that can be pushed back into the

abdomen) becomes non-reducible but there is no pain or tenderness, have the patient rest in bed and see a doctor at the next port.

- If there is pain and tenderness, strangulation may have occurred and you should prepare for evacuation of the patient with a view to urgent surgery.

LIVER AND BILIARY DISEASE

The liver is the largest internal organ of the body. It has many functions but those important in liver disease are:

- processing food that has been absorbed by the bowel;
- making blood clotting substances;
- breaking down toxins absorbed from the bowel;
- processing the pigment bilirubin that is produced when old red blood cells are broken down.

Jaundice

Jaundice, the main symptom of liver disease likely to be encountered on board ship, is a yellow discolouration of the skin and of the white of the eye by bilirubin.

Jaundice can be caused by:

- **excessive destruction of red blood cells** (haemolytic jaundice):
  - more bilirubin is produced than the liver can handle and the excess accumulates in the blood;
  - this occurs in a number of diseases affecting red blood cells;
- **destruction of liver cells** (hepatocellular jaundice):
  - so many cells are lost that there are not enough left to carry out the liver's functions;
  - this is accompanied by loss of other functions of the liver:
    - toxins produced by bacteria in the bowel are not destroyed, so that they accumulate in the blood and affect brain function (hepatic encephalopathy);
    - blood-clotting factors are no longer made by the liver, so that spontaneous bruising and bleeding occur;
- **obstruction of the bile ducts** (obstructive jaundice):
  - the commonest cause of jaundice;
  - can be due either to a gallstone lodged in the common bile duct, to swelling of liver cells that blocks off the tiny bile channels within the liver, or to a tumour of the pancreas.

✔ *What to do in a case of jaundice*

- Use a dipstick to test the urine for the presence of bile.
- Question the patient about:
  - alcohol consumption;
  - risk factors for viral hepatitis;

- symptoms of gallbladder disease;
- medicines the patient has been taking, including over-the-counter drugs, recreational drugs, and herbal and folk remedies.

- Seek medical advice, providing the doctor with this information.
- If the patient is unwell but has no fever or pain, you can delay transfer to an onshore medical facility for 48 hours without danger.
- If there is fever and/or severe pain, arrange for urgent evacuation.
- Meanwhile, give ceftriaxone, 2 g intravenously or intramuscularly, daily; **AND**
  - metronidazole, 500 mg orally, three times daily; **AND**
  - if there is pain, morphine, 10–15 mg intramuscularly.
- If the patient is jaundiced but not at all unwell, treat as for hepatitis A (see Chapter 23, *Infectious diseases*) and have the patient see a doctor at the next port.
- Reassess the patient daily and seek medical advice, again with a view to evacuation, if the patient has:
  - deepening jaundice
  - abnormal mental function
  - fever or pain.

Liver failure

Liver failure is suggested by progressively deepening jaundice together with abnormal bleeding and mental changes, such as confusion and drowsiness. Liver failure usually develops over several days or weeks if the patient has been previously healthy. It is, therefore, unlikely to be a major problem on board ship.

Causes of liver failure include:

- hepatitis B virus infection;
- overdose of paracetamol (acetaminophen), usually in a patient attempting suicide (see Chapter 11, *Poisoning*);
- far-advanced cirrhosis of the liver (see below).

Alcoholic liver disease

There are two main types of alcoholic liver disease: alcoholic hepatitis and cirrhosis of the liver (liver cirrhosis can be caused by many other factors besides alcohol, see below).

ALCOHOLIC HEPATITIS

Alcoholic hepatitis occurs in patients who consume more than 120 g per day of alcohol (roughly equivalent to one and a half litres of wine, four litres of beer, or a third of a bottle of spirits): severe cases often occur after a binge.

Signs and symptoms

- Enlarged, tender liver
- jaundice
- fever, **BUT**:

- fever due to alcoholic hepatitis is rarely over 38°C;
- patients consuming large amounts of alcohol are prone to infection;
- do not attribute fever to alcoholic hepatitis without medical advice;

- nausea
- loss of appetite.

✔ *What to do in a case of alcoholic hepatitis*

- Seek medical advice.
- Allow no alcohol.
- Record an alcohol withdrawal score, repeat it every hour, and treat withdrawal if necessary (see Chapter 22, *Tobacco, alcohol, and drug use*).
- Give Vitamin K, 10 mg subcutaneously.
- Give omeprazole, 20 mg orally, twice daily.
- Warn the patient that alcoholic hepatitis is likely to progress to liver cirrhosis (see below) if abuse of alcohol continues.

CIRRHOSIS OF THE LIVER

Cirrhosis is extensive scarring of the liver as a result of the healing process that the liver undergoes when damage has been inflicted on it for a long time, usually over many years. A diagnosis of cirrhosis usually requires very extensive medical tests. Problems with cirrhosis may arise on board ship, but usually in a patient who has had the diagnosis made on shore.

The commonest causes of cirrhosis of the liver are alcohol abuse and hepatitis C virus infection, which are often present in the same patient: the combination of these two causes is much more likely to lead to cirrhosis than either cause alone.

Less common causes of liver cirrhosis include:

- hepatitis B virus infection;
- haemochromatosis, an inherited disorder in which excessive iron is absorbed from food and accumulates in the body;
- liver inflammation associated with obesity and diabetes mellitus;
- many rare diseases.

► *Signs and symptoms*

- Jaundice;
- portal hypertension (increased pressure in the veins leading to the liver), causing:
  - spleen enlargement and dilated veins around the lower oesophagus (see above, under *Upper gastrointestinal bleeding*);
- bruising and uncontrollable bleeding, because the cirrhotic liver cannot make blood clotting factors;
- fluid accumulation, with:
  - swelling of the legs (oedema);
  - swelling of the abdomen (ascites), which often becomes infected, causing abdominal pain and fever;
- confusion or delirium, and in severe cases coma.

COMPLICATIONS

- Liver cancer develops in some long-standing cases of cirrhosis.

✔ *What to do in a case of liver cirrhosis*

- Seek medical advice with a view to evacuation if a patient known to have cirrhosis also has any one of the these symptoms:
  - fever
  - abdominal pain
  - abnormal bleeding
  - abnormal mental function.

Gallstones

Gallstones are stony lumps that form in the gallbladder or, more rarely, in the bile ducts. They are common in older people. In most cases they produce no symptoms but they can cause three serious problems:

- transient obstruction of the gallbladder outlet, resulting in biliary colic;
- inflammation of the gallbladder (cholecystitis);
- obstruction of the common bile duct resulting in jaundice (see above).

Note

- The gallbladder is a small muscular sac that lies just under the liver.
- The liver secretes bile, which is stored in the gallbladder.
- Bile is made up of water, pigments, and bile salts.
- The bile salts act as detergents in the bowel and break up fat globules in food so that they can be digested.
- Bile leaves the gallbladder via the cystic duct, which joins the gallbladder to the main bile duct (common bile duct) coming from the liver.
- The bile then passes along the common bile duct to the duodenum.

► *Signs and symptoms of biliary colic*

- Pain in the right upper abdomen, that:
  - begins one or two hours after a meal, increases for an hour or two, then subsides over the next four hours or so;
  - is constant (not colicky);
  - is not usually very severe;
  - is not made worse by movement;
- in many cases, a history of similar episodes;
- no fever;
- appearance of the patient not suggestive of severe illness;
- little or no abdominal tenderness on examination.

✔ What to do in a case of biliary colic

- Give a single dose of ibuprofen, 800 mg orally; if this is ineffective:
  - give morphine, 10–15 mg intramuscularly, once, or twice if there is still severe pain three to four hours after the first dose.
- If the pain has not resolved after six hours or if there is fever or marked abdominal tenderness, seek medical advice with a view to evacuation.
- Give only clear fluids until the attack has passed.

► Signs and symptoms of cholecystitis

- Pain that:
  - often begins a few hours after a large fatty meal;
  - is constant;
  - is severe;
  - is felt usually in the right upper abdomen, often radiating to the right lower ribs;
  - is made worse by movement (so that the patient avoids all movement);
  - does not go away in a few hours;
- fever;
- rapid pulse;
- sickly appearance of patient;
- marked tenderness and muscle spasm in the right upper abdomen;
- in some cases, low blood pressure and generalized tenderness of the abdomen, suggesting perforation of the gallbladder.

✔ What to do in a case of cholecystitis

- Seek medical advice with a view to evacuation.
- Insert an intravenous cannula and give normal saline (0.9% sodium chloride), one litre, every eight hours.
- Give nothing by mouth except sips of water.
- To relieve pain, give:
  - ibuprofen, 800 mg orally, then 400 mg every six hours; if this is ineffective after two doses, give
  - morphine, 10–15 mg intramuscularly, every 3–4 hours.
- Give ceftriaxone, 2 g intravenously or intramuscularly, once.
- If evacuation is likely to be delayed for more than 24 hours, give ceftriaxone, 2g intravenously or intramuscularly, daily **AND** metronidazole, 500 mg orally, three times daily.

Kidney and other urinary disorders

DISORDERS OF THE KIDNEY

The kidneys are bean-shaped organs, 10–15cm long, located near the middle of the back, just below the rib cage. The kidneys remove from the blood enough water to keep the body in balance, and the waste products derived from normal tissue activities and from food.

Each kidney contains one million or so tiny units (nephrons) which carry out its functions. Each nephron consists of a knot of tiny blood vessels (glomerulus) joined to a tiny tube (tubule).

There are three main steps in kidney function:

- in the glomerulus, the blood vessels are separated from the tubule by a filter with minute holes, so that some of the water and the small waste molecules are pushed out of the blood into the tubule, forming urine, while blood cells and large molecules are kept in the blood. For this to work, there must be enough blood pressure to force the excess fluid and the molecules of waste substances through the holes in the filter;
- as the urine passes along the tubule it adjusts the salt composition of the urine, and absorbs substances that the body wants, such as glucose;
- further along the tubule the amount of water in the urine is adjusted to match the amount of water the person has had to drink;
- urine leaves the kidneys and passes along the ureters, one on each side, to the bladder.

Acute renal (kidney) failure

Renal failure means that the kidneys are not performing their function of removing wastes from the blood. Acute renal failure is renal failure that develops over a few days to a few weeks. Acute renal failure may produce no symptoms until the level of waste products in the blood becomes dangerously high.

Note

- Acute renal failure can occur because of problems at any of the stages in the formation of urine by the kidney:
  - before the blood enters the kidneys (pre-renal);
  - when the blood is being filtered within the kidneys (renal);
  - when the urine has left the kidneys (post-renal).
- **Pre-renal** failure is due to:
  - in most cases, low blood pressure due to hypovolaemic shock from bleeding (see Chapter 2, *Shock*);
  - rarely, blockage of major blood vessels leading to the kidney.
- **Renal** failure can be due to:
  - inflammation of small blood vessels (vasculitis) in the kidney, in many cases accompanied by a rash or symptoms from other organs, especially the lungs;
  - damage to the nephrons caused by a prolonged period of low blood pressure (acute tubular necrosis);

- inflammation of the kidney (nephritis) caused by an immune reaction to an infection;
- clogging of the urine-collecting tubules in the kidney by protein, especially protein released from damaged muscles in patients with major injuries.

- **Post-renal** failure is due to obstruction:
  - in **both** ureters;
  - in the urethra.

Signs and symptoms

- Low urine output is the main indication of acute renal failure.
- In an ill or injured seafarer **who is receiving adequate fluid** a urine output of:
  - less than 20 ml per hour for 6 hours is probably abnormally low;
  - less than 30 ml per hour for 12 hours is definitely abnormally low;
  - less than 20 ml per hour for 24 hours, or no urine for 12 hours, means acute renal failure.
- A person has the urge to pass urine when the bladder contains 200–400 ml, and feels an urgent need to pass urine when the bladder contains 400–500 ml, so if a patient has not passed urine for 12 hours, it is likely that something is wrong.
- Hourly urine output can only be measured accurately measured when a bladder catheter is in place.
- If a seriously ill patient has not passed urine for 6–8 hours, and feels no urge to pass urine, insert a bladder catheter (see Chapter 26, *Nursing care and medical procedures*) and measure hourly urine output.

What to do

- If you suspect acute renal failure, seek medical advice but first prepare to answer the following questions:
  - Is the patient seriously ill or injured?
  - What is the patient's blood pressure?
  - Have there been periods during the illness or since the injury when the patient's blood pressure was low?
  - How much fluid has the patient drunk over the past 24 hours?
  - What medication (including herbal, natural and folk medicines) has the patient taken?
  - Is there a skin rash?
  - Are there other symptoms, especially coughing up blood?
  - What is the finding of a dipstick test of the patient's urine (see Table 17.1 below)?
- Catheterize the bladder (see Chapter 26, *Nursing care and medical procedures*) before calling for medical advice.
- Insert an intravenous cannula and give one litre of normal saline (0.9% sodium chloride) over 30 minutes:
  - if this produces an increase in urine flow, raise the patient's fluid intake to maintain a urine flow rate of about 50 ml per hour.

Table 17.1 Urinary findings in acute renal failure.

Cause	Urine volume	Urine specific gravity	Blood in urine	Protein in urine	Other signs or symptoms
Pre-renal	Low	High	No	No	Very low blood pressure
Renal	Low or normal	Low or normal	Yes	Yes	Oedema (swelling of hands and feet) and high blood pressure
Post-renal	Low or absent	Normal	Often	No or low (traces)	Pain

Chronic renal failure (Bright's disease)

Chronic renal failure means a failure, developing over many years, of the kidneys to control waste in the blood. The commonest cause of chronic renal failure is diabetes mellitus. With most causes of chronic renal failure the kidney can fulfil most of its normal functions until the disease has destroyed 80–90% of the organ. As a result, symptoms of kidney failure occur very late in the disease. Even then, it can be months or years before wastes in the blood accumulate to dangerous levels (uraemia).

Most cases of chronic renal failure are detected when blood tests are done for reasons unrelated to the kidney. Even blood tests may not detect failing kidney function until half of the kidney is destroyed. For these reasons it is unlikely that problems arising from chronic renal failure will need to be managed on board ship.

Kidney stones (renal colic)

Kidney stones (nephrolithiasis) are common: 10% of men and 5% of women will have a kidney stone at some time in their lives. Stones occur when substances are present in the urine in amounts that cannot be held in solution. The excess amounts form crystals, which gradually grow to form a stone. The stone passes down the ureter, causing an episode of intense pain (renal colic). Most kidney stones are made of calcium or urate (the substance that causes gout). Stones are commoner in hot weather because the urine is more concentrated, and drinking plenty of liquid can reduce the risk of a kidney stone developing. Kidney stones tend to recur: after a first stone, about one patient in 10 will have another stone in the next year; one in three, in the next five years; and three out of four, in the next 10 years.

Signs and symptoms

- Rapid onset of pain, peaking after a few minutes.
- The pain:
  - ranges in intensity from mild to excruciating;
  - lasts a few hours or a few days (depending on how fast the stone travels down the ureter to the bladder);
  - is felt on one side only (the side where the stone is);
  - is felt usually in the side or in the back below the ribs and sometimes also in the groin or scrotum;

    - comes and goes in spasms lasting 30–60 minutes – much longer than intestinal colic but less than biliary colic.
- Blood in the urine is nearly always found on a dipstick test during the first day of pain.

✔ *What to do*

- Encourage the patient to drink plentiful fluids, preferably citrus juices, if available.
- Give ibuprofen, 400–800 mg orally, every six to eight hours.
- If there is vomiting and the patient cannot take medication orally, give morphine, 10 mg intramuscularly, every three to four hours.
- Collect all the urine that the patient passes and strain it through a strainer with holes less than 1 mm in diameter:
    - keep for later analysis any stone or gravel that collects in the strainer: the type of stone affects what can be done to prevent further episodes.
- Take the patient's temperature twice daily.
- If pain is still severe after 48 hours **OR** if fever develops **OR** if urine output is low, seek medical advice with a view to evacuation.
- Otherwise have the patient see a doctor at the next port.

OTHER URINARY DISORDERS

RED URINE

If the urine is red, the cause is nearly always the presence of blood in the urine: this can be confirmed by dipstick testing of the urine. Note that dipsticks need to be used before the expiry date printed on the container in order to achieve reliable results.

Note

- Occasionally, red urine is caused by medication (chloroquine, ibuprofen, rifampicin) or the consumption of large amounts of red food colouring, beetroot, or blackberries: in these cases, dipstick testing will be negative for blood.
- Dipstick testing will give a false positive result for blood if the specimen has been collected after ejaculation and there is semen in the urine.
- Most patients with blood in the urine have no serious disease: usually the bleeding will stop and not recur.
- If there is back pain, a kidney stone (see above) is the most likely cause of red urine.
- Patients over 50 with no pain and, rarely, younger patients may have bladder or kidney cancer.

✔ *What to do*

- If there is blood in the urine and no evidence of a kidney stone (see above), have the patient see a doctor at the next port, because of the risk of bladder cancer.

Urinary tract infection

Urinary tract infections are usually caused by bacteria, which have entered the urinary tract via the urethral opening (at the tip of the penis in men) and which cause inflammation of the urethra (urethritis), bladder (cystitis), or kidneys (pyelonephritis).

Urinary tract infections are uncommon in men but very common in women. In men, infections tend to occur when there is an obstruction somewhere in the urinary tract, either from a stone or an enlarged prostate (see below).

Urinary tract infection in women

In women, most urinary tract infections affect the bladder (cystitis) but not the kidneys. Bacteria gain access to the bladder via the urethra.

Signs and symptoms

- A frequent, urgent need to urinate (frequency).
- A burning or smarting sensation while urinating (dysuria).
- In some cases, discomfort in the lower abdomen.
- No fever or back pain.

✔ *What to do*

- Give amoxycillin/clavulanate, 875/125 mg orally, twice daily for seven days.
- If the patient is allergic to penicillin, give ciprofloxacin, 500 mg orally, twice daily for three days (do not give ciprofloxacin to a woman who is or may be pregnant).
- Suspect kidney infection (pyelonephritis), if there is:
  - fever; **AND**
  - pain or tenderness in the loin; **OR**
  - vomiting.
- Treat as for cystitis, but seek medical advice because septic shock (see Chapter 2, *Shock*) can complicate pyelonephritis.

Urinary tract infection in men

In men, bacteria that ascend the urethra tend to cause infection of the prostate gland (prostatitis) rather than cystitis, as they do in women. Infection of the prostate gland can be acute or chronic.

Prostatitis

Signs and symptoms

- A frequent, urgent need to urinate (frequency).
- A burning or smarting sensation while urinating (dysuria).
- Fever and chills.
- Pain in the lower abdomen or in the area between the scrotum and anus (perineum).
- Difficulty in passing urine (because of the swollen prostate gland), usually:
  - difficulty in starting (hesitancy)

- a weak urine stream
- difficulty in stopping (dribbling).

- Acute prostatitis causes high fever and severe pain.
- Chronic prostatitis causes mild symptoms, mainly dysuria and frequency, and tends to relapse after treatment.

✔ *What to do*

- Give ciprofloxacin, 500 mg orally, twice daily for 28 days; **OR**:
  - amoxycillin/clavulanate, 875/125 mg orally, twice daily for 28 days.
- Septic shock can occur in acute prostatitis: if there is altered mental status or falling blood pressure, seek medical advice with a view to urgent evacuation.
- If the patient cannot pass urine **DO NOT** pass a bladder catheter – seek medical advice with a view to evacuation.
- If you are within three days of the next port of call, or the patient is to be evacuated, take a mid-stream urine specimen, place it in a sterile jar, and refrigerate it.
- To relieve pain, give ibuprofen, 400 mg orally, every six hours.
- If, after 48 hours, fever has not fallen and the patient does not feel better, seek medical advice.

Chronic pelvic pain in men

Pain is the main feature, which is:

- present for months, usually on and off;
- felt between the scrotum and the anus (the perineum), and/or in the lower abdomen and/or testicles;
- often made worse with, or sometimes felt only with, ejaculation.

Dysuria and frequency are also present, usually on and off.

✔ *What to do*

- Give ibuprofen, 400 mg orally, every six hours, for pain relief.
- Have the patient see a doctor in his home port: investigations and treatment are usually prolonged.

Benign prostatic hyperplasia (BPH, enlarged prostate)

- The prostate gland surrounds the urethra immediately below the bladder.
- Enlargement of the prostate gland can interfere with bladder emptying.
- The prostate enlarges with age in all men, and the proportion of men with difficulty passing urine because of an enlarged prostate increases with age: problems are rare below age 40 but affect 20% of men aged 60.
- Symptoms are:
  - frequent urination;
  - more frequent need to get up at night to pass urine (nocturia);

  - inability to delay the need to urinate (urgency);
  - trouble starting (hesitancy) and trouble stopping (terminal dribbling).
- These symptoms start slowly and get very gradually worse over years.
- The main problem caused by BPH on board ship is likely to be acute urinary retention (see below).
- Prostate cancer can cause the same symptoms, BPH is not associated with or a precursor to prostate cancer.
- Patients with troublesome symptoms of prostate enlargement should see a doctor in their home port.

Acute urinary retention

Urinary retention means an inability to urinate despite a full bladder. In men, it is most often due to an enlarged prostate blocking the bladder outlet or, less often, a blockage of the urethra due either to a previous insertion of a bladder catheter or to previous episodes of gonorrhoea. Acute urinary retention is rare in women, except after childbirth or surgery to the uterus.

► *Signs and symptoms*

- An inability to urinate despite feeling the urge to do so.
- Pain, usually in the lower abdomen.
- Enlargement of the bladder, which, on palpation, can be felt as a dome-shaped mass in the lower abdomen.

✔ *What to do*

- If pain is severe, give morphine, 10 mg intramuscularly.
- Have the patient lie in a hot bath and relax before trying to pass urine into a urine bottle (keep the bath water hot).
- If after 30 minutes the patient has still not passed urine, prepare for bladder catheterization (see Chapter 26, *Nursing care and medical procedures*).
- If you are unable to successfully catheterize the bladder, seek medical advice (prolonged bladder distension can cause permanent harm).

Pregnancy and childbirth

PREGNANCY

Signs and symptoms

- One or more periods missed; note:
  - pregnancy is the commonest, but not the only cause of delayed menstruation in a healthy woman whose cycle has previously been regular.
- Nausea and/or vomiting (morning sickness).
- A feeling that the breasts are bigger and heavier than before.
- Darkening of nipples and surrounding pigmentation.
- Frequent need to urinate.

Note

- Abdominal enlargement is rarely noticeable before the 16th week of pregnancy and in obese women may not be obvious even in advanced pregnancy. Any pregnant crew members should be assigned light duties only for the remainder of the voyage.

Drugs in pregnancy

- The risk of harm to the fetus from medications is highest in the first 12 weeks of pregnancy, and low late in pregnancy.
- Avoid giving medicine to a pregnant woman unless:
  - a doctor who knows the woman is pregnant advises it; OR
  - the woman is at risk of serious harm unless she is treated before medical advice can be obtained.
- Common conditions carrying a risk of serious harm to both the fetus and the pregnant woman, for which the treatment recommended in this book is safe in pregnancy include:
  - severe or life-threatening asthma (see Chapter 15, *Respiratory diseases*);
  - anaphylactic shock (see Chapter 33, *Ship's medicine chest*);
  - status epilepticus (see Chapter 13, *Paralysis, strange behaviour, unconsciousness*).
- For analgesic drugs in pregnancy, see Chapter 3, *Pain management*.
- Of the antibiotics available on board ship:
  - amoxycillin/clavulanate and ceftriaxone are safe in pregnancy;
  - doxycycline (and other tetracycline drugs), ciprofloxacin (and other fluoroquinolone drugs), are not safe in pregnancy.

VAGINAL BLEEDING DURING PREGNANCY OR SUSPECTED PREGNANCY

About 20% of pregnant women with normal pregnancies experience vaginal bleeding in early pregnancy. Bleeding sometimes occurs at the time the fertilized egg implants (i.e. becomes embedded) in the womb (uterus). Other important causes of bleeding during the first six months of pregnancy include:

- threatened or "inevitable" miscarriage;
- ectopic pregnancy (see below, *Ectopic pregnancy*).

Bleeding in early pregnancy may or may not be associated with lower abdominal pain.

Remember:

- severe pain with little vaginal bleeding suggests ectopic pregnancy (see below);
- mild pain with copious vaginal bleeding suggests miscarriage (see below).

Bleeding during the seventh to the ninth month of pregnancy may be a sign of an abnormality of the afterbirth (placenta) inside the uterus. In this case:

- the lives of the woman and her baby are at risk;
- seek medical advice and prepare for urgent evacuation.

ECTOPIC PREGNANCY

An ectopic pregnancy occurs when a fertilized egg begins to develop outside the womb, most often in one of the tubes (Fallopian tubes) leading from the ovaries to the womb. In most cases, problems appear six to eight weeks after the last normal menstrual period.

Signs and symptoms

- Moderate to severe lower abdominal pain.
- Scanty vaginal bleeding.
- In more than half of cases, no symptoms until the affected Fallopian tube ruptures, causing severe bleeding into the abdomen, and shock (see Chapter 1, *First aid*, under sections on *Choking* and *Bleeding*, and Chapter 2, *Shock*); note:
  - laboratory tests are needed to distinguish a ruptured ectopic pregnancy from other major abdominal problems, such as appendicitis (see Chapter 12, *Examination of the patient*, and Chapter 16, *Gastrointestinal and liver diseases*).

What to do in a case of vaginal bleeding and shock during pregnancy or suspected pregnancy

- Insert an intravenous cannula, using the largest cannula available.
- Seek medical advice with a view to evacuation of the patient.
- While seeking medical advice, give sodium chloride, 0.9% solution (normal saline):
  - start the infusion to give one litre in the first hour;
  - follow medical advice about the amount of sodium chloride needed (the amount will be based on pulse rate and blood pressure, but very large volumes may be needed).

MISCARRIAGE

Miscarriage is a pregnancy that ends before the fetus has developed to the point where it can live independently. A fetus that has reached this point is defined by WHO as having a body weight of 500 g or a gestation time (gestational age) of about 20–22 weeks. In many countries, you are not required to report a miscarriage to the authorities, but you are required to report births, and the death of a newborn child. Seek medical advice about the regulations that may apply in a particular case.

Note

- About one third of all pregnancies end in miscarriage.
- Miscarriage is unusual in a first pregnancy and also in women whose previous pregnancy was completed normally.
- Many miscarriages occur so early in pregnancy that the woman is unaware that she is pregnant:
  - about 80% of miscarriages occur in the first 12 weeks of pregnancy;
  - early miscarriages are associated with abnormalities of the fetus;
  - miscarriage of a normal fetus is very unusual after 15 weeks.

Signs and symptoms

There may be vaginal bleeding with little or no pain:

- this is called **threatened miscarriage**:
  - most women with threatened miscarriage will stop bleeding and the pregnancy will continue.

If there is increasing bleeding accompanied by crampy lower abdominal pain:

- this is called **inevitable miscarriage**;
- if the increase in bleeding with lower abdominal pain occurs **before** 12 weeks of pregnancy, it is likely that:
  - the contents of the uterus will be expelled quickly;
  - the bleeding and pain will become minimal or cease;
- if the increase in bleeding with lower abdominal pain occurs **after** 12 weeks of gestation, it is possible that:
  - some pregnancy tissue will remain in the uterus;
  - bleeding will continue, with severe, cramping abdominal pain and a high risk of shock.

If symptoms of threatened or inevitable miscarriage are followed by fever over 38°C, abdominal pain, and vaginal bleeding mixed with purulent discharge:

- there is probably infection of the uterus;
- this is called septic abortion.

If there has been vaginal bleeding which has now stopped and the woman says she no longer "feels pregnant":

- it is possible that the fetus has died but remains in the uterus;
- this called a missed abortion.

✔ *What to do*

- If septic abortion is suspected:
  - seek medical advice with a view to evacuation;
  - give ceftriaxone, 2 g intramuscularly;
  - continue to give ceftriaxone, 2 g intramuscularly, twice daily while the patient remains on board.
- If there is severe or increasing bleeding with abdominal pain, but no fever:
  - seek medical advice with a view to evacuation;

  - monitor the pulse and blood pressure every four hours (see *What to do in a case of vaginal bleeding and shock during pregnancy or suspected pregnancy* above).
- If bleeding is diminishing or has stopped and there is no pain or the pain is easing:
  - no treatment is required, but
  - have the patient see a doctor at the next port of call.

SALPINGITIS (INFLAMMATION OF A FALLOPIAN TUBE) (see Chapter 19, *Sexually transmitted infections,* under *Pelvic inflammatory disease*)

PRURITUS VULVAE (EXTERNAL GENITAL ITCHING) (see Chapter 19, *Sexually transmitted infections,* under *Vaginal discharge*)

CHILDBIRTH

A ship at sea is not the best place for a woman to give birth. Most births are normal (Figure 18.1), but in some cases, problems that threaten the lives of mother and child can arise without warning. The more premature the birth, the greater the danger to the child. If, for any reason, the woman cannot be put ashore in time to be hospitalized, every effort should be made to place her under the care of a doctor, midwife, or, failing that, someone on board familiar with childbirth.

Preparing for the birth

- Make ready a cabin that is clean and large enough to allow access from the foot of the bunk and both sides.
- Place a waterproof sheet under the bottom sheet of the bunk in order to protect the mattress.
- Have ready:
  - a plentiful supply of hot water
  - soap
  - flannels
  - towels
  - a bedpan
  - sanitary towels (not tampons)
  - a large bowl for the afterbirth (placenta)
  - a plastic bag in which to put the afterbirth
  - four pieces of non-adhesive tape or strong string, each about 25 cm long
  - two artery forceps
  - surgical scissors

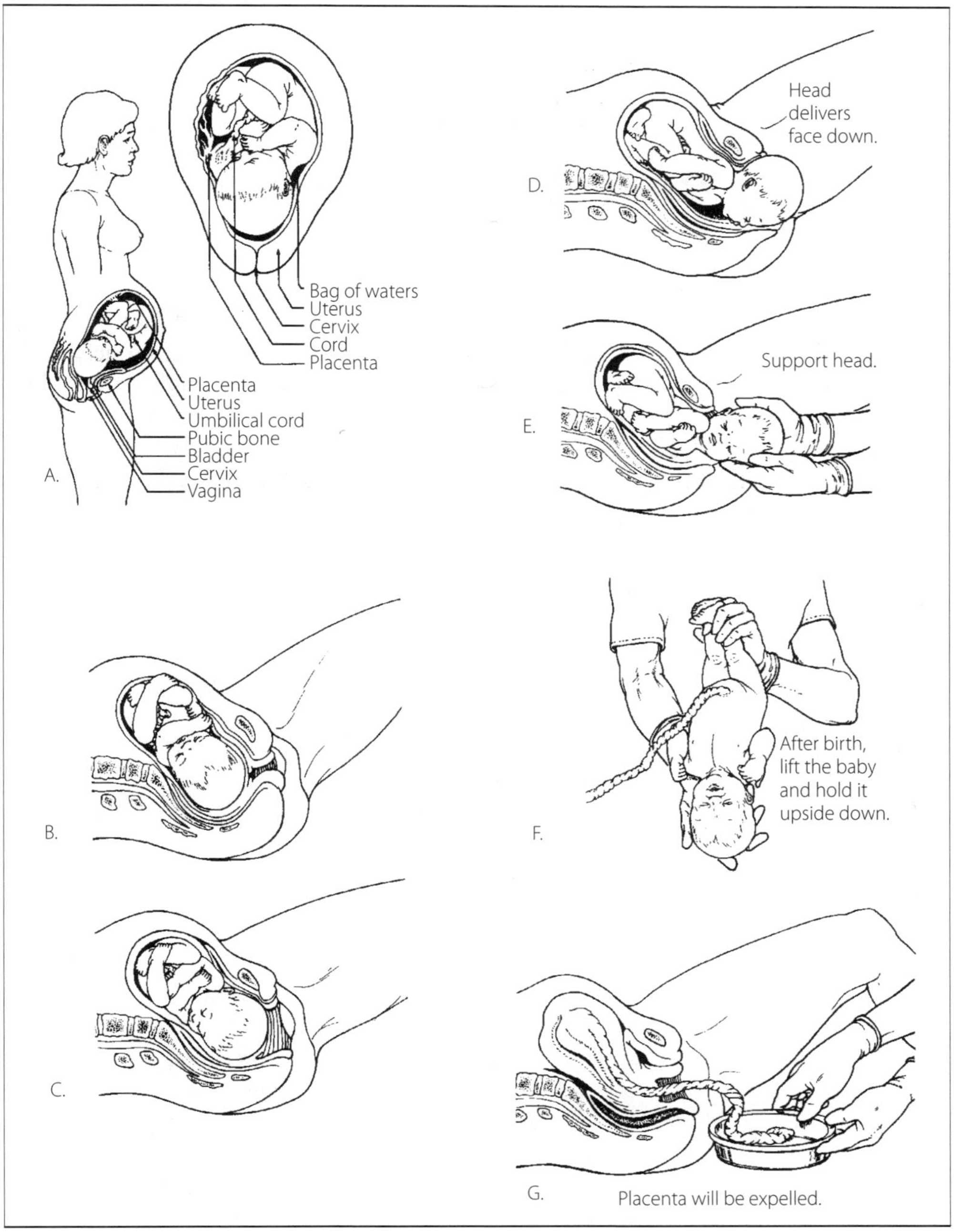

Figure 18.1 Anatomy of pregnancy and normal stages in labour.

  - cotton wool
  - two small sterile dressings
  - bandages
  - surgical spirit
  - an oxygen cylinder and tubing
  - a clean soft blanket in which to wrap the child
  - a suitable box with clean sheets to serve as a cot
  - a clean nightdress and clean sheets for the mother after the birth.
- Sterilize all the instruments by boiling for at least 20 minutes.
- Make sure that no one who will attend the birth or care for the newborn baby is suffering from a cough, cold, diarrhoea, or a skin disease.
- Make sure that all attendants wash and scrub their hands, wrists, and forearms thoroughly with soap and water and have freshly laundered clothes or a freshly laundered overall or gown to wear.

Managing the early stages of childbirth

- **Labour pains:**
  - pain at intervals in the lower part of the back and abdomen signal the start of labour;
  - seek medical advice now and keep in contact with the doctor;
  - prepare for the birth (see above, *Preparing for the birth*);
  - the labour pains become stronger and more frequent over several hours, until they occur every minute or so;
  - if the woman feels more comfortable walking about, encourage her to do so.
- **Passing the show:**
  - at the beginning of labour many women "pass the show", which consists of a small amount of blood and mucus trickling from the vagina.
- **Breaking of the waters:**
  - after the show is passed, the bag of water enveloping the fetus in the womb bursts and a large amount (250–500 ml) of a sticky watery fluid (liquor or amniotic fluid) escapes from the vagina;
  - the delay between the show and the breaking of the waters may be minutes or several hours;
  - inspect the amniotic fluid to see if it contains meconium; this is a thick, greeny-black material with no smell which comes from the rectum of the fetus when it is distressed by conditions in the uterus; inform the medical adviser if you see meconium in the amniotic fluid;
  - encourage the woman to empty her bowels and bladder at this stage (but **do not** use a bladder catheter to empty the bladder).

Managing the birth

- If this is the woman's first experience of childbirth, she is likely to be fearful.
- Encourage her frequently.

- Keep her fully informed about what is happening and about the advice you have received from the doctor.
- Avoid whispered conversations about her progress: they will worsen anxiety.
- Let the woman find the most comfortable position for herself: many women choose to lie on their side, with their head supported on a pillow and their knees drawn up.
- Allow the woman to walk around the cabin if she wants to.
- Keep her warm and give her a warm drink, but no alcohol.
- Make sure she is not left alone.
- Ask her to breathe quickly or pant but not to bear down or to push with the pains: in the early stages of labour, rapid expulsion of the baby can be dangerous.
- When the baby emerges (usually head first), clear any membrane from its nose and mouth.
- As the baby's neck appears, check that the cord is not wrapped around it.
- If the cord is wrapped around the baby's neck:
  - to free the cord, pull it over the back of the baby's head and downwards to the front (Figure 18.2).
- If the cord is too tightly wound around the neck to release it easily:
  - knot two of the non-adhesive tapes tightly around it, 2–3cm apart; OR
  - clip the artery forceps across the cord 2–3cm apart;
  - use the surgical scissors to cut between the tapes or artery forceps; then
  - separate the cut ends of the cord from around the baby's neck;
  - if you used artery forceps, tie tapes tightly around the cut ends of the cord before releasing the artery forceps.

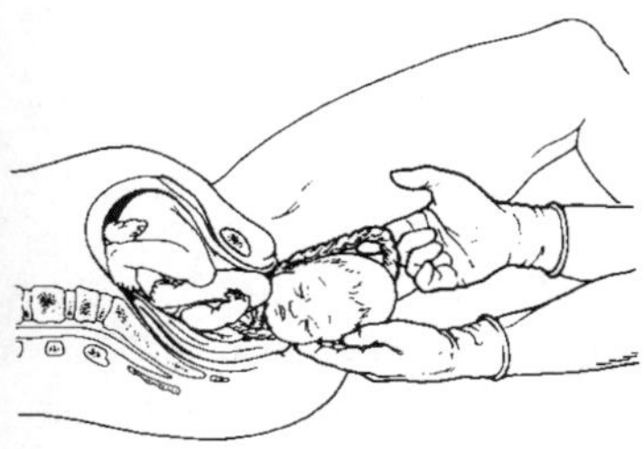

Figure 18.2 Umbilical cord wrapped around the baby's neck.

Caring for the baby after delivery

- As soon as the baby is completely outside the vagina, lift it clear of the mother without pulling the cord, which is still attached to the placenta.
- Make sure that the baby's nose and mouth are not covered by anything that would stop it from breathing.
- **Hold the baby** upside down for a few seconds to allow any fluid to drain out of its throat and nose.
- **Be careful: newborn babies are very slippery**.
- **Hold the baby over the bed, not over the floor**.
- Put the baby on its side on the mother's abdomen.
- If the baby is breathing but not bright red or pink, give oxygen: set the flow rate from an oxygen cylinder to 2 litres per minute and blow oxygen onto the baby's face with the tubing.
- If the baby does not start breathing spontaneously, cover its nose and mouth with your mouth and give gentle artificial respiration, using small puffs of air;
- If the baby is born dead:
  - tell the mother that the baby has been born dead;
  - divide the cord (see below);
  - give the baby to the mother to hold;

- If the baby is breathing and pink, use sterile gauze swabs soaked in potable water to clean the baby's eyes.
- The cord will probably still be pulsating, but after a few minutes it will stop; when it has stopped pulsating:
  - tie two pieces of non-adhesive tape or string tightly around the cord (do not rush this step), with one piece of tape about 5 cm from the baby's abdomen and the other piece of tape about 2½ cm further along the cord towards the mother;
  - cut the cord between the two tapes;
  - put a sterile dressing over the stump of the cord and wrap the child in a soft blanket.
- Give the baby to the mother.
- Over the next five minutes, check whether the baby's stump is bleeding: if it is, tie a third piece of tape round the cord.
- Put the baby to the mother's breast as soon as possible, covering mother and baby with a blanket.
- The baby should be put to the mother's breast at frequent intervals.
- Milk flow is usually established by the second or third day.
- Both breasts should be used at each feed, allowing seven to 10 minutes for each breast.
- Over the first few days of life a baby usally loses weight but should regain its birth weight by the tenth day.
- At a convenient moment, weigh the baby, measure the circumference of its head above the ears with a tape measure, and record your findings.
- Wash the baby a couple of hours after birth:
  - let the mother take the leading role if she is well enough;
  - prepare a bowl of warm water, some toilet soap, and a clean flannel;
  - lay the baby on a towel and gently wash the scalp, face, and body so as to remove the white, wax-like material that covers it;
  - leave the area around the cord unwashed and keep it dry by covering it with a sterile dressing;
  - carefully dry the baby by patting it gently with the towel;
  - put a new sterile dressing on the cord and renew the dressing every two to three days;
  - normally the cord shrivels up and comes away in about 10 days.

Caring for the mother after delivery

- Give misoprostol, 600 micrograms orally, as soon as the baby has been delivered.
- About 15–20 minutes after the birth of the baby, the mother will experience more pains like labour pains and the afterbirth (placenta), with the cord attached to its centre, will be expelled together with some blood.
- Catch the afterbirth in a bowl.
- Do not attempt to hasten expulsion of the afterbirth by pulling on the cord.
- If the afterbirth does not appear within 30 minutes, massage the uterus (Figure 18.3).
- The cord, placenta, and membranes, with any other material that comes out of the mother, should be placed in the plastic bag.

- Seal the plastic bag and store it in a refrigerator until it can be taken with the mother and child to a hospital or doctor for examination.
- There may be a slight trickle of blood and water from the mother's vagina: this is normal.
- Wash the mother and give her a clean sanitary towel and a clean nightdress.
- Have the bed made up with clean sheets.
- If the mother's vulva has suffered any external tears as a result of the birth, seek medical advice about whether any tear should be stitched.
- Make sure the mother is comfortable and give her a warm drink.
- Make sure that someone stays near the mother in case of severe vaginal bleeding.

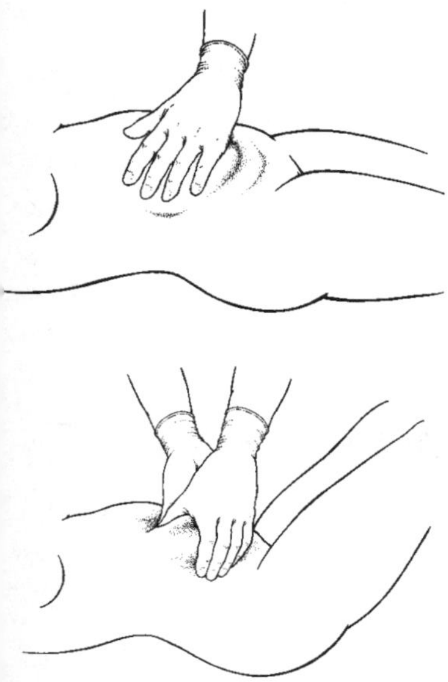

Figure 18.3 How to massage the uterus when the placenta is delayed.

Post-partum haemorrhage

Post-partum haemorrhage, which occurs in about one birth in 30, is the commonest cause of death of women in childbirth. It is defined as bleeding from the uterus or vagina that causes symptoms of blood loss. There are a number of causes, the commonest being the failure of the uterus to contract and thereby shut off the blood vessels in the uterine wall.

Signs and symptoms

- Light-headedness
- dizziness
- rapid pulse rate
- in severe cases, low blood pressure.

What to do

- Seek medical advice.
- Insert an intravenous cannula.
- Give 0.9% sodium chloride (normal saline) solution:
  - the doctor will advise how much to give based on pulse rate and blood pressure;
  - **pending advice allow the fluid to flow at the fastest rate possible**.
- Massage the uterus (Figures 18.4, 18.5).

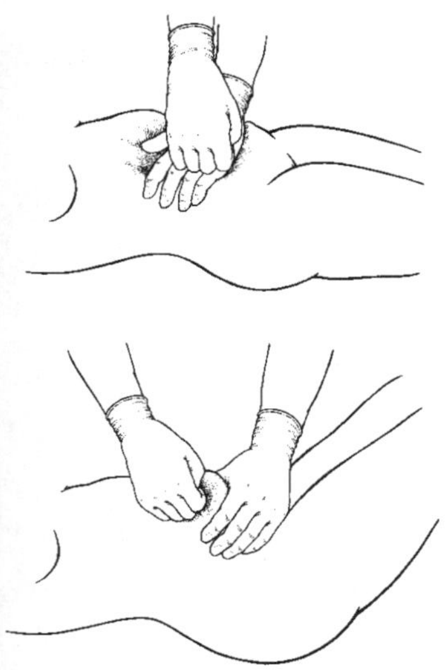

Figure 18.4 How to massage the uterus if the mother is losing blood.

Other possible problems after childbirth

POST-PARTUM CHILLS

Up to 50% of women have post-partum chills, which start within 30 minutes of delivery and last from a few minutes to an hour. There is no fever and no treatment is needed.

DISCHARGE OF THE LOCHIA

In the first few days after delivery there is normally a reddish-brown vaginal discharge, which becomes clear and watery over the next month. This discharge is called the lochia.

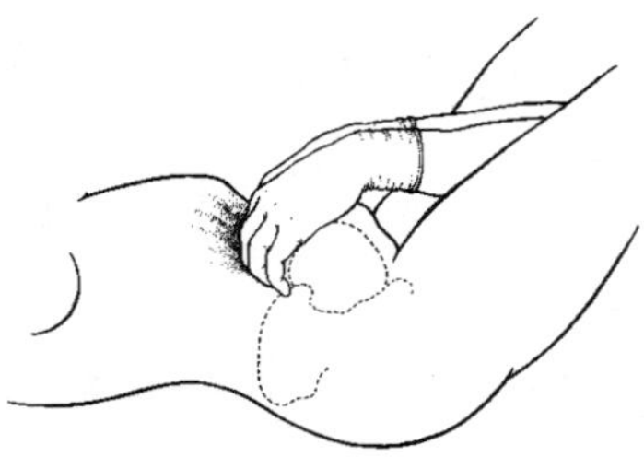

Figure 18.5 How to compress the uterus if the bleeding continues.

AFTER PAINS

The mother may experience pain similar to labour pain: these after pains may be felt more often during breast feeding.

DIFFICULTY PASSING URINE

This is common after delivery. If the woman has not passed urine within six hours of delivery examine the abdomen. If the bladder feels like a dome or sphere in the lower abdomen below the uterus (which is about the level of the navel at this time) pass a catheter to withdraw urine (see Chapter 26, *Nursing care and medical procedures*).

PUERPERAL SEPSIS (PUERPERAL FEVER OR CHILDBIRTH FEVER)

Puerperal sepsis is an infection of the uterus after childbirth.

► *Signs and symptoms*

- Fever, abdominal pain, and abdominal swelling developing over the first 12 hours after childbirth.

✔ *What to do*

- Seek medical advice.
- Give ceftriaxone, 1 g intramuscularly, twice daily until the temperature is normal or the patient is evacuated.

Chapter 19

Sexually transmitted infections

Seafarers generally acquire sexually transmitted infections through unprotected casual sexual contact, often with prostitutes. Multiple infections are common and some may not produce symptoms. All seafarers with a sexually transmitted infection should, even if they have been given effective treatment on board, receive prompt specialized medical attention by an onshore physician to be sure they have not picked up other infections, such as AIDS.

The following infections are transmitted by sexual contact: gonorrhoea, chlamydial infections, chancroid, genital herpes (*Herpes simplex* virus), syphilis, lymphogranuloma venereum, granuloma inguinale, genital warts, pubic lice, viral hepatitis B and C (see Chapter 23, *Infectious diseases*), human immunodeficiency virus (HIV, the cause of AIDS), and trichomoniasis. Some other infections not always transmitted sexually (scabies, candidiasis and bacterial vaginosis) are included in this chapter because they have symptoms similar to those of sexually transmitted infections.

Some sexually transmitted infections affect only a single organ, whereas others may spread throughout the body. Clinical and laboratory facilities are necessary for accurate diagnosis of sexually transmitted infections. Since such facilities are not likely to be available on board, the officer responsible for medical matters can make only a tentative diagnosis based on the symptoms.

Note

- Compared to common infections such as chicken-pox or the common cold, which are highly contagious, sexually transmitted infections are difficult to catch other than by direct sexual contact between an infected part of the patient – a skin ulcer, for example – and broken skin or internal (mucosal) surfaces, such as the rectum or pharynx, in the uninfected partner.
- Infection cannot normally be acquired through intact skin.
- Routine nursing care of a patient with a sexually transmitted infection is, therefore, not dangerous, provided gloves are worn and universal blood and body fluid precautions followed.

✔ *What to do in a case of sexually transmitted infection*

- Make a careful record of the symptoms and signs, the treatment given, and the response to treatment.
- Wear disposable gloves when examining any infected site in a patient suspected of having a sexually transmitted infection.
- If you accidentally touch a genital ulcer or discharge, or any material contaminated with pus from ulcers or a discharge, immediately wash your hands thoroughly with soap and water.
- If you have any doubt concerning diagnosis or treatment, obtain medical advice.
- If there is a sore on the penis or discharge from the tip of the penis, keep a clean gauze dressing on the penis and change the dressing frequently.
- In female patients suffering from genital ulcers or vaginal discharge, use gauze or sanitary pads.
- Discard contaminated materials in plastic bags, so that they will not be touched or handled by others.

- Have the patient examined and, if necessary, treated at a port where a specialized centre for sexually transmitted infections is available.
- If possible, trace all sexual contacts of the patient and treat them (see below) or urge them to seek medical advice.
- Urge the patient to avoid all sexual contact until a medical specialist confirms that there is no risk of transmitting infection.
- Have the patient make a special effort to practise good personal hygiene, using only personal toilet articles (toothbrush, razor, towels, washcloth, etc.), clothes, and linen.
- Use the medical examination and treatment as an opportunity to inform the patient about the condition, about sexually transmitted infections in general, and about the precautions to be taken to minimize the risk of acquiring them (see below).

Note on preventing sexually transmitted infections

- Because sailors are often outside their normal environment and in circumstances that allow for promiscuity, they are at special risk of contracting sexually transmitted infections.
- Avoiding commercial and promiscuous sex is the best way of minimizing the risk of infection.
- Failing this, a condom properly used gives heterosexual and homosexual men and women a worthwhile degree of protection against a number of sexually transmitted infections.
- Crew members should have access to a supply of condoms on board ship and when going ashore on leave.
- Some individuals develop allergy to latex, from which most condoms are made. This results in a red itchy rash on the penis after condom use. If this occurs the penis should be washed with soap and water; give cetrizine, 10 mg orally, at night if the itch disturbs the patient's sleep (do not use hydrocortisone cream on the penis).
- Latex-free condoms are readily available for those with latex allergy.
- To use a condom:
  - open the package containing the condom and unroll the condom;
  - before sexual contact, pull the condom over the tip of the erect penis, holding the tip of the condom to form a pocket to receive the ejaculated semen;
  - unroll the rest of the condom to cover the entire penis;
  - after ejaculation, withdraw the penis from the vagina before the penis softens, causing the condom to loosen and exposing the penis to possible infection;
  - remove the condom by grasping the open end and pulling it down quickly so that it comes off inside out;
  - discard the condom without handling it further, in case it contains infectious material.

URETHRITIS

Urethritis is an inflammation of the urethra, the tube from which urine is passed. It may be caused by the gonococcus (*Neisseria gonorrhoeae*) or by other organisms, most often *Chlamydia* (also called non-gonococcal urethritis).

It is not possible to tell from the symptoms whether urethritis is due to gonorrhoea or *Chlamydia*. In addition, about 25% of men who have gonococcal urethritis also have chlamydial infection without symptoms, and often other infections as well. For this reason, **treatment must always cover both gonorrhoea and chlamydial infection.**

The incubation time for gonococcal urethritis ranges from one to fourteen days but is usually two to five days.

Signs and symptoms

- Discharge from the urethra, typically abundant, yellow and creamy in gonorrhoea and scanty and watery in chlamydial infection.
- In some cases, a burning sensation and pain on urination.
- In some cases, itchiness at the opening of the urethra.
- Fever and blood in the urine are **not** signs of urethritis: if they are present, another cause should be sought.

✔ *What to do*

- In male patients, distinguish between urethritis and balanitis (see below, *Balanitis*):
  - in balanitis, there is an inflammation of the skin around the tip of the penis, which sometimes involves the opening of the urethra and causes a discharge from the tip of the penis and the prepuce, whereas in urethritis the discharge comes from within the penis;
  - if there is doubt about the source of the discharge, milking the penis from its base will produce a marked increase in the discharge in urethritis but not in balanitis.
- Give a single intramuscular injection of ceftriaxone, 250 mg, **PLUS**:
  - **EITHER** azithromycin, 1 g orally, as a single dose;
  - **OR** doxycycline, 100 mg orally, twice daily for seven days.
- For patients allergic to ceftriaxone (or to the beta-lactam class of drugs, that includes penicillin), or as an alternative if an oral treatment is preferred, give azithromycin, 2 g orally:
  - this treatment often causes nausea and vomiting.
- As a second alternative for patients infected in Africa or Europe give a single oral dose of ciprofloxacin, 500 mg, **PLUS**:
  - **EITHER** a single dose of azithromycin, 1 g orally;
  - **OR** doxycycline, 100 mg orally, twice daily for seven days; note:
    - this may not cure gonorrhoea in patients infected in Asia, Israel or North America (including Hawaii); and
    - **do not** give ciprofloxacin to women who are or may be pregnant.
- After completion of treatment, have the patient attend a specialized clinic to check for persistent infection and to be screened for syphilis and HIV infection.

URETHRITIS IN WOMEN

- In women, the same organisms that cause urethritis can cause infection of the cervix and urethra.

- If a female sexual contact of a crew member whom you have treated for urethritis is on board treat her as well, using the same drugs and doses as for men.
- In more than 60% of women with cervical or urethral infection there are no symptoms.
- In the remaining 40% of women with cervical or urethral infection the only sign is unusually copious vaginal discharge.
- Impress on the crew that these facts mean that:
  - the client of an infected female sex worker cannot know that the sex worker is infected;
  - the fact that a female sexual contact of the patient has no symptoms does not mean that she is not infected.

GONOCOCCAL PROCTITIS

Gonococcal infections of the rectum (gonococcal proctitis) can occur in both men and women. They result, in both sexes, from rectal intercourse with an infected partner or, in women, from a vaginal infection that has spread to the rectum. Many patients with gonococcal proctitis do not have urethritis. Gonococcal proctitis is associated with an increased risk of HIV infection and requires careful follow-up by a doctor.

Signs and symptoms

- Pain on passing faeces.
- Discharge of pus from the rectum, sometimes mixed with blood.

GONOCOCCAL PHARYNGITIS

The throat can also be infected with the gonococcus (gonococcal pharyngitis), usually in homosexual men and women. Most people who have this infection do not have any symptoms in the throat and do not have urethritis.

The importance of this is that **treatment for gonorrhoea should be given to a sexual contact of a patient with gonorrhoea, even if the sexual encounter involved only oral-genital sex**.

GENITAL ULCERS

Genital ulcers are common. They are caused by a wide range of sexually transmitted infections, non-infectious disorders, cancer, and trauma but the great majority are caused by three sexually transmitted infections: genital herpes (*Herpes simplex* infection), syphilis, and chancroid (*Haemophilus ducreyi* infection).

Signs and symptoms of genital ulcers

- One or more sores on or around the penis.
- Penile discharge or inability to retract the foreskin (in an uncircumcised male), suggestive of an ulcer on the glans penis or on the inside of the foreskin.

✔ *What to do in a case of genital ulcer*

- Wear disposable gloves to examine the ulcers.
- Note the number of ulcers, whether they are painful or tender, and whether there is pus in the ulcer base; note:
  - a single, painless, clean ulcer with a firm edge (a chancre) is almost certainly due to syphilis:
    - but syphilitic ulcers may also be multiple or painful or contain pus;
  - a single, painful, soft-edged ulcer with pus is almost certainly chancroid:
    - but chancroid often causes multiple ulcers;
  - multiple, shallow, clean, tender ulcers are typical of genital herpes.
- Examine the lymph nodes in the groin; note:
  - they are generally swollen in syphilis and chancroid;
  - they are generally (but not always) painless in syphilis and tender in chancroid.
- Because diagnosis is difficult and multiple infections are common, you need to treat for both syphilis and chancroid, **and also** for gonorrhoea and chlamydial infection.
- Give azithromycin, 2 g orally, in a single dose; note:
  - this will treat all common infections (except genital herpes) but often causes nausea and vomiting.
- Some patients with syphilis develop fever, malaise, and swelling of the syphilitic ulcer and of lymph nodes a few hours after treatment. This is called the Jarisch-Herxheimer reaction, and is a response to large numbers of dead bacteria. It passes quickly and is not dangerous.
- Since genital ulcers increase the risk of acquiring HIV infection, arrange for follow-up and screening for HIV.
- If the enlarged lymph nodes (buboes) of a patient with chancroid liquefy, it may be necessary to aspirate the liquid with a needle and syringe to prevent ulceration. This is best done by a doctor, but if this is impossible seek medical advice before attempting aspiration.
- There is no cure for genital herpes, but acyclovir, 400 mg orally, three times daily for seven days can shorten episodes, reduce the likelihood of repeated episodes, and interrupt spread of the infection, BUT:
  - treatment **must** begin within 24 hours of the first symptoms to be of any use;
  - it is not usually possible to start treatment this early in the first episode of genital herpes, but treatment of recurrent episodes is worthwhile if they come to attention early.

Note on syphilis

- Untreated, a genital ulcer (chancre) of primary (first stage) syphilis will heal in a few weeks. The patient will think that the infection is cured, but in about 25% of patients it continues and within a few weeks or months secondary (second stage) syphilis develops.
- Occasionally, secondary syphilis occurs without a primary chancre having been noticed (for example, if it was under the foreskin).

- Secondary syphilis causes:
  - fever, headache, and feeling unwell;
  - a rash consisting of red spots or blotches, 0.5–2 cm across, found on the **whole** body, **including** the palms of the hands and soles of the feet;
  - rashes with this distribution are likely to be syphilis.
- Secondary syphilis is treated in the same way as primary syphilis.
- As with primary syphilis, secondary syphilis resolves without treatment; but again, untreated, the infection continues, leading to "latent syphilis" and to the possibility of complications affecting the heart and major blood vessels or the brain and spinal cord.

ACUTE PAIN IN THE SCROTUM

Among ships' crews most episodes of acute scrotal pain are the result of epididymitis, or inflammation of the epididymis, the duct in which sperm are stored. Pain in the scrotum can also occur with testicular torsion, a blow to the testicles, and mumps (see below).

Epididymitis

Epididymitis in younger men is caused by sexually transmitted organisms, most often *Chlamydia* but occasionally the gonococcus. It can sometimes occur after prolonged sitting (as on long plane flights) or bicycle riding, but it is safer to regard all cases of epididymitis as due to infection and to treat accordingly.

In older men, and in men who practice receptive anal intercourse, epididymitis is more often due to the same bacteria that cause urinary tract infections, and associated with prostatitis (see Chapter 17, *Kidney and other urinary disorders*).

Signs and symptoms

- If associated with prostatitis:
  - onset usually over a 24–48-hour period
  - severe pain in the epididymis (behind and above the testicles)
  - marked swelling and tenderness of the scrotum
  - high fever.
- If due to *Chlamydia*:
  - onset gradual
  - fever absent or mild
  - scrotal swelling mild
  - tenderness of the epididymis mild or moderate.

✔ *What to do*

- In mild illness, treat as for urethritis (see above).
- In severe, acute illness give ciprofloxacin, 500 mg orally, twice daily for 28 days.

Testicular torsion

Epididymitis must be distinguished from testicular torsion, which is caused by the testicle twisting on the spermatic cord. The spermatic cord carries the sperm duct, blood and lymph vessels, nerves, and other structures from the abdomen to the scrotum. The result of the torsion is that these blood vessels and other structures are twisted and blocked. The testicle is pulled upwards and lies with its long axis parallel to the ground rather than pointing downwards. The blood supply to the testis is blocked and the testis can die within a few hours if the blockage is not removed. This condition occurs most frequently in children and adolescents and is less common in adults.

Signs and symptoms

- Marked swelling and extreme tenderness of the testis.
- In many cases, fluid collection around the testis.

What to do

- Seek medical advice with a view to urgent evacuation: surgical treatment is needed and a delay longer than 12 hours is likely to result in loss of the testicle.
- If urgent evacuation is not possible, you may be able to untwist the cord manually: seek medical advice before attempting this.
- Apply ice packs to the scrotum and give pain-killing medication appropriate to the severity of pain (see Chapter 3, *Pain management*).

Trauma to the scrotum

Trauma to the scrotum, due to a kick or falling astride a beam or pipe, is common. Severe injury to the testicle, however, is rare, even with high-impact blows.

What to do

- Have the patient rest and use scrotal support.

Testicular inflammation (orchitis)

The only common cause of testicular inflammation without inflammation of the cord or epididymis is mumps (see Chapter 23, *Infectious diseases*).

BALANITIS

Balanitis is an inflammation of the skin around the tip of the penis, sometimes involving the opening of the urethra. Poor hygiene in uncircumcised males is usually the cause, although the presence of diabetes mellitus may play a role.

Signs and symptoms

- Mild-to-profuse discharge at the tip of the penis.
- Itching and irritation.
- Swelling of the penis in some cases, especially after repeated episodes of balanitis, making retraction of the foreskin difficult and painful (phimosis).
- Redness of the skin at the tip of the penis, sometimes with scaling or small breaks in the skin.

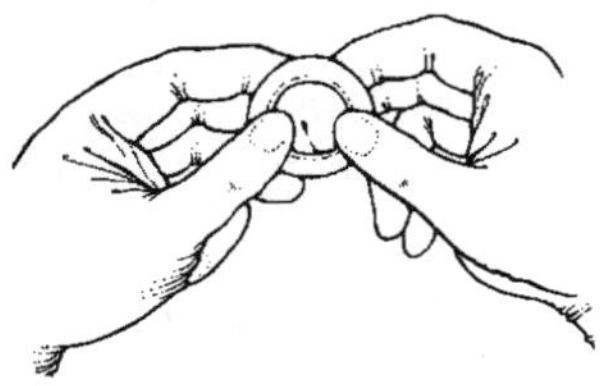

Figure 19.1 How to retract the foreskin.

✔ *What to do*

- Wearing disposable gloves, retract the foreskin (Figure 19.1) in order to determine the origin of the secretion and distinguish between balanitis and urethritis.
- In balanitis, there is an inflammation of the skin around the tip of the penis, which sometimes involves the opening of the urethra and causes a discharge from the tip of the penis and the prepuce, whereas in urethritis the discharge comes from within the penis.
- If there is doubt about the source of the discharge, milking the penis from its base will produce a marked increase in the discharge in urethritis but not in balanitis.
- If the penis is swollen, do not try to retract the foreskin by force: you may not be able to replace it because of the swelling and this can cause a blockage of blood flow to the tip of the penis.
- If you are unable to retract the foreskin because of scarring, symptoms are likely to persist, and you should have the patient see a doctor as soon as convenient.
- Have the patient wash the glans and foreskin thoroughly with water three times a day.
- Have the patient apply 2% miconazole cream twice daily for two weeks.
- If there is no improvement within a week or there are repeated episodes, have the patient see a doctor at the next port.

LYMPH NODE SWELLING IN THE GROIN

The lymph nodes in the groin can be enlarged as a result of infection or of a disease in a lower limb or in the scrotum. Table 19.1 lists the sexually transmitted infections that cause lymph node swelling and the corresponding clinical characteristics of the swelling.

✔ *What to do*

- Retract the foreskin.
- If you see genital ulcers or scars of genital ulcers, proceed as described above for *Genital ulcers*.
- Consider whether the lump could really be a hernia (see Chapter 16, *Gastrointestinal and liver diseases*). Ask the patient to cough: if the swelling gets bigger, it is a hernia.

Table 19.1 Sexually transmitted infections causing lymph node swelling.

Disease	Characteristics of swelling
Chancroid	Painful, tender, sometimes suppurating
Genital herpes	Tender
Primary syphilis	Rubbery, painless
Secondary syphilis	Rubbery, painless, generalized
Lymphogranuloma venereum	Not felt as separate lumps, sometimes painful, sometimes suppurating, often divided by inguinal ligament, with one swelling above the ligament (the groin fold) and one below
AIDS	Usually painless, generalized

VAGINAL DISCHARGE

A change in the amount, colour or odour of vaginal secretions is a very common complaint in women. It does not always indicate an abnormality. The commonest cause is inflammation of the vagina (vaginitis) and the commonest cause of vaginitis is replacement of the normal bacterial population of the vagina with bacteria not normally found there (bacterial vaginosis).

Infections with *Trichomonas* (a protozoan) and with *Candida* (a yeast) are also very common. The organisms that cause urethritis (the gonococcus and *Chlamydia*) can infect the cervix in women, producing a white or yellow watery discharge. However, most women with gonorrhoea and chlamydial infection have no symptoms. Infection with herpes virus usually produces painful reddish blisters and ulcers on the area around the vagina (vulva). More than one infection may be present.

Fever and abdominal pain are not present in vaginitis, and an unusual vaginal discharge suggests urinary tract infection or pelvic inflammatory disease (see below).

Bacterial vaginosis

A bacterial infection of the vagina (vaginosis) is commonest in women with new or multiple sexual partners but can also occur in women who have never had sexual intercourse.

Signs and symptoms

- Abnormal discharge, usually grey, sometimes of foam- or paste-like consistency and fishy odour.
- Itching around the vagina.
- Burning on urination (dysuria) in some cases.

Vaginal candidiasis

A yeast infection of the vagina (vaginal candidiasis) is very common, particularly in pregnant women. It is not sexually acquired. It often follows a course of antibiotics given for another infection and may be a clue to the presence of diabetes mellitus.

Signs and symptoms

- Severe itch and soreness over the whole vulva.
- Redness and swelling of the vulva.
- Discharge usually absent, but if present it is white and semi-solid, resembling cottage cheese.

Trichomoniasis

Trichomoniasis is almost always sexually acquired. Male sexual partners are infected, but they have no symptoms and the infection eventually disappears without treatment.

Signs and symptoms

- A thin, foul-smelling discharge from the vagina, sometimes frothy and yellow-green.
- Burning and itching around the vagina.

✔ What to do

- Give metronidazole, 2 g orally, in a single dose; this will treat trichomoniasis and bacterial vaginosis.
- Give the woman's male sexual partner, if available, metronidazole, 2 g orally, in a single dose.
- Advise patients to abstain from alcohol for 48 hours after treatment with metronidazole.
- If there is no improvement or if symptoms are severe, treat candidiasis, by having the patient apply miconazole cream, 5 g daily for seven days, to the vulva and vagina.
- If these symptoms occur in a woman who is a sexual contact of a patient whom you have treated for urethritis, treat her for gonorrhoea and *Chlamydia*, as described above for *Urethritis*.

PELVIC INFLAMMATORY DISEASE

Pelvic inflammatory disease is a general term covering infections of the pelvic organs in women. The infections are caused by microbes in the vagina that have invaded the normally sterile inner surface of the uterus, fallopian tubes, or ovaries. Pelvic inflammatory disease usually begins with a gonococcal or chlamydial infection but at a later stage several organisms may be present. The illness caused by pelvic inflammatory disease ranges in severity from mild pain and low fever to life-threatening peritonitis. Without facilities for gynaecological examination and laboratory analysis, it is difficult to differentiate this disease from other causes of acute abdominal pain.

► Signs and symptoms

- Mild-to-severe lower abdominal pain and tenderness
- fever
- vaginal discharge.

✔ What to do

- Seek medical advice.
- If you suspect pelvic inflammatory disease, give:
  - ceftriaxone, 250 mg intramuscularly, in a single dose; **AND**
  - azithromycin, 1 g orally, in a single dose; **AND**
  - **EITHER** doxycyline, 100 mg orally, twice daily for 14 days;
  - **OR** amoxycillin/clavulanate, 875 mg orally, twice daily for seven to 10 days.
- If there is no improvement in two to three days, evacuation is likely to be needed.
- If male sexual partners of women with pelvic inflammatory disease can be traced, suggest they be tested or treated for gonorrhoea and chlamydial infection (see above).
- Suggest that women with pelvic inflammatory disease be screened for other sexually transmitted infections, especially HIV.

ANO-GENITAL WARTS

Ano-genital warts are caused by the human papilloma virus and occur most frequently in young adults. In males they can appear on the penis, around the anus, and in the rectum. In females, the usual sites of infection are the vulva, the area surrounding the anus, and the vagina.

Signs and symptoms

- Soft, flesh-coloured, broad-based or pedunculated (on stems) warts of variable size, often with a cauliflower-like appearance; note that:
  - there may be only a single wart or many warts forming a large coalesced mass.
- Ulceration, secondary infection, and, with very large warts, bleeding.

✔ *What to do*

- Since treatment can be prolonged and requires appropriate equipment and expertise not generally available on board, have the patient see a doctor at the next port where appropriate medical facilities are available.

PUBIC LICE (see Chapter 20, *Skin diseases*)

ACQUIRED IMMUNODEFICIENCY SYNDROME (AIDS)

The acquired immunodeficiency syndrome (AIDS), first recognized in 1981, has become a major public health problem throughout the world. In Western Europe and North America, the disease has been observed mainly in male homosexuals and intravenous drug users. In central, eastern and southern Africa and in some countries in the Caribbean, it is seen primarily in heterosexuals. AIDS is caused by the human immunodeficiency virus (HIV), which damages the immune system. Most AIDS-related diseases are due to loss of immune cells and a consequent lowering of immune defences. The virus can also infect specific organs directly, notably the brain.

- Nearly all cases of HIV infection result from contact with the semen, vaginal and cervical secretions, blood, or blood products of a person infected with the virus.
- HIV cannot be transmitted through social or workplace contact with an infected individual and there are no documented cases of transmission through kissing.
- The risk of acquiring HIV infection after a single episode of sexual intercourse with a person infected with HIV, but without a condom, is about 1/1000 for vaginal or insertive anal intercourse and about 2/100 for receptive anal intercourse.
- The risk if acquiring HIV after rape by a person infected with HIV is higher than after consensual intercourse, but still less than a few per cent.

Signs and symptoms of acute (primary) HIV infection

- Within two to four weeks after infection and over a 24–48-hour period, onset of an illness lasting 10–14 days and consisting of:

  - fever
  - nausea
  - loss of appetite
  - headache, often behind the eyes and made worse by eye movement
  - sore throat
  - non-tender enlarged lymph nodes in the neck.
- The acute stage of HIV infection lasts 10–14 days: it is usually disabling and many patients describe it as the "worst flu they have ever had".
- It is important to recognize this illness as an HIV infection, because patients are at their most infectious at this time: being unaware of having an HIV infection, they may continue high-risk behaviour and infect others.

Later stages of HIV and AIDS

- After the acute illness, the infection enters a latent period lasting between six months and several years.
- During the latent period, the only abnormality may be enlarged lymph nodes, but loss of immune cells continues.
- After the latent period most infected patients enter a phase formerly called "AIDS-related Complex" or ARC and now called Class B infection.
- During the period of Class B infection, patients are abnormally prone to acquire infections, but these are infections that also occur in healthy people, so that firm diagnosis can only be made by laboratory tests.
- After an average interval of 10 years, damage to the immune system is extensive enough to allow infections that rarely affect healthy people (called *opportunistic infections*) to occur: this is the condition called AIDS.
- The commonest infections in AIDS patients in developed countries are a form of pneumonia caused by an organism called *Pneumocystis carinii* and *Candida* infection of the oesophagus. Neither of these infections can spread to healthy people.
- Tuberculosis is very common in AIDS patients in poor countries, and it can infect healthy people who come in contact with it.
- Once AIDS has developed, life expectancy is one to two years on average.
- About 5% of HIV-infected individuals show no evidence of disease progression at all.
- About 20% of HIV-infected individuals survive more than 20 years.

Treatment of HIV Infection

- Since 1996, relatively effective drug treatment has become possible for HIV infection. For many, if not most, patients who receive the treatment, the infection has turned from an acute into a chronic condition.
- Treatment is usually begun when damage to the immune system has reached a potentially dangerous level. There is, at present, no evidence that treatment at the time of the early or acute stage of the infection is useful.
- Cure of HIV infection is not possible with current treatment, which calls for constant monitoring of the patient's response and strict adherence to treatment.

Post-exposure prophylaxis

- Drugs effective against HIV, given soon after exposure or suspected exposure to the virus, are believed to lower the risk of HIV infection.
- If a caregiver or any other person on board has been exposed to the blood of a patient not known to be free of HIV infection, or has been raped by someone not known to be free of HIV infection, see *Needle-stick injuries*, in Chapter 23, *Infectious diseases*.

Skin diseases

Many diseases can affect the skin. A patient with a skin problem should, therefore, be questioned about his or her general state of health and, if necessary, an appropriate examination should be made.

Some skin diseases remain localized. Others may spread without the patient realizing it. It is always essential to inspect all of the patient's skin.

The following questions may help in identifying the underlying disease. However, there are many skin diseases and a good number are uncommon.

Consider sending a digital photograph by e-mail to an onshore medical facility together with a completed medical history form (see Chapter 25, *External assistance*). Seek medical advice before taking photographs on the best way to use the photographic equipment you have available and the best way to transmit the image. In order to compare images, ships with Internet access may find it useful to consult one of the many online atlases of skin diseases, such as *http://dermatlas.org/derm/*.

QUESTIONS TO ASK A PATIENT

- When did the skin problem first appear?
- What did it look like at first and how has it changed since?
- Where on your body did it first appear?
- Is it still in the same place?
- Does it affect any other part of your body?
- Have you used any treatments?
- Did the treatments make the problem better or worse?
- Is there any itching?
- Is there any pain?
- Does anyone you have regular contact with have a similar problem?
- Have you ever had this kind of skin problem before?
- If so, how long did it last?
- Are you doing anything different now that might expose you to anything new, including:
    - medications
    - soaps and detergents
    - shaving cream
    - deodorants
    - perfumes
    - different work
    - new hobbies or sports?

BARBER'S RASH

Barber's rash covers several conditions affecting the beard area. These conditions need to be distinguished from one another, and from acne.

Folliculitis

This is an infection of the hair roots (follicles) of the beard area that spreads from person to person via shared razors or shaving brushes.

Signs and symptoms

- Rash consisting of red spots, each spot centred on a hair follicle, some with a bead of pus around the hair.

Pseudofolliculitis (also called "razor bumps")

This inflammation of the skin (not the hair follicles) occurs mainly in men who shave frequently, particularly black men and men with thick, curly beards. It is due to hairs curling over and re-entering the skin, causing inflammation. Shaving makes the hairs sharper and more able to penetrate the skin.

Signs and symptoms

- Rash similar to folliculitis (above).
- The neck often more severely affected than the cheeks or lips, and in white men often the only area affected.
- The rash is often itchy at first, and scratching can lead to secondary infection with bacteria.
- Close inspection reveals curved hairs re-entering the skin.

✔ *What to do in cases of folliculitis and pseudofolliculitis*

- Advise the patient to stop shaving for at least one month, and to keep facial hair short only by clipping with scissors.
- In a case of folliculitis:
  - the patient can resume shaving when the rash has cleared, using a new razor or the same one after the cutting head has been sterilized in boiling water;
  - advise the patient not to share razors or towels with other crew members.
- In a case of pseudofolliculitis:
  - if the patient does not wish to grow a beard advise him to let the beard grow to 5 mm or longer before resuming shaving, and then to shave as infrequently as possible (longer hairs are less likely to curve over and re-enter the skin);
  - hairs cut by an electric razor are less sharp than those cut by a blade and less likely to re-enter the skin;
  - advise the patient to search the beard area after shaving, preferably using a magnifying mirror, and to use fine tweezers to pluck out any hairs re-entering the skin before inflammation develops.
- If there is secondary infection (i.e. a new infection caused, for example, by the patient scratching an itchy rash):
  - give doxycyline, 100 mg twice daily, for five days, note:
    - › if there is no secondary infection, antibiotic treatment is of no value in folliculitis or pseudofolliculitis.

Tinea barbae

This is a fungal infection of the beard area that often occurs in men who have a beard and do not shave.

Signs and symptoms

- Rash of pustules in a limited area;
- greater redness and scaling than in folliculitis and pseudofolliculitis (above);
- very itchy.

What to do in a case of tinea barbae

- Have the patient apply miconazole cream twice daily until the rash disappears.

ACNE

Acne (acne vulgaris) is probably the commonest of skin conditions. It is due to blockage and inflammation of the sebaceous glands of the skin, which produce sebum, an oily lubricant for skin and hair.

Although acne occurs to some degree in nearly everyone during adolescence, severe acne should not be neglected, since it can lead to severe scarring and pigment changes, especially in dark-skinned individuals.

Signs and symptoms

- Whiteheads, or clogged hair follicles beneath the skin.
- Later, blackheads, clogged hair follicles reaching to the skin surface.
- Blackheads occur only in acne vulgaris and so are important for diagnosis.
- Inflamed sebaceous glands:
  - due to overgrowth of *Propionibacterium acnes*, a bacterium that normally inhabits the skin surface.
- Pustules and nodules:
  - due to rupture of a blocked sebaceous gland within the skin and spread of inflammation into the skin close to the ruptured gland; BUT
  - no redness of the skin between the pustules – another important diagnostic sign.

What to do

- Have the patient seek medical advice at an appropriate time if the acne is severe or the appearance of the rash unacceptable.

CHAPS

Chaps are cracks on the backs of the hands, feet, lips, ears, or other parts of the body. They are caused by exposure to cold wind or salt water, or by washing in cold weather without the skin being dried properly.

Signs and symptoms

- Irritation and pain.

What to do

- Have the patient smear the affected parts with a copious layer of petroleum jelly.
- Have the patient wear gloves when exposed to the elements.
- See *Cold exposure injuries* in Chapter 28, *Medical care for survivors at sea*.

DERMATITIS

Most cases of dermatitis seen on board ship arise from irritation of the skin by substances that have been handled or misused. Occasionally, the cause is allergy.

DO NOT allow the use of "medicated" soaps containing disinfectants or antiseptics in any form of dermatitis. Use only plain soap, preferably of pure vegetable origin.

Irritant contact dermatitis

Dermatitis due to contact with an irritant involves physical or chemical damage to the skin. It can affect anyone and can occur the first time a person uses the substance. The hands, especially the webs between the fingers, are nearly always affected first and most severely.

Common irritants that cause dermatitis include:

- detergents
- soap
- bleaches
- cleaning powders
- solvents
- oil
- petrol
- kerosene
- paraffin.

Note

- Using petrol or kerosene to clean grease or paint from the hands is a common cause of irritant dermatitis and should be discouraged.
- A substance, for instance a detergent, with which the patient has been in contact for some time without any adverse effect, may suddenly become an irritant.
- Rubber glove dermatitis is an irritant dermatitis caused by prolonged exposure of the hands to detergents and moisture inside the gloves followed by repeated harsh drying.

Signs and symptoms

- Diffuse redness of the affected skin;
- small blisters on the reddened area that later break, releasing a watery, yellowish fluid which forms crusts;

- in most cases, severe itch;
- skin of the hands often cracked and painful.

✔ *What to do*

- Advise the patient to avoid contact with a known cause of irritation.
- If you suspect allergy because of a previous medical test or because the reaction occurs regardless of the amount of exposure, have the patient smear a small amount of 1% hydrocortisone ointment on the affected part three times daily **but for no more than 10 days**.
- In cold climates, if the patient's exposed skin often becomes dry and itchy, tell the patient to:
  - avoid repeated hand washing with soap;
  - use alcohol-based cleansers, if possible;
  - avoid washing and bathing in hot water.

Eczema (atopic dermatitis)

Most patients with eczema are first affected before the age of seven: a skin problem appearing for the first time in an adult is, therefore, not likely to be eczema. Most patients with eczema are allergic to several things in their environment, any of which can trigger an episode of eczema. Secondary bacterial infection is very common in eczema.

► *Signs and symptoms*

- A red, very itchy rash, with scales and crusts;
- neck, elbows, and back of the knee most affected;
- armpits and groin not affected.

✔ *What to do*

- If the patient's rash is troublesome, apply a 1% hydrocortisone ointment three times daily **but for no more than 10 days**.
- Advise the patient to see a doctor when convenient, because long-term or frequent treatment with steroid ointments and creams may have adverse effects on the skin.

Allergic contact dermatitis

To cause allergic contact dermatitis, the allergen, i.e. the substance causing the allergy, must come into direct contact with the patient's skin (unlike eczema, in which direct contact is not necessary to cause the allergy). Moreover, the allergic reaction takes longer to develop – from two days to two weeks – compared with hours or days in eczema.

Common causes of allergic contact dermatitis are poison ivy, mango skin, nickel (found in cheap jewellery), perfumes, and preservatives. Allergic contact dermatitis goes away over a period of two to four weeks if the patient can avoid contact with the allergen.

► *Signs and symptoms*

- Red, itchy rash;
- pattern of distribution of rash clearly related to the area of skin contact with the allergen.

✔ What to do

- To relieve symptoms, apply a 1% hydrocortisone ointment three times daily **but for no more than 10 days**.

FUNGAL SKIN INFECTIONS

Several types of fungi can affect different parts of the skin. The fungi feed on keratin, the protein that makes up dead skin, nails, and hair. The fungi live only on these dead tissues and do not invade living tissues. Untreated, the disease persists indefinitely.

Tinea pedis (athlete's foot)

Athelete's foot is a fungal infection of the skin of the feet. It spreads in community, or group, showers or in other wet areas where people walk barefoot: infected individuals shed fungi on the floor and others become infected.

► Signs and symptoms

- Rash, often appearing suddenly and often after heavy exercise that has caused the feet to sweat.
- Rash, slowly expanding over weeks or months.
- Red, scaly, very itchy skin between the toes:
  - especially between the fourth and fifth toes, with possible spread to other toe webs and also to the tops and soles of the feet.

✔ What to do

- Have the patient apply miconazole cream twice daily.
- If the infection affects only the skin between toes, one week of treatment may be enough.
- If the soles or tops of the feet are affected, continue treatment for four weeks.
- Tell the patient to avoid sweating of the feet by wearing sandals, using talcum powder, and changing socks frequently to keep the feet dry.

Tinea corporis (ringworm)

Ringworm can occur alone or accompany a fungal infection elsewhere in the body. Ringworm can spread by close direct contact.

► Signs and symptoms

- A roughly ring-shaped reddish rash, often on exposed areas of the arms, legs, face, or trunk.
- Healing at the centre, leaving a rim of red, scaly, itchy skin a few millimetres wide.

✔ What to do

- Have the patient apply miconazole cream to the affected skin for two to three weeks.

Tinea cruris (Jock itch, Dhobie itch)

Jock itch is a fungal infection of the groin. It often begins after heavy exercise that has caused the groin to sweat. It is much commoner in men than in women, and especially common in obese men. Tinea pedis is usually present as well.

Signs and symptoms

- An itchy, red, scaly patch of skin, first appearing on the inner thigh at the level of the scrotum then, if untreated, spreading downwards over the thigh and upwards onto the abdomen.
- Central healing as patch grows, leaving a red, scaly, itchy line over the upper thigh and lower abdomen.

What to do

- Have the patient apply miconazole or a similar antifungal cream twice daily for two weeks, not only in the area of the groin but also on the feet (otherwise the rash will return when treatment stops).
- Have the patient keep the groin dry with talcum powder and avoid close-fitting underwear.

BACTERIAL SKIN INFECTIONS

Impetigo

This is an infection of the skin that occurs most frequently in warm, humid settings. Crowding and poor personal hygiene often play a role. Impetigo usually begins as an infection of a minor scratch, burn or insect bite on the face or arms. The infection can spread to several parts of the body and to other people coming into close contact.

Signs and symptoms

- Appearance of a thin-walled blister, which soon bursts and becomes covered with a thick honey-coloured crust;
- no fever or pain;
- rapid spread of sores, especially over the beard area of face and neck.

What to do

- To prevent the infection spreading, tell the patient not to touch the sores.
- If the face is affected, advise the patient not to shave.
- Remove the crusts on the sores by washing and gentle scrubbing with one part povidone-iodine to 10 parts potable water.
- Have the patient use only disposable paper tissues or towels.
- Ensure that the patient's bedding, clothing, and equipment likely to have been in contact with the sores are thoroughly boiled after use.
- Have the patient wash the hands thoroughly after touching the affected area.

- Use a dry dressing to protect sores on the hands or any part of the body covered by clothing and change the dressing frequently.
- Leave sores on the face uncovered.
- If the area affected is large give azithromycin, 250 mg orally, daily for six days.

Carbuncles and furuncles (furunculosis)

Carbuncles and furuncles are bacterial infections of hair follicles. A furuncle is a single affected follicle and a carbuncle is a group of several follicles close to one another. The infections appear most commonly in the armpits, face, and the back of the neck. They are spread by close contact and often occur when personal hygiene is poor. Patients with recurrent infections often carry the causative bacterium (*Staphylococcus aureus*) in their noses.

Signs and symptoms

- Painful red nodules, usually covered with broken skin, from which pus trickles;
- in most cases, no fever or malaise.

✔ What to do

- Apply warm wet compresses to promote drainage of pus: often no other treatment is necessary.
- If the patient is feverish or has extensive lesions, give amoxycillin/clavulanate, 875 mg orally, twice daily.
- Have the patient pay careful attention to personal hygiene.
- Patients with repeated episodes of furunculosis may be carrying the responsible organism in their nose, and cure may require special antibiotics: have them see a doctor when convenient.

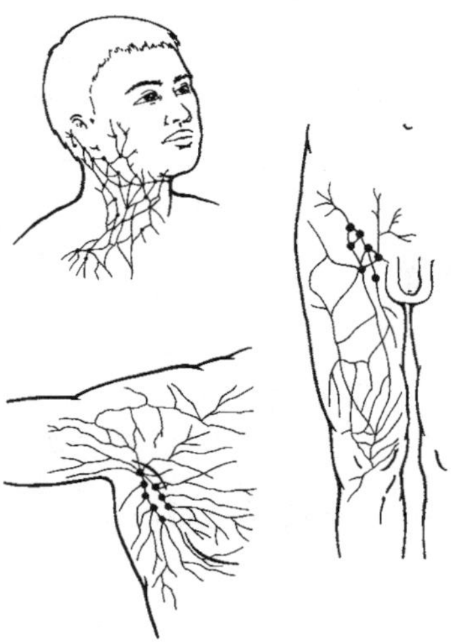

Figure 20.1 Lymph nodes in the neck, groin and axilla.

SKIN ABSCESS

Abscesses in the skin are spaces filled with pus. They are the result of a bacterial infection that goes deeper into the skin than an infection of hair follicles. Pain, swelling and tenderness are more severe than in carbuncles and furuncles, and the patient often has fever and feels unwell. The commonest sites for abscesses are in the armpit, the groin, and near the anus.

Signs and symptoms

- At first, a red, hot, hard, very tender swelling;
- after a day or two, swelling filled with pus and increasingly painful;
- skin stretched thinly over the swelling and often purplish in colour;
- the swelling "gives" slightly when pressed;
- usually a rise in temperature to 38–40 °C;
- swelling around the abscess;
- lymph nodes draining the area enlarged and painful (Figures 20.1, 20.2).

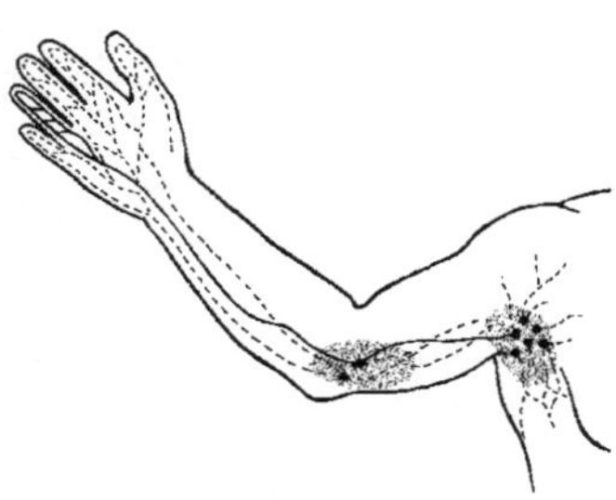

Figure 20.2 Lymphangitis caused by an infected wound on the finger.

✔ What to do

- Have the patient rest and apply hot-water compresses to the abscess area:
  - the patient can use hot saline solution (two level teaspoonfuls of table salt to one litre of tap water), at a temperature of around 45°C, for the compresses;
  - if the compresses are too hot for you to handle comfortably, they are too hot for the patient.
- If you cannot feel the movement of pus in the abscess when you press gently on it and if the patient has a fever, give:
- amoxycillin/clavulanate, 875/125 mg orally, twice daily; **OR**
  - if the patient is allergic to penicillin, give azithromycin, 500 mg orally, once daily.
- As soon as you can feel the presence of pus, cut the abscess (see section below, *How to incise and drain a pus-filled abscess*) and drain the pus from it.

✗ What not to do

- Do not wait for the abscess to burst.
- Do not give antibiotics for abscesses that have been drained or are ready to drain, except for:
  - abscesses in the area between the bridge of the nose and the corner of the mouth (see next point);
  - abscesses in the palm of the hand (see second point below).
- **DO NOT INCISE** abscesses in the area between the bridge of the nose and the corner of the mouth: there is a danger of infection spreading to blood vessels around the brain, with serious consequences:
  - treat with warm compresses and antibiotics;
  - seek medical advice.
- **DO NOT INCISE** abscesses on the palm of the hand: you can easily damage important structures; also, the abscess may spread and drainage will be difficult to achieve without anaesthesia:
  - treat with warm compresses and antibiotics;
  - seek medical advice.

How to incise and drain a pus-filled abscess

- Assemble the following items:
  - gloves, preferably sterile;
  - morphine, 10 mg for injection, if the abscess is causing severe pain;
  - equipment for intramuscular injection;
  - local anaesthetic (lignocaine 1%, 5 ml) and injection equipment;
  - a scalpel;
  - tissue forceps;
  - dressing forceps.
- Boil these instruments for 20 minutes.

- Place the sterilized instruments (with the water drained off) on a clean towel and allow them to cool.
- Assemble the following items:
  - a bowl of povidone-iodine;
  - cotton wool swabs;
  - a bowl to collect the pus;
  - a container for disposal of soiled swabs and dressings;
  - a 30 cm strip of sterile ribbon gauze.
- If the abscess is in the armpit, groin, or neck **make sure you are familiar with the location of major blood vessels and nerves in the area**: seek medical advice if necessary.
- Wash your hands.
- Have an assistant arrange the patient so that he is comfortable and the abscess is in a good light.
- Put on the gloves.
- If the abscess is causing severe pain, give morphine, 10 mg intramuscularly, and wait 15 minutes.
- Inspect the area and decide where to make the incision:
  - you should make the incision at the site where you can feel the greatest amount of pus under the skin;
  - since blood vessels and nerves generally run vertically, a vertical incision is less likely than a horizontal (or transverse) incision to cut a vessel or nerve: (an anal abscess is an exception, see next point);
  - in the case of an abscess near the anus, the incision should be made as close as possible to the anus itself.
- Paint the abscess and a wide area of skin around it with povidone-iodine solution **and wait for it to dry**.
- Inject lignocaine under the skin along the line you have chosen for the incision and wait 5 minutes.
- Take a scalpel and make a single incision at least 1.5 cm long in the area you anesthetized:
  - **do not make a cross incision.**
- If the abscess is on an arm or leg, have your assistant hold the limb steady.
- Pus should drain freely from the incision.
- If pus does not drain freely from the incision, wrap gauze around a pair of forceps and carefully probe the abscess (this may be very painful); note:
  - do not probe an abscess either with your finger, in case there is a foreign body inside it, or with a scalpel.
- Withdraw the forceps and, with a swab in each hand, press gently on each side of the abscess to help evacuation of the pus; note:
  - vigorous squeezing is unnecessary and may spread infection.
- Use dressing forceps to pick up a length of sterile ribbon gauze and insert it into the wound.

- Pack the gauze in lightly and leave a length of about 10 cm on the surface of the wound; note:
  - the object is to keep the wound open so that it drains and heals from the bottom up.
- Clean the skin area with a sterile swab.
- Apply a gauze dressing.
- Check the wound after 24 hours, by which time all the pus should have drained out and the pain and tenderness should be much less severe. If this is not the case, you have probably not drained all the abscess cavities.
- Remove the ribbon gauze drain after 48 hours.
- Have the patient apply warm, wet compresses to the wound four times a day to keep the abscess cavity open:
  - in the case of an abscess near the anus, instead of warm compresses, have the patient sit in a warm bath or use a hand-held shower.
- Since an anal fistula can develop following an anal abscess, **have the patient see a doctor at the next port**.
- After a further 48 hours, if there is only a slight discharge, if the patient is free from pain, and if the temperature is normal, apply a simple gauze dressing to the wound and change it daily until the wound heals (usually in seven to 10 days).
- If fever, local redness, pain, or swelling returns, re-open the wound and drain the abscess again.

PEDICULOSIS (LICE INFESTATION)

HEAD AND BODY LICE

Lice live on the outside of the body, often in clothing, but feed on blood by biting. The bites cause itching, usually around the trunk and neck. Scratching may lead to secondary infection.

✔ *What to do*

- Maintain personal hygiene by bathing and by laundering clothing and bedding frequently.
- Keep cabins clean by vacuuming floors, rugs, and upholstered furniture weekly.
- Watch for and eliminate lice introduced with luggage, clothing, bedding, or furniture.
- Have the patient wash thoroughly.
- To relieve itching, have the patient apply a 1% hydrocortisone cream three times daily **but for no more than 10 days**.
- Hot-wash and dry, or dry-clean, all clothing and bedding.
- To treat head lice:
  - have the patient use a lotion containing permethrin 1%; note:
    - lindane is not effective against head lice;
    - crew members do not need to be isolated once treatment has been given;
    - eggs are not always killed: after seven days give a second treatment.

PUBIC LICE

Pubic lice are usually transmitted by sexual contact or other forms of close contact.

Signs and symptoms

- Moderate-to-severe itching, mainly in the pubic area, but sometimes also in the armpits.
- Redness, irritation, and bleeding from scratching.
- Lice can be seen as small brown spots in the groin or around the genitals and anus.
- Nits (louse eggs) attached to hairs are visible through a magnifying glass.

✔ *What to do*

- Apply permethrin lotion to dry hair and massage it into the hair for four minutes.
- Add small amounts of water to the hair until a lather forms, then rinse the hair thoroughly and comb it with a fine-tooth comb to remove the nits.
- Treat all close contacts (especially sexual contacts) of the patient at the same time to prevent reinfection.
- Machine-wash sheets, towels, and clothing and dry them in a hot tumble dryer or have them dry-cleaned.

SCABIES

Scabies is caused by the mite *Sarcoptes scabiei*. It is spread mainly by close contact, often sexual, but also by indirect contact, such as hot-bunking.

Signs and symptoms

- Itching:
  - between the fingers
  - under the wrist
  - at the back of the elbows
  - in the axillary folds (skin folds at the base of armpits)
  - around the navel
  - on the penis, scrotum, buttocks, and the back of the upper thighs
  - not usually on the back of the head.
- Itching often severe and worse at night.
- The skin looks normal except for scratch marks.
- If more than one crew member is affected with severe itching in normal looking skin a diagnosis of scabies can be made with certainty.

✔ *What to do*

- Have the patient apply a thin layer of permethrin lotion, 1%, to the entire trunk and extremities and leave it on for 8–12 hours.

- At the end of this period, have the patient take a shower or a bath, and change clothes and bed linen.
- Apply treatment to any close contacts on board.

SHINGLES (HERPES ZOSTER AND VARICELLA ZOSTER) (see Chapter 23, *Infectious diseases*)

URTICARIA (HIVES)

Urticaria are welts, or swellings, that can appear on any area of the skin. Common causes are drugs (especially penicillin and related drugs), foods (most often fish, shellfish, and nuts), insect stings, and latex (in surgical gloves and condoms). In about two-thirds of cases urticaria occurs once or as a series of attacks over a few weeks. In the remaining third of cases, episodes continue to occur for months or years.

Signs and symptoms

- Reddish or pinkish, extremely itchy raised areas (welts) on the skin that quickly expand, then disappear after a few hours, leaving no trace except scratch marks.
- Itching is often severe enough to interfere with sleep and work.

✔ *What to do*

- To alleviate the itching, give cetirizine, 10 mg orally, twice daily until the urticaria subsides; **NOTE**:
  - this drug may cause drowsiness; while taking it the patient should not:
    - operate machinery
    - take watch
    - consume alcohol.

CELLULITIS AND ERYSIPELAS

CELLULITIS

Cellulitis is a potentially serious bacterial infection of the skin that can occur in almost any part of the body but most often on the face or lower legs. In many patients, cellulitis appears at the site of a minor skin wound, scratch or insect bite: instead of remaining localized, the infection spreads. It may be superficial but can also affect the tissues lying under the skin and can even spread to lymph nodes and the blood stream. Cellulitis can be very difficult to cure and many patients have repeated episodes. Often patients with cellulitis have diabetes, or are obese, or have other skin conditions such as tinea pedis (see above).

Signs and symptoms

- Sudden appearance of a swollen, warm, tender, red area on the skin.
- Transition between affected skin and the surrounding normal skin is gradual.
- The area of affected skin grows noticeably over 24–48 hours but rarely over 4–8 hours.
- The skin appears "tight" and glossy.
- In some cases, fever, chills, sweating, fatigue, muscle aches.
- Patient feels unwell.

What to do

- If a leg is affected, have the patient elevate it.
- Give amoxycillin/clavulanate, 875/125 mg orally, twice daily; note:
  - response to treatment may take two to three weeks.
- If the cellulitis spreads while the patient is taking this antibiotic medication:
  - add ceftriaxone, 1 g intramuscularly, twice daily;
  - seek medical advice.

Cellulitis arising from wounds exposed to estuary or seawater

This can be much more severe than the usual form of cellulitis described above. There is often high fever and the infection can spread rapidly, with extension over a whole limb in a few hours.

What to do

- If cellulitis develops following wounds from shells or fish spines anywhere, or from fish-hooks or propellers in estuarine waters:
  - give amoxycillin/clavulanate, 875 mg orally, twice daily; **AND**
  - ciprofloxacin, 500 mg orally, twice daily; **AND**
  - doxycycline, 100 mg orally, twice daily.
- Seek medical advice as soon as possible.

ERYSIPELAS

Erysipelas is a form of cellulitis that usually occurs in older adults in poor health. In most cases it involves the legs but can also appear on the face.

Signs and symptoms

- Redness and swelling of the skin much severer than with cellulitis.
- Affected area much more sharply demarcated than with cellulitis.
- Fever often high.
- Patients much sicker than with cellulitis.

✔ *What to do*

- Seek medical advice.
- If a leg is affected, have the patient elevate it.
- Give amoxycillin/clavulanate, 875 mg orally, twice daily.

Bone, joint, and muscle disorders

JOINT INFLAMMATION

If only one joint is affected, the likely cause is gout (see below) or septic arthritis (see below) or injury (see Chapter 6, *Bone, joint and muscle injuries*). If several joints are affected, the likely cause is rheumatoid arthritis (see below). Joint pain without inflammation is probably due to osteoarthritis (see below) or to chronic joint problems related to injury or to over-use of the joint: in such cases pain is made worse by activity and relieved by rest.

Signs and symptoms

- Joint pain, warmth, redness, swelling:
  - inflammation of joints covered by large muscles, such as the shoulder and hip joints, can be difficult to detect because there may not be much redness, warmth, or swelling.
- Joint stiffness, worse after rest (e.g. on waking).

GOUT

Gout can affect many organs, but in most cases it results in acute arthritis.

Signs and symptoms of arthritis due to gout

- Severe pain of rapid onset, peaking in a few hours and lasting a few days if untreated.
- Marked redness, warmth, swelling, and tenderness of the affected joint or joints.
- Nearly all first attacks of gout affect only one joint, most often at the base of the big toe.
- Subsequent attacks most often affect small joints in the leg.
- Fever can be due to gout but could also be due to septic arthritis (see below).

✔ *What to do*

- Have the patient rest, with the affected joint elevated.
- Give ibuprofen, 800 mg orally, three times daily: this high dose is needed to control the intense inflammation.
- As the pain begins to subside, reduce the dose to 400 mg every six hours and continue this treatment for 7–10 days.
- If ibuprofen cannot be used because of a contraindication, such as peptic ulcer, give prednisone, 50 mg orally, at once, then daily for seven days.
- Have the patient see a doctor at the next port.
- To reduce the risk of further attacks advise the patient to:
  - lose weight;
  - limit alcohol consumption to one or two glasses of wine daily and avoid beer;
  - limit meat intake and avoid eating fish and offal (liver, etc.).

✗ What not to do

- DO NOT use acetylsalicylic acid (Aspirin®) for acute gout.

SEPTIC ARTHRITIS

Septic arthritis usually occurs when bacteria enter the bloodstream from an external source, such as an unsterile intravenous injection or a penetrating injury, and accumulate in a joint.

► Signs and symptoms

- Pain, warmth, redness, and swelling of a single joint, the knee in half the cases, less often the hip, wrist, or ankle.
- In some cases, mild-to-moderate fever.

✔ What to do

- If you suspect septic arthritis, seek medical advice.
- Give ceftriaxone, 2 g intravenously (preferably) or intramuscularly, once daily.
- To relieve pain, give ibuprofen, 400 mg orally, every six hours, or 800 mg orally, every eight hours.

RHEUMATOID ARTHRITIS

Rheumatoid arthritis is one of the commonest joint diseases. It can affect any joint but most often involves small joints (especially of the fingers) and in a symmetrical fashion (i.e. affecting the same joints on both hands or both feet). It can cause joint destruction and deformed hands. The problems rheumatoid arthritis is likely to cause on board ship would not usually require urgent attention and could wait until a doctor is consulted at the next port.

Note

- Rheumatoid arthritis is usually treated with non-steroidal anti-inflammatory drugs, such as ibuprofen, although severe cases may require a variety of specialized medicines.
- Unwanted effects of medication, especially the specialized medicines, are common and may be serious.

✔ What to do

- If a patient known to have rheumatoid arthritis requires treatment give ibuprofen, 400 mg orally, every six hours.
- If a patient taking specialized medicines for rheumatoid arthritis develops new symptoms, seek medical advice.

OSTEOARTHRITIS

Osteoarthritis tends to affect joints subject to wear and tear and repeated injury, especially the end joints of fingers, knees, and hips. It occurs, therefore, most often in patients over 50 years of age.

Signs and symptoms

- Joints mildly tender but not warm.
- In some cases, morning stiffness but lasting less than 30 minutes.
- Joint pain made worse by activity and relieved by rest.
- Grating of joint edges against one another as the joint moves (crepitus).
- Growth of bone around the edge of the affected joint, leading to a hard, enlarged joint with irregular edges.

Note

- Osteoarthritis rarely affects the elbow, wrist, or ankle joints: pain in these joints should not be diagnosed as due to osteoarthritis.

✔ *What to do*

- Advise the patient to lose weight, especially if weight-bearing joints such as the hip and knee are affected.
- To relieve pain, apply a water bottle filled with hot (not boiling) water to the painful joint for 20 minutes.
- If you believe medication is needed, start with paracetamol, 1000 mg orally, every six hours.
- If pain persists, try ibuprofen, 400 mg orally, every six hours; it is more effective than paracetamol but increases the risk of unwanted effects.

PROBLEMS IN SPECIFIC JOINTS

The knee

First points to verify:

- where exactly around the knee the pain is located;
- whether there is swelling of the knee joint, how severe it is, and where exactly it occurs;
- whether there are mechanical problems affecting the joint, such as:
  - giving way and locking;
  - weakness;
- whether the problem causes the patient to limp;
- pain on the inner side of the knee suggests medial collateral ligament damage (see Chapter 6, *Bone, joint, and muscle injuries*) or osteoarthritis;
- pain on the outer side of the knee suggests lateral collateral ligament damage (see Chapter 6, *Bone, joint, and muscle injuries*);

- pain at the front of the knee suggests damage to the kneecap (patella) or patellar bursitis (see below):
  - in patients under 45, pain at the front of the knee, especially if it affects both knees, is most often due to repetitive knee bending and straightening that causes the patella to rub against the femur;
  - this pain tends to subside over a few months without treatment;
- pain, swelling, and tenderness of the bursa – the thin-walled sac lying immediately under the skin in front of the patella – is due to patellar bursitis (inflammation of the bursa, or "housemaid's knee"), which is due to repetitive injury, such as from prolonged kneeling:
  - movement of the knee is normal in bursitis (if it is not, the problem may not be bursitis but rather a problem with the knee joint);
  - there is no swelling of the knee joint itself in bursitis;
  - bursitis can be complicated by infection (septic bursitis): if there is evidence of bursitis but the patient has fever and there is marked warmth around the knee, medical advice should be sought;
- locking and giving way of the knee associated with pain and swelling suggest tearing of a cartilage (meniscus). The meniscus often tears when the knee is twisted with the patient bearing weight on the foot:
  - the injury may appear quite minor when it occurs, and the patient may not remember it when symptoms appear;
  - pain, swelling, locking and giving way can begin immediately after the injury or days or weeks later.

✔ *What to do*

- To relieve pain, give ibuprofen, 400 mg orally, every six hours, and have the patient see a doctor at the next port.
- Assess the severity of the problem as described in *Knee injuries*, in Chapter 6, *Bone, joint, and muscle injuries*.
- If you suspect a tear of a meniscus in a patient whose knee locks and gives way, have the patient taken off work that requires kneeling and squatting and arrange for the patient to see a doctor at the next port.

The shoulder

The most frequent complaint relating to the shoulder is pain at the front and top of the shoulder that is made worse by raising the arm above the head.

- If the patient has suffered a fall onto the point of the shoulder within the previous two weeks, trauma is the most likely cause of the pain (see Chapter 6, *Bone, joint, and muscle injuries*).
- If there has been no recent injury in a patient under 30, the most likely cause is a problem with the tendons of the rotator cuff muscles:
  - the rotator cuff muscles are on the shoulder-blade (scapula);
  - the rotator cuff muscle tendons pass forwards into the shoulder: with the upper arm at the side and the elbow at an angle of 90°, these tendons rotate

  - the arm so that the forearm lies across the chest or points sideways away from the body;
  - the shoulder pain is made worse by lifting with the arm away from the body or by working with the arms above the head.
- The term "frozen shoulder" refers to an inability to move the shoulder joint following an injury or other possibly painful condition: the inability is neither due to the pain itself nor to muscle weakness (the actual cause is unknown), and it can appear after:
  - any painful shoulder condition;
  - use of a sling for more than two weeks.

✔ *What to do*

- In a patient with shoulder pain, give ibuprofen, 400 mg orally, every six hours and have the patient taken off duties requiring work with the arms raised.
- Pain may be relieved by "weighted pendulum exercises":
  - have the patient lie face down, or bend over, so that the affected arm hangs straight down;
  - place 3–4 kg weight in the patient's hand, and have him swing the arm gently from left to right for 1–2 minutes;
  - this exercise can be repeated as often as needed.
- Have the patient see a doctor at the next port.

✘ *What not to do*

- DO NOT have the patient wear a sling for longer than three days in a case of muscle and tendon injuries around the shoulder: frozen shoulder may result (see above).

The back

Low back pain affects 80% of people at least once in their lives. About 25% of workers have an episode of low back pain each year and 10% cannot work for some period each year because of back pain.

- Most cases of low back pain are due to muscle or ligament damage, which causes a dull aching pain in the back and buttocks (lumbago).
- Pain may start suddenly or gradually – sudden onset with a definite injury suggests that recovery will be relatively speedy and complete.
- Pain starting in the buttock and radiating down the back of the leg to the calf, sometimes with numbness, is called sciatica;
  - sciatica is caused by a tear in one of the discs (slipped disc) that separate the vertebrae;
  - the tear allows the jelly-like centre of the disc to bulge out and compress one of the nerves leaving the spinal cord (of which several join up to form the sciatic nerve);
  - the pain, which may begin suddenly or gradually, is often sharp or burning;
  - the pain is worse when standing or sitting.

- With simple treatment, about 90% of patients, including those with sciatica, recover in about four weeks.

✔ *What to do*

- Look for red flags (see below).
- Encourage the patient to be as active as is possible: bed rest is not helpful unless the patient cannot stand without pain.
- Make sure bed rest does not continue for more than five days: if the patient still has severe pain after five days, seek medical advice.
- Have the patient relieved of duties that require prolonged sitting, bending or lifting.
- Give paracetamol, 1000 mg orally, every six hours, **OR**:
  - ibuprofen, 400 mg orally, every six hours; **OR** in severe cases
  - tramadol, 50–100 mg orally, twice or three times daily.

Red flags

If any **ONE** of the following is present, seek medical advice at once:

- back pain that is not relieved when the patient lies down;
- constant pain all night;
- changes in bowel or bladder function;
- difficulty with erection;
- back pain for the first time in a patient over 50;
- fever;
- a history of cancer;
- recent weight loss;
- use of intravenous recreational drugs.

The neck

About 10% of adults have neck pain at any time, although lost time at work is less common than with back pain.

Most neck pain is due to tears or strain and soreness in muscles and ligaments around the neck vertebrae.

Common activities that cause such an injury are carrying heavy loads in one hand (e.g. heavy luggage), prolonged hand work on a bench that is too high, sitting hunched forward when writing or using a computer, sleeping in a chair (as on a long plane flight), sleeping on pillows that are thicker or thinner than usual. In these conditions neck pain is usually short-lived and recovers without treatment beyond avoiding the activity that caused it.

"Whiplash" injury occurs when a person is pushed forward from behind; this typically happens in a rear-end motor vehicle collision, but it can be due to any accident that causes the head to jerk backwards then forwards. Pain in this condition is often prolonged and hard to treat.

Neck pain can also be due to osteoarthritis (see above) of the joints between vertebrae in the neck, and this pain tends to come and go over a long period.

Fractures of the neck vertebrae can occur with falls onto the head (see Chapter 4, *Head injuries*).

In most cases, whatever the cause, pain is felt in the midline of the neck, often going down into the back of the shoulder and upper back. Pain is made worse by rotating the head, or by bending the neck forwards or sidewards. Spasm of the muscles around the neck and shoulders is often easily felt.

✔ ***What to do:***

- Look for red flags (see below).
- If there are no red flags:
  - give paracetamol, 1000mg orally, every six hours;
  - modify the work or living environment to reduce strain on neck muscles.

Red flags

- Pain or tingling in the arm or hand;
- muscle weakness in the arm or hand (ask not only about weakness but also about "clumsiness", such as dropping cups of liquid);
- difficulty walking;
- fever;
- a history of cancer;
- recent weight loss;
- use of intravenous recreational drugs;
- a recent fall onto the head.

Tobacco, alcohol, and drug use

When a ship's medical officer is confronted with a patient under the influence of alcohol or narcotic drugs, or who has a history of alcohol or drug use, the main issue is not to judge whether the patient's drinking or drug taking habits are "right" or "wrong" but rather to determine to what extent those habits are responsible for the patient's health problems. The *International Convention on Standards of Training, Certification and Watchkeeping for Seafarers* should be consulted for guidance on the use of breathalyzers and the interpretation of alcohol levels.

FOUR MAIN QUESTIONS TO CONSIDER

What adverse effects does a patient's use, or abuse, of alcohol or drugs have on the patient's everyday life?

- **Use** is likely to have become **abuse** if **ONE** of the following situations has occurred **MORE THAN ONCE**:
  - failure to meet important obligations:
    - example: a senior officer unable to take watch following an alcoholic binge;
  - using the substance in a physically hazardous situation:
    - example: handling cargo while drunk;
  - legal problems caused by substance use:
    - example: arrested for driving while intoxicated;
  - continued use of the substance despite serious social or inter-personal problems:
    - example: repeated fights with fellow crew members.

To what extent is the patient psychologically dependent on alcohol or a narcotic drug?

- A patient is likely to have become psychologically dependent if **MORE THAN TWO** of the following conditions apply:
  - compulsive use, so that the substance is consumed in larger amounts or for longer than intended in a session:
    - example: agreeing to have one drink with friends, then staying on alone until drunk;
  - repeated unsuccessful attempts to stop or cut down on consumption;
  - a lot of effort is spent to obtain the substance:
    - example: making an expensive or inconvenient journey merely to replenish alcohol supplies;
  - consuming the substance has priority over social, work, or recreational activities:
    - example: refusing a promotion because the job would require abstaining from alcohol during working days;
  - use of the substance continues despite awareness of the harm it is causing:
    - example: continuing to smoke after being diagnosed as having a chronic lung disease.

To what extent is the patient physically dependent on alcohol or a drug?

- A patient is likely to have become physically dependent on a substance if there are physical symptoms (withdrawal symptoms) when attempting to stop consuming the substance. Each substance is associated with a specific set of withdrawal symptoms.

To what extent has the patient become tolerant to alcohol or a drug?

- A patient is likely to have become tolerant to a substance if increasing amounts of the substance are needed to obtain the desired effect or if the same amount has less and less effect.

ALCOHOL INTOXICATION

Death can result directly from over-consumption of alcohol or indirectly, for example, by falling from wharves and gangways while drunk. A seafarer brought on board in a semi-comatose condition may simply be put to bed and a few hours later be found dead either from having absorbed a fatal amount of alcohol or from choking on vomit or from head injuries sustained while drunk. A drunken seafarer should always be treated as a sick person requiring close observation and careful nursing.

As with any drug, the effect of alcohol increases with the dose taken. The relation between the blood level of alcohol and its effect is roughly described below under *What to do* and in Table 22.1.

✔ *What to do*

- In a patient whose breath smells of alcohol and whose condition – coma, mental confusion, slurred speech, etc. – suggests over-consumption of alcohol, always consider the possibility of the condition being due to:
  - injuries, especially head injuries;
  - illness, such as from low blood sugar due to medication for diabetes mellitus;
  - potentially fatal combinations of alcohol and narcotic drugs or of alcohol and other chemicals – chloral hydrate ("Mickey Finn") in the past, but more likely flunitrazepam (trade name: Rohypnol) or gamma-hydroxybutyrate (GBH) today;
  - consumption of "moonshine alcohol" containing methanol and/or ethylene glycol, both of which are poisonous.

Table 22.1 Effects of blood alcohol levels.

Blood alcohol concentration, g/100 ml	Number of drinks	Effects
0.02–0.03	1–2	Mild sedation, normal behaviour
0.04–0.05	2–5	Euphoria and reduced self-control, impaired performance of skilled tasks
0.06–0.10	5–10	Impulsive and uninhibited behaviour, reduced reaction time, reduced memory, impaired coordination
0.2–0.3	20	Disorientation, difficulty walking, emotional outbursts
0.4–0.5	30	Hard to rouse, incontinent, unable to stand
> 0.5	40 and over	Coma, risk of death

- In a patient who has a fit following a drinking bout, suspect:
  - head injuries sustained during a robbery or a fight, or when falling;
  - epilepsy, which can result from alcohol withdrawal within a few hours of the last drink.
- In individuals tolerant to alcohol, dangerous intoxication can occur without making them obviously drunk.
- Remember that it can take hours for the blood alcohol concentration to return to zero after a drinking bout: a crew member waking up in the morning after a drinking bout may not feel or act drunk but may still have a high blood alcohol concentration and be unfit for skilled or dangerous tasks.
- In an unconscious patient who is not known to have consumed large amounts of spirits (not beer or wine) over a very short period of time, suspect a cause other than alcohol.

Alcohol withdrawal

Alcohol depresses the brain, and when alcohol is withdrawn the brain undergoes a period of over-activity.

Minor withdrawal symptoms do not usually progress to severe or complicated symptoms (called delirium tremens, or DTs). Delirium tremens occurs in about 5% of patients who have minor withdrawal. The likelihood and severity of delirium tremens is related to the duration of heavy drinking, and the risk is low with a once-a-year binge lasting "only" one or two days.

Minor withdrawal symptoms always precede severe or complicated withdrawal by 48 hours or so, and the key to avoiding severe withdrawal is to identify and treat early withdrawal during this window of opportunity. To determine the risk of delirium tremens always use the withdrawal assessment scoring system (see below) in any patient who drinks heavily and then stops suddenly.

Even with hospital care, severe delirium tremens is often fatal: assess for the risk of severe withdrawal early, treat early, and seek medical advice early.

Minor withdrawal ("the shakes")

- Onset of symptoms within a few hours of the last drink, even if the patient still has alcohol in the blood:
  - insomnia
  - trembling
  - nervousness or edginess
  - rapid pulse
  - sweating.

Major withdrawal (delirium tremens, DTs)

- Onset of symptoms 2–4 days after the last drink
- duration: 2–3 days
- in mild cases:
  - tenseness

  - guardedness
  - easily startled
  - sweating
  - rapid pulse rate;
- in severe cases:
  - extreme agitation
  - writhing in bed
  - pacing back and forth
  - frequent intrusive hallucinations (that the patient "hears", "sees", or "touches")
  - drenching sweats;
- mental confusion and disorientation, combined with:
  - tremulousness
  - agitation
  - jumpiness;
- hand tremors (especially when patient holds hands in front of body)
- rapid pulse
- high blood pressure
- sweating
- headache
- nausea
- non-productive vomiting (dry heaves).

✔ *What to do*

- Have the patient rest in a quiet cabin, with only one attendant.
- As most patients undergoing alcohol withdrawal are dehydrated, encourage oral fluid intake.
- Determine the severity of the patient's alcohol withdrawal by scoring the symptoms according to the following scheme:
  - **nausea and vomiting**:
    - 0 = absent
    - 1 = slight and occasional
    - 4 = marked, intermittent nausea and dry heaves (non-productive vomiting)
    - 7 = constant nausea and dry heaves;
  - **sweating**:
    - 0 = absent
    - 1 = barely detectable moistness of the palms
    - 4 = beads of sweat on the forehead
    - 7 = whole body sweating;
  - **anxiety**:
    - 0 = absent
    - 1 = slightly edgy
    - 4 = obviously anxious and guarded
    - 7 = in a panic;

- **agitation**:
  - 0 = absent
  - 1 = slightly agitated
  - 4 = obviously restless
  - 7 = pacing back and forth continuously;
- **tremor**:
  - 0 = absent
  - 1 = fingertips trembling slightly
  - 4 = obvious trembling with arms held straight out in front
  - 7 = obvious trembling with arms resting;
- **headache**:
  - 0 = absent
  - 1 = present
  - 4 = moderately severe
  - 7 = very severe;
- **disturbed hearing**:
  - 0 = absent
  - 2 = easily startled by ordinary noises
  - 4 = evident sound hallucinations
  - 7 = continuous sound hallucinations;
- **disturbed vision**:
  - 0 = absent
  - 2 = bothered by light but no apparent hallucinations
  - 4 = evident visual hallucinations
  - 7 = continuous visual hallucinations;
- **disturbance of sense of touch**:
  - 0 = absent
  - 2 = the touch of ordinary objects – bedclothes, for example – feels mildly abnormal
  - 4 = hallucinations about things moving on the skin
  - 7 = continuous hallucinations about things moving on the skin;
- **orientation**:
  - 0 = knows the date and place and can perform serial calculations (e.g. subtracts 7 from 100, then 7 from the result, and 7 from that result, and so on; replace 7 by 3 for a less educated person);
  - 1 = knows the date and place but cannot do serial calculations;
  - 2 = knows the place, but cannot do serial calculations and knows the date only to within two days;
  - 3 = knows the place, but cannot do serial calculations and does **not** know the date to within two days;
  - 4 = does not know the place or the date and cannot do serial calculations.

- Add up the total score for all nine symptoms: less than 10 indicates very mild withdrawal; 10–20, significant but not dangerous withdrawal; over 20, serious withdrawal.

- For a patient with a score less than 8, do nothing, but reassess the withdrawal score in an hour.
- If the score is 8 or more, give diazepam, 5 mg orally.
- Repeat the score assessment every hour and give diazepam, 5 mg orally, each time it is over 8.
- You may have to give large amounts of diazepam in a patient who has developed tolerance to diazepam and alcohol.
- In a patient who has had episodes of delirium tremens before or if you are too short-handed to manage frequent reassessment with alcohol withdrawal scores an alternative is:
  - give diazepam, 10 mg orally, every six hours for the first day;
  - then give diazepam, 5 mg orally, every six hours for the next two days;
  - record the withdrawal assessment score twice daily and, if the patient appears to be getting worse, add an extra 5–10 mg dose of diazepam if the score is over 8.
- Consider other possible conditions that produce symptoms resembling those of delirium tremens, such as:
  - infections (see Chapter 23, *Infectious diseases*);
  - head injury (see Chapter 4, *Head injuries*);
  - liver failure (see Chapter 16, *Gastrointestinal and liver diseases*);
  - kidney failure (see Chapter 17, *Kidney and other urinary disorders*);
  - psychiatric illness (see Chapter 13, *Paralysis, strange behaviour, unconsciousness*).

✗ What not to do

- Do not use haloperidol for alcohol withdrawal: this drug promotes convulsions and is dangerous in a patient going through alcohol withdrawal.
- Do not use alcohol to treat withdrawal unless you have no alternative: alcohol suppresses early withdrawal symptoms but is difficult to use and dangerous in delirium tremens: doses are hard to predict but may be very large, the effect is short-lived, and it is easy to give too much or too little.

CANNABIS INTOXICATION

After alcohol and tobacco, cannabis is the third commonest drug used by seafarers. Legal constraints on the use of cannabis vary: in some countries use and possession of small quantities are permitted; in others, tacitly tolerated; and in yet others, heavily punished.

Cannabis is derived from the hemp plant *Cannabis sativa*. There are two main forms of cannabis: marijuana, which consists of the dried leaves and seeds of the plant, and hashish, a resin made from the flowers. Both are usually taken by smoking, either as cigarettes ("joints") or through a pipe ("bong"). Cannabis can be taken orally, usually as cakes or cookies (hash brownies, space cake), but is rarely injected intravenously. With smoked cannabis, intoxication is apparent within minutes.

Signs and symptoms

- Rapid pulse
- rapid respiratory rate

- dry mouth
- red eyes
- increased appetite ("the munchies")
- reduced reaction time
- mood changes – usually euphoria, but sometimes depression or panic
- distortion of time perception – time passes very slowly.

Note

- The euphoria and marked changes in mental function caused by cannabis last 3–4 hours.
- Impairment of judgement and concentration, and distortion of time perception (and therefore estimation of speed), continue for several hours more.
- The active ingredient of cannabis accumulates in the body, so that in heavy users concentration and judgement may be impaired for 24 hours after use without their feeling intoxicated or displaying intoxicated behaviour.
- Absorption of the active ingredient after oral use is unpredictable, and can be slow:
  - this can lead the user to take more drug-containing food in an effort to achieve a "high", so that, when the drug is eventually absorbed, the effect is very intense and prolonged;
  - a seafarer who takes a dose of cannabis orally may go on watch unaffected, but become dangerously intoxicated in the course of the watch.

✔ *What to do*

- Discourage cannabis use in seafarers who have responsibilities calling for precision skills and judgement.
- Discourage especially the simultaneous use of alcohol and cannabis: the combination increases the negative effect on judgement.

OPIOIDS, OPIATES, AND RELATED DRUGS

Opioids are a broad class of drugs that have morphine-like (tranquilizing, sedative, or painkilling) effects on the body. They include synthetic drugs, such as the painkiller pethidine, and substances produced by the human brain, such as endorphins.

Opioids also include the **opiates**, drugs extracted from the opium poppy: morphine is the most commonly used.

Heroin intoxication

Heroin is the most widely abused opioid. It enters the brain more quickly and in higher concentrations than morphine, giving users a sudden effect (the "rush") that they find intensely pleasurable.

Historically, heroin has nearly always been taken intravenously, the route that ensures a strong rush, even when heroin of low purity is used. The intravenous route, however, is the most dangerous.

Heroin can also be injected under the skin ("skin-popping"). In recent years heroin has become widely available in a form pure enough to give a rush when smoked ("chasing the dragon") or applied to the inside of the nose ("snorting"). These routes are much safer than intravenous injection.

Signs and symptoms

- Drowsiness
- a sense of relaxation and dissociation
- small pupils
- reduced respiratory rate
- slurred speech
- impaired mental function.

Note

- The effects of heroin intoxication last 3–4 hours.
- Users may have other symptoms from drugs used to dilute ("cut") heroin or taken to counteract the sedative effect of heroin (amphetamine is often used for this purpose, see below).

Heroin overdose

Overdose is an important hazard of intravenous heroin use. It is much less common with smoking and snorting. Most deaths from heroin overdose occur in users who have injected heroin regularly for five to 10 years and are dependent on the drug. The most dangerous effect of heroin in overdose is depression of breathing.

A young person who is unconscious and not breathing but whose pulse is strong and regular is very likely to be suffering a heroin overdose.

Heroin bought from a dealer usually consists only partly of the active drug: the rest may be sugar, powdered milk, aspirin, or another white powder. The amount of active drug varies from day to day and dealer to dealer, so that users can easily inject more than they intended to.

Tolerance to the effects of heroin on mental function develops after one to two weeks of daily intravenous use, so that the dose has to be increased progressively to obtain a rush. However, there is little or no tolerance to the depression of breathing. For this reason, periods of frequent use often culminate in the depression of breathing characteristic of heroin overdose.

✔ What to do

- Give naloxone, 0.4 mg intravenously, (preferably) or subcutaneously, repeated as necessary.
- Note that naloxone acts for only one to two hours, much less than heroin, so that overdose patients may respond well at first and then relapse.

Infection in heroin users

Three bloodborne viruses – HIV, the AIDS virus, hepatitis B, and hepatitis C – are common in intravenous heroin users.

Bacteria can also infect heroin injection users via a poorly sterilized injection needle. The most important complication resulting from a bacterial infection is an infection of the heart valves (infective endocarditis).

Signs and symptoms of infective endocarditis

- If the infection affects the valves of the right side of the heart, between the veins and the lungs, it can spread to the lungs, causing:
  - fever
  - breathlessness
  - cough, with blood-stained sputum.
- If the infection affects the left side of the heart, between the lungs and the arteries, it can destroy the heart valves, causing heart failure, which produces:
  - sudden onset of severe breathlessness
  - inability to lie flat
  - cough with profuse, watery, blood-tinged sputum
  - low blood pressure.

Heroin withdrawal

It takes as little as two weeks of daily heroin use for withdrawal symptoms to appear when the user tries to stop the habit. Withdrawal symptoms are less common in heroin users who smoke or snort the drug. Heroin withdrawal is very unpleasant but rarely dangerous (unlike alcohol withdrawal).

Signs and symptoms

- Onset soon after the last dose has worn off of:
  - craving for the drug
  - anxiety.
- About **12 hours** later:
  - restlessness
  - insomnia
  - yawning
  - runny nose
  - sweating
  - stomach cramps
  - dilated pupils.
- About **24 hours** later:
  - vomiting
  - diarrhoea
  - cramps
  - fever and chills
  - tremor
  - "goose-bumps" (caused by erection of hair follicles, hence the term "cold turkey").

✔ *What to do*

- Consider whether to relieve the withdrawal symptoms with morphine or to allow the patient to go through the withdrawal.
- To alleviate withdrawal symptoms, give morphine, 30 mg orally, every four hours or 10 mg intramuscularly, every four hours.
- After one day reduce the oral dose to 20 mg orally, every four hours, or the intramuscular dose to 7.5 mg intramuscularly, every four hours.
- If the symptoms recur to an intolerable degree you may have to increase the dose, in which case reduce the dose again on the following day.
- Reduce the dose progressively to zero over three to four days.
- Encourage the patient to enter a programme in which methadone, a long-acting synthetic opioid, is given to replace heroin. Note that patients on methadone can drive and operate machinery safely.

OTHER OPIOIDS

All opioids are occasionally abused. The commonest, apart from heroin, are pethidine (meperidine) – an opioid usually abused by health professionals – and fentanyl. Morphine is not commonly abused.

A number of highly potent synthetic derivatives of fentanyl and pethidine have been made. The first to appear was called "China White" and its potency led to an epidemic of overdose deaths. Current names for fentanyl derivatives include "Mexican Brown" and "Persian White".

All these drugs cause intoxication and overdose effects similar to those of heroin, which can be reversed with naloxone in the same doses as for heroin (see above).

COCAINE ("COKE", "SNOW", ETC.)

Cocaine is the active component of coca leaves and one of the oldest stimulants known to man. Some indigenous population groups in South America chew coca leaf for its stimulant effects but this practice is not generally associated with problems of abuse. In the 19th century cocaine was widely used in the United States (also as a component of Coca-Cola®, from which cocaine was removed only in 1903). Cocaine is also a local anaesthetic used in several countries by eye surgeons.

Today, cocaine is used mainly by young men in North American and western European cities. Unlike heroin, regular daily use of cocaine is rare and most cocaine users are not dependent (and therefore do not experience withdrawal symptoms).

Note

- There are two forms of cocaine: the free base ("crack"), which can be smoked but not injected, and the salt, which can be injected and snorted.
- Intoxication with cocaine occurs within seconds if smoked or injected intravenously and after 30 minutes if snorted.

- The effects of cocaine last 15–30 minutes after injection or smoking and one hour after snorting.
- Desired effects of cocaine include:
  - euphoria
  - increased alertness
  - energy
  - sociability
  - reduced appetite.
- Undesired effects of cocaine include:
  - mental changes closely resembling schizophrenia
  - suspiciousness
  - grandiose delusions (false beliefs) and hallucinations (perceptions not perceived by others)
  - stroke
  - heart problems:
    - abnormal heart rhythm
    - cardiac arrest
    - myocardial infarction.

✔ *What to do*

- You rarely need to treat the problems associated with intoxication because the duration of the effect is so short.
- If psychotic symptoms do not subside after an hour or so and there is extreme agitation or a risk of violence treat as for psychosis (see Chapter 13, *Paralysis, strange behaviour, unconsciousness*).

AMPHETAMINES

Amphetamines are now among the most widely used illicit drugs, particularly in Africa, Asia, Australia and eastern Europe. Amphetamines resemble cocaine in that they stimulate the brain and can produce schizophrenia-like behaviour. The effects of intravenous amphetamine are similar to those of intravenous or smoked cocaine, except that heart rhythm is less affected and the mental and behavioural effects last much longer (up to eight hours, vs. 15–60 minutes for cocaine).

Most amphetamines are obtained from clandestine production sources and are taken by intravenous injection. Amphetamines also exist as tablets, which were used fairly widely in the past to counteract sedation from barbiturates or opioids.

Like cocaine, amphetamine is popular among young men, who tend to indulge in intermittent binges, with daily use for a few days followed by a period of abstinence. Rebound depression and somnolence often follow a binge. Some long-distance truck drivers use oral amphetamine to enable them to drive for long periods without sleep. Its use for a similar purpose may also occur among seafarers.

Note

The main amphetamine-like drugs are:

- amphetamine itself ("bennies", after the trade-name Benzedrine) and dexaphetamine (Dexedrine, "dex", "dexies", "speed");
- methylphenidate, widely used for:
  - the treatment of Attention-Deficit Hyperactivity Disorder in children;
  - the treatment of narcolepsy in adults;
  - illicit use, often by students as a "cramming drug";
- methamphetamine ("crank", "crystal meth", "uppers", "speed"), a synthetic form of amphetamine, which exists also in a smokeable form ("ice"):
  - produced legally in some countries for:
    - the treatment of Attention-Deficit Hyperactivity Disorder in children;
    - the treatment of narcolepsy in adults;
  - produced illegally in clandestine laboratories;
- two illicit drugs related to methamphetamine, widely used among young people for their euphoric and stimulant effects, particularly in a sexual context, are:
  - methylenedioxymethamphetamine (MDMA, "ecstasy", "E");
  - methylendioxyethamphetamine ("Eve"), which is closely related chemically to MDMA.

Desired effects of amphetamine and related drugs include:

- increased alertness, energy, endurance, and self-confidence;
- enhanced mental and physical performance (hence, its wide popularity, in the past, among athletes).

Undesired effects of amphetamine include:

- suspiciousness
- aggressiveness
- impulsiveness
- exaggerated self-confidence and risk-taking
- increased heart rate
- high blood pressure, increasing the risk of stroke or heart failure
- life-threatening increase in body temperature (particularly with MDMA).

✔ *What to do*

- Activated charcoal 1 g/kg body weight will reduce the absorption of the drug if it has been taken orally.
- Agitation and aggression should be treated as directed for psychosis (see Chapter 13, *Paralysis, strange behaviour, unconsciousness*).

HALLUCINOGEN INTOXICATION

The hallucinogens most widely available commercially are LSD and phencyclidine. The drugs are often mixed when sold illicitly, and many users who believe they are taking LSD have been given another hallucinogenic drug, usually phencyclidine (see below).

Lysergic acid diethylamide (LSD)

LSD is the prototype hallucinogen.

The LSD "trip" is variable and can include:

- hallucinations
- sensory distortions (i.e. of sight, touch, hearing, smell, taste)
- feelings of "oneness with the universe"
- intense fear (in a "bad trip").

Phencyclidine ("PCP", "angel dust")

This is now the most widely used hallucinogen, because it is easily manufactured and cheap. It is related to the anaesthetic agent ketamine, which is also used as a hallucinogen in its own right.

- Phencyclidine produces reactions that resemble schizophrenia, including an impression that the body and soul are separated or that the user has met God.
- Only about half of users find the phencyclidine experience pleasant.
- Some phencyclidine users become violent; others can become immobile.
- In high doses, phencyclidine may cause a dangerous increase in blood pressure, body temperature, or both.

Plant hallucinogens

Hallucinogens found in plants are used widely in some communities. The commonest are psilocybin ("magic mushrooms") and mescaline (found in some types of cactus). The effects are similar to those of other hallucinogens. Psilocybin is usually taken as cooked mushrooms. The cactus containing mescaline is extremely bitter and cannot be consumed directly, so the cactus flesh is dried, ground and placed in capsules; commercially sold capsules often contain phencyclidine because it is cheaper than mescaline.

✔ *What to do*

- Put the patient in a quiet place, together with a person familiar to the patient, until the effects of the drug wear off.
- Attempt to keep the patient calm by soothing reassurance and gentle contact.
- If the patient is highly agitated give midazolam, 5–10 mg intramuscularly or intranasally.

"FLASHBACKS"

- A flashback is a "replay" in the user's mind of an episode experienced during a hallucinogen trip.
- Flashbacks can intrude into the consciousness long after the drug has been consumed and its effects have worn off.
- Flashbacks last from a few seconds to a minute or so and become less frequent and vivid with time.

- Anxiety is often associated with flashbacks.
- Flashbacks can be dangerous if they occur while the user is driving or operating machinery.

KAVA KAVA

Kava kava (*Piper methysticum*) is a plant native to the South Pacific. It is widely taken as a tea in traditional Polynesian society and is now used in developed countries, either as capsules or tea. It causes relaxation, which its users claim is not associated with impaired memory or judgement. However, high doses are definitely sedating and kava use should be discouraged in crew members required to perform skilled work.

Infectious diseases

Communicable, or infectious, diseases are diseases caused by infectious agents (microorganisms, microbes, or germs), such as bacteria, viruses, fungi, and parasites. Illness results when the infectious agent enters a person's body and multiplies in it, producing poisons (toxins) that damage the body or weaken its defences against other infectious agents, or provoking an immune response that, in trying to kill the invading organism, damages the host. Some infections can be caught from another person who has the infection; some from infected animals or insects; yet others from contaminated food, water, or inanimate objects.

An epidemic of an infectious disease, affecting many people during the same period of time, could endanger the operation and safety of a ship.

For many infections the risk of disease can be reduced or eliminated by immunization. This involves exposing a person to the organism which causes the disease, after it has been killed or modified so that it cannot cause illness but so that the person develops immunity. Immunizations are most effective against diseases caused by viruses and toxins. Whether a particular immunization is needed depends on how common and how dangerous the disease is, how effective the immunization is, and the area in which the ship is sailing. A list of immunizations available for seafarers is given in Chapter 30, *Preventing disease and promoting health in seafarers*.

INFECTIOUS AGENTS

Organisms that produce disease in man range in size from the tiny microscopic virus to the tapeworm, which may attain a length of several metres. For a list of common families of infectious agents and the diseases they cause, see Table 23.1.

HOW INFECTIONS SPREAD

- **By direct contact** with the infected person, as in sexual intercourse, which is the route of transmission of:
    - sexually transmitted infections (see Chapter 19, *Sexually transmitted infections*), including:
        - HIV/AIDS
        - gonorrhoea
        - syphilis
        - some cases of hepatitis B and C.

Table 23.1 Infectious agents and some of the diseases they cause.

Bacteria	Pneumonia, tuberculosis, gonorrhoea, dysentery, cholera
Viruses	Common cold, influenza, dengue, yellow fever, rabies, measles
Rickettsiae	Typhus, spotted fever
Protozoa	Malaria, amoebic dysentery
Metazoa	Filariasis, hookworm and tapeworm infection
Fungi	Ringworm and tinea (athlete's foot)

- **By droplet spread**, when an infected person sneezes or coughs, which is the route of transmission of:
  - whooping cough
  - influenza.
- **By faecal–oral contamination**, when faeces are transferred from an infected person to the mouth of a non-infected person, usually via the hands, which may pick up an infectious microorganism from soiled clothing, bedding, and towels, etc.; this is the route of transmission of:
  - hepatitis A
  - rotavirus disease.
- **Via nonliving vehicles**, such as:
  - **water**, which may be polluted by faeces containing an infectious agent, especially of diarrhoeal diseases, such as cholera;
  - **milk**, that can carry some diseases of cattle that spread to humans, such as bovine tuberculosis;
  - **food**, the main vehicle for typhoid and paratyphoid fever and for most diarrhoeal diseases (see Chapter 16, *Gastrointestinal and liver diseases*);
  - **air**, which carries the tiny particles produced when droplets from a cough or sneeze lose water and become small and light enough to be suspended in air currents that may carry them for long distances; this is the route of transmission of:
    - tuberculosis
    - chicken pox
    - measles;
  - **soil**, that can carry the agents of:
    - tetanus
    - hookworm infection
    - gas gangrene;
  - **fomites**, which include all inanimate objects or substances other than water, milk, food, air, and soil; examples of fomites are:
    - bedding
    - clothing
    - books
    - cutlery
    - door-knobs.
- **Via living vehicles (vectors)**, such as through:
  - **mechanical transfer**, as when:
    - human hands contaminated by infected respiratory secretions spread infection;
  - **carriage in the intestines**, as in the case of certain insects that:
    - harbour disease-causing microorganisms in their intestinal tracts; then
    - pass the organisms in their faeces or regurgitate them; then
    - pass the organisms to a human through a bite-wound, as in epidemic typhus;
  - **biological transmission**, as in malaria, which is transmitted when a mosquito:

› bites a human with malaria and in the process picks up in the human's blood the malaria parasite, which
› develops in the mosquito's body, and
› is transferred to another human when the mosquito bites again.

COMMON TERMS USED IN CONNECTION WITH INFECTIONS

- **Carrier**: a person carrying a disease-causing microorganism without becoming ill but able to pass the microorganism to others.
- **Contact**: a person who has been in contact with an infected person and who may, or may not, have picked up the infection.
- **Incubation period**: the time it takes a disease-causing microorganism to produce symptoms and signs of the disease after entering a person's body: this period varies in length from a few hours to many years, depending on the species of microorganism.
- **Isolation period**: the time during which a patient suffering from an infectious disease should be isolated from others.
- **Segregation period**: the time during which a patient who may be incubating an infectious disease following infection should be segregated from others.
- **Quarantine period**: the time during which port authorities may require a ship to be isolated from contact with the shore: usually only because patients with serious epidemic diseases, such as plague, cholera, and yellow fever, are present or have recently been present on board.

Signs and symptoms of infectious disease

Onset

Many diseases caused by bacteria and viruses begin with non-specific features: this stage is often called a "flu-like prodrome" and consists of some combination of:

- feeling unwell
- poor appetite
- lack of energy
- mild fever
- aches and pains
- headache.

Note

- The flu-like initial (prodromal) period may last only a few hours but could last for several days.
- In some infections, onset is slow, whereas in others (e.g. bacterial meningitis) it can be dramatic.
- During the prodromal phase it is usually not possible to make a diagnosis and nearly all patients who seem to have an ordinary viral "cold" do.

Fever

Fever is a common feature of infectious disease. In most cases it develops as part of the body's defence against infection. Taking the temperature is important not only to diagnose an infection but also to follow its course: whether or not the fever goes away is often the best indicator of whether or not treatment is working.

Note

- Not all patients with fever feel unwell: a classic example is tuberculosis, in which fever is present without the patient being aware of it.
- Not all infectious diseases produce fever: infections, such as cholera and tetanus, which are caused by bacterial toxins in the bowel or in a wound, generally do not cause fever.
- Fever can have many other causes besides infection: medicines, including antibiotics, are one example.
- Fever is part of the body's mechanisms for fighting infection: do not try to lower the fever unless:
  - the patient is distressed by fever;
  - the fever is over 40°C.
- Paracetamol 1000 mg orally every four hours can be given if necessary to lower fever.
- **NEVER give acetylsalicylic acid (Aspirin®) to anyone under 18 years with fever.**

Rash

Some infectious diseases produce a characteristic rash from which a diagnosis can be made.

✔ *What to do in a case of rash and fever*

- When examining a patient with a possible infectious disease, examine the whole body in order to get a full picture of the rash and how it is distributed.
- In examining a rash, note:
  - its pattern: round spots or irregular blotches;
  - its size: 1–2 mm, 1–2 cm, or several centimetres;
  - its colour: pale-pink or dark red;
  - its form: raised or flat (i.e. whether it can be felt when the fingers pass lightly over the skin);
  - whether, when you press it with a finger, it goes pale for a time;
  - whether there are any pustules.

Note

- A rash is often due to drugs, especially antibiotics:
  - of the penicillin family (with names ending in –cillin, such as amoxycillin);
  - of the sulfonamide family (e.g. co-trimoxazole);
  - a drug rash is usually itchy and appears on the back and legs (in a patient lying in bed) after the patient has been taking the drug for a few days.

MANAGEMENT OF INFECTIOUS DISEASES – GENERAL PRINCIPLES

Isolation (see also Chapter 26, *Nursing care and medical procedures*)

Isolation of a patient with an infectious disease is time-consuming and makes caring for the patient much more difficult. Isolation is generally required with diseases such as tuberculosis and whooping cough that spread via droplets. By contrast, there is no reason to isolate patients with sexually transmitted infections or with infections carried by vectors, such as malaria. With many infections, particularly viral infections, the patient is most likely to transmit the infection before becoming obviously ill: isolating such a patient once symptoms have appeared may not stop transmission.

✔ *What to do – precautions against spread of infection*

- Hand-washing is the best way to reduce the risk of infection being transmitted from one person to another:
  - hands should be washed before and after every contact with a patient, using alcohol-based gels or liquids rather than soap to disinfect the hands;
  - the use of gloves does not replace the need for hand-washing.
- Masks prevent spread of infection via droplets:
  - cloth and paper masks become ineffective if they are worn long enough to be dampened by the wearer's breath.
  - The precautions needed to prevent infection depend on the way each infection is spread (see Table 23.2).

Table 23.2 Precautions required to reduce risk of spreading infection on board.[1]

How transmitted	Infection	Precautions required
By air	▪ tuberculosis ▪ varicella	Isolation in a single-berth cabin with door closed; mask for anyone entering the patient's cabin
By droplet	▪ meningitis ▪ pertussis ▪ plague ▪ diphtheria ▪ rubella ▪ mumps	Isolation in a single-berth cabin: door may be open; masks to be worn within one metre of patient
By direct (human) contact	▪ enteric (gastrointestinal) infections ▪ scabies ▪ impetigo	Contacts to wear disposable gloves; for close contact (e.g. to bathe or turn the patient); plastic overalls or aprons also essential

Needle-stick injuries

Doctors, nurses, and other caregivers can be infected by disease-causing microorganisms, particularly viruses, when they accidentally prick themselves with a needle that has been used in treating infected patients. The most common infections that are spread through such needle-stick injuries are hepatitis B, hepatitis C, and HIV/AIDS.

Many needle-stick injuries occur when a caregiver tries to replace the cover on a needle after using it for an injection or when a needle is left in a towel or sheet. **After injections, ALL needles, with the syringe attached, MUST be placed immediately in an approved sharps container**.

Viruses that can be transmitted by needle-stick injury include the following:

- **Hepatitis B virus (HBV)**:
  - HBV is the most infectious of the three viruses discussed here but infection is preventable by immunization;
  - anyone likely to be providing medical or nursing care on board ship should be immunized against HBV;
  - if an unimmunized person is exposed to HBV, the risk of infection can be reduced by starting immunization straight away; this is most effective if started within 24 hours, so seek medical advice as soon as possible.
- **Hepatitis C virus (HCV)**:
  - there is about a 2% risk of acquiring HCV infection after a needle-stick injury;
  - there is no vaccine against HCV and no treatment that can prevent infection after exposure to the virus;
  - crew members who suffer a needle-stick injury from a patient known to have HCV infection or from a patient whose HCV status is unknown should be seen by a doctor at the next port;
  - if the patient whose blood was in the needle agrees, they can be tested in the next port, and a negative result will save extensive testing of the crew member who has received the needle-stick.
- **Human immunodeficiency virus (HIV)**:
  - transmission of HIV after a needle-stick injury is uncommon;
  - the risk of acquiring an infection is less than 0.5% after a single needle-stick injury involving a patient known to have HIV/AIDS in a health-care setting (hospital, clinic, health centre, etc.);
  - if the HIV status of the patient is not known, as is likely to be the case on board ship, the risk of transmission will be 0.5% of the prevalence rate (the percentage of people with HIV infection) in the patient's home community;
  - the risk of HIV transmission from an infected patient's blood or other body fluid splashed into a caregiver's eyes or mouth is much lower than for needle-stick injuries;
  - treatment to prevent HIV infection in a person who has suffered a needle-stick injury involving a patient whose HIV status is unknown should not usually be given unless the patient is known to belong to a group with a high risk of HIV infection, such as intravenous drug users or men who have sex with men;

- if a crew member who has suffered such a needle-stick injury wishes to receive preventive treatment, that wish should be respected;
- the recommended treatment to prevent HIV infection in a person who has suffered a needle-stick injury involving a patient who may or may not be infected with HIV is:
  - zidovudine, 300 mg, plus lamivudine, 150 mg, combined in a single tablet (Combivir (R)), one tablet twice daily for four weeks;
  - see Chapter 33, *Ship's medicine chest* for unwanted effects and precautions;
  - if the person who was the source of the blood agrees to an HIV blood test, this can be performed at the next port: if the test result is negative, treatment can be stopped.

TREATING INFECTIOUS DISEASES

Many infectious diseases have no specific treatment. Even where an antibiotic exists that will kill the microorganism causing an infection, the body's own response to the infection is usually essential to curing the disease. It is, therefore, essential to maintain or improve the patient's own defence mechanisms against the infection.

✔ *What to do – basic principles*

- Strip the patient and make a thorough examination, looking particularly for rash or a wound or bite mark that may help to establish the diagnosis.
- Put the patient to bed and appoint someone to provide nursing care and to organize any preventive procedures that might be required regarding utensils used by the patient for eating and drinking (see Chapter 26, *Nursing care and medical procedures*).
- If the patient's temperature is more than 39.5 °C, sponge him all over with cold water.
- If the patient shows signs of prostration (complete lack of energy) or has a high temperature, arrange for the patient to receive help in using a bedpan and urine bottle.
- If the patient is seriously ill or if you suspect a serious disease likely to affect the rest of the crew, seek medical advice.

Food

Decisions about the best diet for a patient with an infectious disease will depend on the type of infection and the severity of the fever it causes. A patient with fever from an infectious disease usually has a poor appetite and this may limit the diet to fluids, such as water flavoured with lemon juice and sugar, sweet tea, or any similar drink that appeals to the patient.

✔ *What to do*

- Allow the patient to eat as desired, except where there is specific advice to the contrary below (usually in the case of a diarrhoeal disease).
- If the patient has no appetite, do not insist: a few days' fasting will do no harm, as long as fluid intake is maintained.
- Advise a patient who is not eating to take at least some sugar in the form of fruit juice or soft drinks or sweetened tea: in the absence of sugar, the body breaks down muscle protein to provide energy.

SOME COMMON OR IMPORTANT INFECTIONS THAT COULD OCCUR ON BOARD (presented here in alphabetical order; for HIV/AIDS, see Chapter 19, *Sexually transmitted infections*)

Anthrax

Anthrax is caused by *Bacillus anthracis*. It is primarily a disease of cattle, goats, and sheep. The "spores" of the bacillus are dormant but infectious forms of the organism that can remain alive in soil for many years. Human infection occurs through contact with infected animals or their hides, meat, or hair. Human infection can affect the skin, lungs, or gastrointestinal tract, depending on whether the infection is acquired by a skin prick, by inhalation, or by eating contaminated meat. The skin is affected in most cases because of contact with hides or hair containing anthrax spores. Anthrax is common in Iraq, the Islamic Repubic of Iran, Pakistan, Turkey, and sub-Saharan Africa.

Signs and symptoms

- A history of exposure to animal hair or hides.
- At onset, a small, itchy but painless lump on exposed areas, such as the hands, arms, or face.
- Over the next two days, the lump becomes an ulcer.
- Marked swelling around the ulcer.
- Little or no pain or tenderness.

✔ What to do

- Even if you only suspect anthrax of the skin (cutaneous anthrax) but are not sure, treat the patient anyway: delaying treatment could risk the patient's life.
- Give ciprofloxacin, 500 mg orally, twice daily for five days; **OR**:
  - doxycycline, 100 mg orally, twice daily for five days.
- Since the discharge from the ulcer is infectious, have the patient isolated from contact with others: attendants should wear gloves and a disposable plastic apron.
- Cover the ulcers with a gauze dressing until they heal.
- Use instruments to handle used dressings and sterilize the instruments by vigorous boiling for not less than 30 minutes: anthrax spores are difficult to kill.
- Seek medical advice about dealing with potentially infective cargo.

Chickenpox and shingles (varicella-zoster virus)

The varicella-zoster virus (VZV) causes both chickenpox (varicella) and shingles (herpes zoster). Chickenpox occurs when a person is infected with the virus for the first time. The patient recovers fully but the virus remains in the body and, when re-activated years later, can cause shingles.

CHICKENPOX

Chickenpox is spread by airborne particles. It is highly contagious: if a case occurs on board ship at least two-thirds of crew members who have not already had the disease or been vaccinated against it can be expected to become infected if precautions are not taken. Infection is likely if a susceptible person spends more than one hour in the same room with an infected person. Most adults from the more developed countries have had chickenpox as children but roughly one third of adults from poor or tropical countries have not and are likely to be susceptible. Because adults who are infected with chickenpox can become seriously ill, an outbreak on board could seriously impair the ship's operation.

Signs and symptoms

- Onset within 15 days of exposure to an infectious patient;
- fever;
- feeling unwell;
- within a day, a rash of red spots, rapidly becoming fluid-filled blisters (vesicles), that are often intensely itchy;
- appearance of new vesicles over three to four days, as older lesions form crusts and heal.

COMPLICATIONS

- Bacterial infection of the skin lesions causing:
  - renewed fever;
  - redness and swelling of skin around infected areas.
- Pneumonia, an uncommon complication that occurs while there is an active chickenpox rash, and causes:
  - breathlessness;
  - a dry cough;
  - a sharp rise in respiratory rate;
  - death in a significant proportion of patients, even with the best hospital care.

✔ *What to do*

- You can only treat the symptoms of chickenpox: there is no treatment for the underlying infection.
- Have the patient nursed by a crew member who has had chickenpox or been vaccinated against it.
- You do not need to confine the patient to bed but arrange for isolation in a single-berth cabin.
- Ensure that visitors who have not had chickenpox or been vaccinated against it do not come in contact with the patient.
- Tell the patient not to scratch the rash: it could introduce bacterial infection.
- Have the patient wash the hands often and trim the fingernails very short because scratching during sleep is common.
- To relieve itching, give cetirizine, 10 mg orally, in the evening.
- It is not usually necessary to reduce fever but, if required, you can give paracetamol, 1000 mg orally, every six hours.

- If you suspect a secondary bacterial infection of chickenpox skin lesions, give amoxycillin/clavulanate, 875/125 mg orally, twice daily.
- If you suspect chickenpox pneumonia, arrange for urgent evacuation.
- Note:
  - patients are no longer infectious to others when the last lesion has crusted over (it does not need to have healed completely);
  - vaccination within three to five days of exposure to the virus will prevent most cases of chickenpox;
  - if a crew member develops chickenpox while in port, or a susceptible crew member is exposed to a case, consider vaccinating all susceptible crew members to prevent an outbreak.

SHINGLES (HERPES ZOSTER)

Shingles occurs years after a person has recovered from chickenpox. In the course of chickenpox, the varicella-zoster virus hides from the immune system in the nerves that supply sensation to the skin. Years later, as a person's immune defences weaken, the virus can escape from the nerves and affect the skin in the area served by the nerve. Most cases occur in patients over 55.

Signs and symptoms

- In most cases, a deep burning pain felt in a narrow band around one side of the chest or abdomen.
- In some cases, fever and feeling unwell.
- A few days or a week after the start of pain, a rash appears in the painful area; note:
  - the rash resembles that of chickenpox rash but is found only in the area affected by pain.
- After a week to 10 days, crusting of the lesions (and the patient is no longer infectious).

COMPLICATIONS

- Pain of long duration in the area of the rash (post-herpetic neuralgia) in about 10% of cases of shingles.
- Involvement of the eye, with possible loss of sight, if the nerve serving the forehead is affected.

✔ *What to do*

- If the patient is seen within 72 hours of the appearance of the rash give aciclovir, 800 mg orally, five times daily for seven days.
- The pain of shingles can be very distressing and hard to treat: and morphine, 10–20 mg, preferably orally, every three to four hours may be required;
- If the patient has a shingles rash affecting the skin around the eye, seek medical advice with a view to evacuation; begin aciclovir as above while awaiting evacuation.
- Cover the rash with clothing or a light non-adherent dressing.

- Note:
  - you do not need to isolate the patient;
  - anyone who is susceptible to varicella-zoster virus and who comes in contact with fluid from a patient's vesicles (blisters) may develop chickenpox but not shingles;
  - unlike chickenpox, shingles is not transmitted by airborne particles.

Cholera

Cholera is caused by the bacterium *Vibrio cholerae*, which is spread mainly by water but sometimes by food contaminated by the faeces of a cholera patient. Direct person-to-person transmission does not occur. The main manifestation of cholera is severe diarrhoea, which can cause dehydration and death within hours of onset. The diarrhoea is the result of a *Vibrio cholerae* toxin that causes the bowel to secrete very large amounts of fluid. Since the bacterium does not damage tissues, it does not cause fever.

Signs and symptoms

- Onset of diarrhoea one to three days after infection.
- Diarrhoea severe for two days and lasting six to eight days; the diarrhoea is:
  - frequent, copious, very watery ("rice-water"), but not blood-stained
  - mild in most cases
  - not accompanied by fever
  - indistinguishable from diarrhoea from other causes.
- If an outbreak is in progress in a port city, most cases of watery diarrhoea will be due to cholera.

What to do

- Since a healthy adult can die of cholera in 24 hours, give cholera treatment to any patient with severe watery diarrhoea.
- If you can prevent dehydration, no other treatment is necessary: the infection will get better on its own.

Table 23.3 Guide to the severity of dehydration in a patient with diarrhoeal disease.

	Mild hydration	Moderate dehydration	Severe dehydration
Mental status	alert	restless	lethargic or comatose
Eyes	normal	sunken	sunken and dry
Tears	present	absent	absent
Mouth and tongue	slightly dry	dry	very dry
Thirst	increased	greatly increased	drinks little
Skin pinch test	skin goes back rapidly (to normal)	goes back slowly	goes back very slowly or not at all

- Seek medical advice; evacuation is appropriate for moderate and severe dehydration.
- Treat according to the severity of dehydration (see Table 23.3):
  - **mild dehydration**:
    - give one cup of Oral Rehydration Solution for each diarrhoeal stool; **PLUS**
    - as much plain water as the patient wants;
  - **moderate dehydration**:
    - give 1000 ml of Oral Rehydration Solution every hour for the first four hours; **PLUS**
    - one cup of Oral Rehydration Solution for each diarrhoeal stool; **PLUS**
    - as much water as the patient wants;
  - **severe dehydration**:
    - while awaiting evacuation, start intravenous rehydration;
    - insert the largest intravenous cannula available and give normal saline solution (0.9% sodium chloride), one litre every 30 minutes until the pulse is easily felt and has returned to the normal range (less than 100 beats per minute);
    - as soon as the patient can drink, start oral rehydration therapy as for moderate dehydration (see above).
- If you are uncertain about the severity of dehydration, treat as you would for moderate dehydration.
- If the patient is hungry, allow a normal diet but with no sugary or fatty foods.
- If Oral Rehydration Solution is not available, make a substitute using:
  - a mixture of four teaspoons of sugar, a pinch of salt, a pinch of sodium bicarbonate, and the juice of an orange (or a bottle of fruit juice) in half a litre of water.
- You do not need to give antibiotic treatment but if crew members need to return to duty quickly you may give one dose of azithromycin, 1000 mg orally, which slightly reduces the duration of diarrhoea.
- It is not necessary to isolate a patient with cholera, but enteric precautions should be followed: stools and vomited matter should be flushed into the ship's sewage treatment system or retention tank.
- Since cholera is transmitted by water and food and has a short incubation period, cases that develop more than two days after leaving port are likely to have been acquired on board: the ship's water supply must be thoroughly treated.
- Cholera is a notifiable disease: as soon as practicable, the ship's master must notify any case to the health authorities at the next port of call and take such measures as the authorities require to prevent spread of the disease.

Dengue

Dengue is caused by a virus transmitted by the *Aedes aegypti* mosquito. The mosquito breeds in or close to houses, never flies far from where it was born, and bites mainly in the daytime. Dengue is primarily a disease of tropical and sub-tropical cities and is one of the commonest diseases acquired by visitors to cities in Africa, Asia and Central America.

There are four sub-types of the dengue virus. Infection with one sub-type gives life-long immunity against that sub-type but not against the others.

Signs and symptoms

- Fever lasting five to seven days;
- headache;
- pain behind the eyes;
- severe pain in muscles and joints (so severe that dengue is sometimes called "break-bone fever");
- marked fatigue that can last for weeks;
- in about half of cases, onset of a rash about two days after the fever;
- in about half of cases, nausea and vomiting;
- in about a third of cases, diarrhoea.

COMPLICATIONS

- Occasionally, dengue hemorrhagic fever or dengue shock syndrome occurs – both life-threatening illnesses, characterized by:
  - abdominal pain
  - bleeding, usually into the skin
  - vomiting of blood
  - blood in the faeces
  - nose bleeds.

✔ What to do

- Seek medical advice with a view to evacuation.
- For fever and for muscle and joint pain, give paracetamol, 1000 mg orally, every six hours **but never acetylsalicylic acid (Aspirin®)**, which may worsen bleeding if dengue hemorrhagic fever develops.
- Encourage the patient to take fluids but otherwise to eat normally.
- Note:
  - there is no specific treatment for dengue, which usually resolves spontaneously with complete recovery of the patient;
  - there is no vaccine against dengue;
  - isolation of the patient is not required.

Diphtheria

Diphtheria is caused by the bacterium *Corynebacterium diphtheriae*. Infection is acquired from an infected person, most often a healthy carrier. The severe illness it causes is due to a toxin that the bacterium produces. Infection with diphtheria can result in two forms of disease, one affecting the skin, the other, the respiratory tract, or it can result in a healthy carrier state. The disease has practically disappeared from the more developed countries but remains common in poorer countries and in the countries of the former Soviet Union.

Diphtheria is preventable by immunization. However, people who were immunized as children may be susceptible as adults because of waning immunity. Reimmunization every

10 years up to the age of 50 is recommended (a combined diphtheria-tetanus vaccine is available for adults).

Signs and symptoms

- Gradual onset;
- feeling unwell;
- low fever;
- in respiratory infection, sore throat followed in one or two days by the appearance in the throat of the characteristic "membrane" – a grey, sharp-edged membrane, firmly stuck onto the throat, so hard to scrape off that attempts at removal cause bleeding;
- in skin infection, ulcers covered with a grey membrane.

Note

- In patients with sore throats from other bacterial infections (see below), fever is high and the tonsils are covered with pus, which wipes off easily.

What to do

- Give azithromycin, 500 mg orally, twice daily for 14 days.
- In the case of respiratory diphtheria:
  - isolate the patient in a single-berth cabin;
  - have the patient wear a mask except when eating;
  - sterilize by boiling or incinerate any cutlery and other utensils that may have been contaminated with the patient's oral secretions;
  - allow only fully immunized crew members to have contact with the patient;
  - allow no other visitors, such as passengers, even if immunized, because they may still become carriers;
  - continue isolation of the patient until cure of infection is confirmed by laboratory testing at the next port;
  - give all close contacts of the patient azithromycin, 500 mg orally, twice daily for seven days;
  - diphtheria infection does not confer immunity: have the patient immunized at the next port of call if they have not had primary immunization and a booster within 10 years.

Ear infections

INFECTION OF THE OUTER EAR (otitis externa)

Infection of the outer ear is common in hot weather or after swimming, especially in the tropics and subtropics. Most cases are due to bacteria.

Signs and symptoms

- Pain in one ear
- scanty discharge

- in mild cases:
  - discomfort
  - itch
- in severe cases:
  - redness of the ear
  - swelling severe enough to block the ear canal
  - pain when the ear is pulled upwards.

✔ *What to do*

- Gently clean out the ear passages with cotton-wool swabs.
- In mild cases, apply 2% acetic acid (a solution of one part wine vinegar to three parts potable water), four to six drops, three times daily for 7–10 days.
- In severe cases, apply 1% tetracycline ointment: fill a 5 ml syringe with ointment, inject it gently into the ear canal, and leave it for a week.
- Advise the patient not to swim or to allow water into the ears when washing until a doctor has examined the ears or until the ears have been normal for two weeks:
  - to keep the ears dry during showering, have the patient use a plug of cotton wool moistened with petroleum jelly.
- To relieve pain, give paracetamol, 1000 mg orally, every six hours, or ibuprofen, 400 mg orally, every six to eight hours.

INFECTION OF THE MIDDLE EAR (otitis media)

Otitis media is common in small children and rare in adults. Infection occurs when the eustachian tube is blocked by inflammation, often during a viral upper respiratory tract infection. The fluid produced by the lining of the middle ear cannot drain into the nose: it accumulates and becomes infected by bacteria which colonize the nose, most often pneumococcus and *Haemophilus influenzae*.

Signs and symptoms

- Earache
- hearing loss
- in some cases, impaired balance
- mild fever
- in a small percentage of patients, discharge of pus from the ear canal from perforation of the eardrum.

COMPLICATIONS

- Infection of the mastoid air cells (in the bone behind the ear), which communicate with the middle ear: in a few cases, the mastoid infection does not resolve when the otitis media improves and the mastoid air cells become chronically infected;
- spread of infection to the skull or brain, particularly in poorer countries.

✔ What to do

- To relieve pain give paracetamol, 1000 mg orally, every six hours.
- Give amoxycillin/clavulanate, 875/125 mg orally, twice daily for seven days.
- Note:
  - antibiotic treatment has little impact on the duration of illness and the risk of complications;
  - decongestant nose drops are of little use.

Hand infections in seafarers and fishers

Many infections of the hands can be prevented by simple measures that are often neglected. Small scratches, cuts, abrasions, or pricks caused by fish spines should never be ignored.

✔ What to do

- Have the patient wash the hands thoroughly in soap and water.
- Swab the affected site with alcohol or povidone–iodine solution.
- Cover with a waterproof dressing.
- Take special care in cleaning wounds caused by shells or fish spines, which can be infected by unusual organisms that cause rapid tissue destruction.
- For a hand or finger wound caused by a hook or knife, give amoxycillin/clavulanate, 875 mg orally, twice daily.
- For a wound caused by a shell or fish spine, give ciprofloxacin, 500 mg orally, twice daily, and have the patient remain at rest with the hand elevated above shoulder height.
- If redness, heat and pain spread rapidly in the skin after a wound caused by a shell or fish spine seek medical advice and treat as directed under *Cellulitis* in Chapter 20, *Skin diseases*.

Infectious mononucleosis (glandular fever)

Glandular fever, or infectious mononucleosis, is caused by the Epstein-Barr virus (EBV), which is also the cause of a common form of cancer in children in tropical Africa. Infection is spread by close contact with an infected person. In poor countries, children are infected with EBV at a young age but rarely develop glandular fever. In the more developed countries, where there is less crowding, infection is often delayed until adolescence or early adulthood, and it is then that glandular fever occurs. In virtually all countries, nearly everyone older than 45 has been infected with EBV and has immunity to the virus.

► Signs and symptoms

- A combination of moderate or high fever and sore throat, lasting one to two weeks, with swelling of the neck lymph nodes.
- Often, swelling of lymph nodes in the armpit and groin (not seen in most patients with sore throat due to other causes).
- In many cases, severe fatigue, that may continue for months.
- Nausea and vomiting if the liver is affected, as it often is in glandular fever, although this can only be verified by laboratory tests.

✔ *What to do*

- To reduce fever and relieve sore throat give paracetamol, 1000 mg orally, every six hours.
- Allow the patient to eat a normal diet, although in some cases the throat is so sore that only fluids can be taken.
- Isolation is not necessary.

✘ *What not to do*

- Do not give amoxycillin or amoxycillin/clavulanate to a patient who has glandular fever: it will cause an unpleasant rash.

Influenza

HUMAN INFLUENZA

Influenza, or "flu", is an acute infectious disease caused by the influenza virus, which is spread by respiratory droplets from a person with influenza. Most people with influenza get better in two to five days.

The disease tends to occur in epidemics or small outbreaks. There are two types of influenza virus: influenza A, which sometimes causes major epidemics, and influenza B, which does not. Major epidemics (called pandemics when patients in many countries are affected), occur when the virus undergoes a major change, so that few people have any immunity to it. Between pandemics, the influenza virus changes only slightly from year to year, so that most people have at least some immunity and illness is less widespread and less severe than in pandemics. Outbreaks occur in winter in temperate zones but can occur at any time of the year in the tropics. They begin quite suddenly and reach a peak in two to three weeks, then decline over two to three months.

During outbreaks in cities one tenth to one fifth of the population is affected but in a closed community such as a ship nearly everyone may be affected at the same time, with potentially disastrous effects on the efficiency and safety of shipboard operations. For these reasons, aggressive measures to control an outbreak on board ship must be taken as soon as a case occurs or if the ship enters a port in which an outbreak is underway.

A vaccine to prevent infection exists. It is recommended for people over 50 and those with chronic illnesses. It must be given every year because of the constant change in the influenza virus. It takes two weeks for immunization to provide protection, so it is best to immunize before an outbreak occurs.

► *Signs and symptoms*

- Sudden onset one to two days after exposure to the virus
- fever
- cough
- feeling unwell
- headache
- weakness and fatigue.

Note

- **The diagnosis is very likely to be influenza if**:
  - during an outbreak of influenza, the patient has had fever and cough from the very beginning of the illness.
- **The diagnosis is unlikely to be influenza if the patient has**:
  - symptoms of a head cold, such as blocked and runny nose and sneezing;
  - enlarged lymph nodes;
  - respiratory symptoms, when there is no influenza outbreak in the area.

COMPLICATIONS

- The main complication of influenza is bacterial pneumonia, which is most likely to occur in patients over 50 or in patients who have another disease affecting the lungs or heart.
- The commonest cause of pneumonia in an influenza patient is infection with the pneumococcus bacterium or the *Staphylococcus aureus* bacterium.
- Bacterial pneumonia should be suspected if a patient with influenza begins to improve but then experiences a return of high fever, with a cough producing opaque and possibly blood-stained sputum, and breathlessness.
- In a small percentage of cases severe pneumonia can be caused by the influenza virus itself: the patient does not improve after three or four days but has rising fever and worsening of breathlessness and cough.

✔ *What to do*

- To relieve the symptoms of influenza, notably fever, give paracetamol, 1000 mg orally, every six hours.
- Isolate the patient.
- Ensure that attendants wear masks, gloves, and disposable plastic aprons or a similar covering which can be hot-washed and that they wash their hands after being in the patient's cabin.
- Treat pneumonia associated with influenza as your would for any other case of pneumonia (see Chapter 15, *Respiratory diseases*).

AVIAN INFLUENZA (INFLUENZA H5N1, "BIRD FLU")

Birds, especially aquatic birds such as ducks, have always been subject to infection with influenza viruses. Most of these viruses cannot infect humans. However, the influenza pandemics of 1918, 1957, and 1968 appear to have been caused by avian influenza viruses that had acquired the ability to infect, and spread among, humans. Pigs, which can be infected by both human and bird influenza viruses, may play a role in enabling the avian influenza virus to infect humans.

A strain of avian influenza virus, called H5N1, has recently become widespread among birds in Asia and Europe and has infected some humans who had close contact with infected birds.

- At the time of writing, there has not been transmission between humans via respiratory droplets, as occurs with ordinary influenza.
- The illness caused by H5N1 in humans can be very severe, with a high mortality rate.
- If this virus does acquire the capacity to pass easily from human-to-human, there could be a pandemic with many deaths, as was the case in the 1918 flu pandemic.
- For up-to-date information on avian influenza infections see:
  - www.cdc.gov/flu/avian/outbreaks/current.htm; **OR** www.who.int/csr/disease/avian_influenza/en/.

✔ *What to do*

- Seek medical advice at once if a person who has had contact with domestic poultry within the past 10 days, in a country where cases of H5N1 infection have appeared, develops:
  - a fever of over 38 °C; **AND**
  - a cough or a sore throat or breathlessness.
- Isolate the patient and apply strict contact precautions.

Malaria

Malaria is caused by a protozoan, or single-cell, parasite that infects humans when they are bitten by the female *Anopheles* mosquito. There are four types of malaria parasite, but two, *Plasmodium falciparum* and *Plasmodium vivax*, account for most malaria in humans. Falciparum malaria is the commonest type in tropical Africa, the Amazon basin, Papua New Guinea and South-East Asia, while vivax infections predominate in Central America, India and the Middle East. Most deaths caused by malaria are the result of falciparum infections. There is no vaccine against malaria.

Note

- Malaria is widespread in tropical and sub-tropical regions.
- *Anopheles* mosquitoes are more common in rural areas than in cities, so that major urban ports tend to carry a low risk of malaria infection even in countries with a high overall risk.
- Broadly, the risk of malaria is greatest in sub-Saharan Africa, intermediate in India and South-East Asia, and low in Central and South America.
- For up-to-date information about the risk of acquiring malaria in a given port, see www.cdc.gov/travel/regionalmalaria/index.htm.

✔ *What to do to reduce the risk of malaria infection*

For short-term visitors to urban areas of South-East Asia and South America

- Since the *Anopheles* mosquito carrying malaria parasites usually bites between dusk and dawn, advise crew members to remain indoors at night, in a screened or air-conditioned area.
- Advise crew members who are out-of-doors between dusk and dawn to wear long-sleeved shirts and trousers and to use insect repellent on exposed skin (see Chapter 29, *Environmental control and hygiene*).

- Advise crew members who do not sleep in air-conditioned areas to sleep under insecticide-treated bed nets.

For short-term visitors to rural areas of South-East Asia and South America, and for all visitors to Africa and New Guinea

- Carry out the measures above meticulously.
- Before leaving your home port, consider providing the crew with antimalarial drug prophylaxis (prevention) as recommended by:
  - the World Health Organization (see www.who.int/malaria/publications.html); **OR**
  - the Centers for Disease Control and Prevention in the United States (see www.cdc.gov/travel/regionalmalaria/index.htm).

Signs and symptoms

- Onset of symptoms 12–14 days after infection in the case of falciparum malaria and up to several months after infection in the case of vivax malaria.
- Fever, typically in paroxysms, or crises, occurring daily in falciparum malaria, every second day in vivax malaria, with;
  - at first, shaking chills as fever rises;
  - then headache, muscle pain, vomiting, and diarrhoea;
  - after an hour or two, drenching sweat, with a rapid fall in fever.
- Few or no symptoms between paroxysms.

COMPLICATIONS

- **Cerebral malaria**, the main complication of falciparum infection:
  - more common in short-term visitors to malarial areas than in long-term residents, who are likely to have some degree of immunity to the malaria parasite;
  - if severe and/or untreated, may cause:
    - drowsiness
    - confusion
    - coma
    - fits (convulsions)
    - death
    - note that the most important alternative cause of fever and impaired consciousness is meningococcal infection, which causes neck stiffness and a rash, both of which are absent in malaria patients (see below, under *Meningitis and meningococcal infection*).
- **Kidney failure**, a possible complication of falciparum infections, causing:
  - reduced output of urine;
  - very dark urine ("blackwater fever");
  - in some cases, severe breathlessness and cough that produces frothy blood-stained sputum.

What to do – basic principles

- Put the patient to bed.
- Every four hours take the temperature, pulse, and respiratory rate.

- Continue recording the temperature every four hours until the attack has passed.
- Take a blood sample for later examination to confirm the diagnosis.
- Examine a urine specimen for blood once a day.
- Record the Glasgow Coma Scale score (see Table 26.3, Chapter 26, *Nursing care and medical procedures*) twice daily or whenever you suspect that the level of consciousness is declining.
- You do not need to isolate the patient but provide an air-conditioned cabin if possible.
- To reduce fever give paracetamol, 1000 mg orally, every six hours.
- If the body temperature rises to 39°C, cool the patient (see Chapter 26, *Nursing care and medical procedures*).
- Make a slide with the patient's blood for later examination for malaria parasites (see below, *How to take a blood slide*).
- Suspect malaria in a patient who has fever but no other symptoms of severe illness and who:
  - in the past 9–30 days, has visited an area where malaria transmission is known to occur; **OR**
  - is known to have had attacks of malaria and has a fever but no features of other severe illnesses;
  - do not discount malaria as a possibility because the patient has taken anti-malarial prophylaxis.
- Start treatment as soon as possible: delay increases the risk of serious complications:
  - if the illness is not malaria, little or no harm will result from the treatment;
  - if the illness is malaria, failure to treat can result in a death which could have been prevented.
- Once you decide to treat, make sure the patient takes the full recommended course, even if:
  - there is reason to believe that the patient has partial immunity to malaria; **OR**
  - you are not certain that the patient has malaria.
- Note that patients with vivax malaria may need additional treatment which cannot be given on board ship: therefore, ensure that all patients treated for malaria see a doctor at the next port.
- If there are symptoms consistent with either cerebral malaria or meningococcal disease, give antimalarial drugs for malaria and antibiotics for meningococcal disease (see below, under *Meningitis and meningococcal infection*), since both diseases can be rapidly fatal if untreated.
- Obtain medical advice urgently and prepare to evacuate the patient to a hospital if:
  - the symptoms are severe; **OR**
  - you are concerned about the patient's progress; **OR**
  - any one of the following conditions is present:
    - level of consciousness below normal (Glasgow Coma Scale score below 13, see Table 26.3 in Chapter 26, *Nursing care and medical procedures*)
    - blood found in the urine
    - severe breathlessness
    - jaundice

Table 23.4 Dose regimen of artemether-lumefantrine antimalarial tablets adjusted to patient's body weight or age.

Body weight in kg (age in yrs)	Number of tablets and approximate timing of doses					
	0 h	8 h	24 h	36 h	48 h	60 h
5–14 (<3)	1	1	1	1	1	1
15–24 (3–8)	2	2	2	2	2	2
25–34 (9–14)	3	3	3	3	3	3
>34 (>14)	4	4	4	4	4	4

› bleeding with no evidence of injury
› the patient is a pregnant woman.

✔ *What to do in treating uncomplicated malaria*[2]

- For the treatment of uncomplicated falciparum or vivax malaria, acquired in any part of the world, give six doses of artemether-lumefantrine over three days (to calculate the number of tablets required for each dose and the timing of administration of these doses, see Table 23.4).
- **Note that artemether-lumefantrine must be given with full-cream milk or fatty food**.
- Remember that patients with vivax malaria may need additional treatment to prevent late relapse.

✔ *What to do in treating severe (complicated) malaria*

- Remember that, untreated, severe malaria is nearly always fatal: even with the best hospital care the mortality rate is still high.
- You should always aim at evacuation of the patient if this is possible.
- You must give the first dose as early as possible and you must always give full doses:
  - **DO NOT "wait and see"**;
  - **DO NOT delay giving treatment** because evacuation has been arranged;
  - **DO NOT reduce the dose** because the diagnosis is uncertain.
- Start an intravenous fluid infusion if the patient cannot swallow; give one litre of 0.9% sodium chloride (normal saline) every 6–8 hours.
- If consciousness is impaired, place the patient in the coma, or recovery, position (see Chapter 1, *First aid*).
- Insert a bladder catheter and keep a record of fluid input and output (see Chapter 26, *Nursing care and medical procedures*).
- Give artemether, 3.2 mg/kg body weight, intramuscularly, as soon as the decision to treat is made; **THEN**:

- 1.6 mg/kg body weight intramuscularly, every day, beginning 24 hours after the first dose, if the patient is still on board.

- Continue intramuscular artemether until the patient can swallow.
- If the patient remains on board, begin a full course of artemether-lumefantrine, as for uncomplicated malaria (see above), as soon as the patient can swallow.

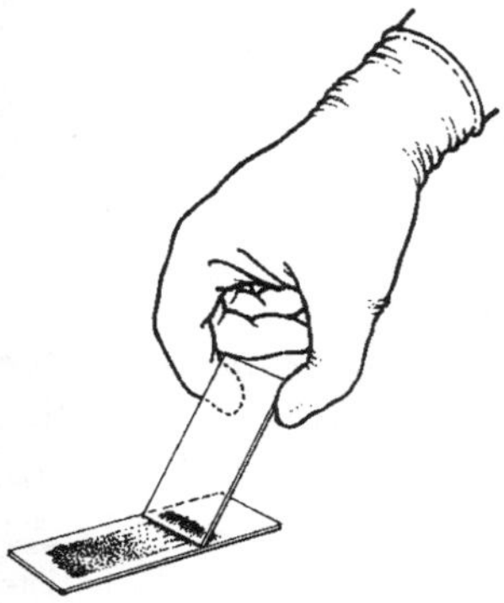

Figure 23.1 How to make a blood slide.

How to take a blood slide

- Obtain a sterile disposable lancet or, if one is not available, a sterile disposable syringe needle.
- Take two microscope slides and polish them with a clean cloth.
- Wash the patient's left thumb, dry it, swab it with surgical spirit, and allow it to dry.
- Wrap a small length of bandage around the base of the thumb tightly enough to congest the blood vessels.
- Wash your hands.
- Stab the ball of the patient's thumb lightly with the lancet or needle so that a drop of blood oozes out.
- Take one of the microscope slides and place one end gently on the drop of blood.
- Remove the bandage from the base of the thumb.
- Place the slide on a flat surface and hold it steady with your left hand.
- Take the other microscope slide with your right hand, incline it at an angle of 45°, and place the edge in the centre of the drop of blood in the first slide, allowing the blood to spread along the width of that slide.
- With a steady continuous movement draw the inclined slide along the length of the other slide to make a fine smear (Figure 23.1).
- Allow the smeared slide to dry in the air.
- Place the dry slide in an envelope labelled with the date, time, and patient's name.
- Seal the envelope and tape it securely to a page of the patient's medical record.

Meningitis and meningococcal infection

Meningitis is an inflammation of the membranes surrounding the brain and spinal cord. The cause can be an infection with bacteria, viruses or fungi, but a noninfectious cause is also possible. Only bacterial meningitis will be discussed here, as it is the most life-threatening form of meningitis. Several types of bacteria can cause meningitis but most cases in adults are due to pneumococcus, the organism that also causes most cases of pneumonia, or to *Neisseria meningitidis*, also called meningococcus.

Meningitis caused by meningococcus (meningococcal meningitis) can occur in epidemics. The infection is spread by respiratory droplets: household contacts of an infected person are at a high risk of infection and disease. Meningitis due to other bacteria does not cause epidemics and does not spread among contacts.

Immunization against meningococcal infection is recommended for anyone travelling to areas where meningococcal disease is common – mainly sub-Saharan Africa – but epidemics occur from time to time in many other areas. Immunization does not prevent meningitis caused by other bacteria and does not prevent infection with all strains of meningococcus.

Signs and symptoms

- Abrupt onset, with:
  - high fever
  - headache
  - confusion
  - drowsiness.
- Without treatment, coma and shock within 24–48 hours of first symptoms: an illness continuing for several days without treatment is unlikely to be bacterial meningitis.
- Neck stiffness (difficulty placing the chin on the chest when lying flat) is strongly suggestive of meningitis.
- In about half of cases, a pink, blotchy rash initially similar to rubella rash but later consisting of small dark-red spots, mainly on the trunk and legs; **this rash in a patient with headache and fever makes meningococcal infection very likely**.
- Meningococcal infection of the bloodstream (without meningitis) is suggested by:
  - fever
  - drowsiness
  - leg pain
  - cold hands and feet
  - pale, mottled skin.

What to do

- **Treat as soon as you suspect meningitis**: early treatment saves lives and a delay of even one hour increases the risk of death.
- Give ceftriaxone, 2 g intramuscularly, at once and then every 12 hours for as long as the patient remains on board.
- Seek medical advice and prepare to evacuate the patient but **DO NOT delay treatment** while awaiting advice.
- If the patient remains on board, treat for a total of 14 days.
- Isolate the patient and apply strict precautions against droplet transmission (see Chapter 26, *Nursing care and medical procedures*).
- Give a single dose of ceftriaxone, 250 mg intramuscularly, to **all** crew members who have shared accommodation or work space with the patient.

Mumps

Mumps is mainly a disease of children. It is caused by a virus that spreads through direct contact with the respiratory secretions or saliva of an infected person. In the more developed countries immunization has confined the disease to a small number of adults who have not been effectively immunized or who have not been infected earlier in their lives. There is no specific cure: treatment is given to relieve symptoms.

Signs and symptoms

- Onset with:
  - low fever
  - feeling unwell;

- within two days:
  - swelling of both parotid glands (the salivary glands in front of and below the ear);
- within one to two weeks of onset, inflammation of the testicles (orchitis) in about a third of infected men, causing:
  - high fever
  - severe pain in the testicles
  - swelling of the scrotum.

✔ *What to do*

- Apply precautions against droplet transmission (see Chapter 26, *Nursing care and medical procedures)* and isolate the patient.
- Note that patients are most infectious before the parotid gland swelling appears but remain infectious for about seven days after onset of the swelling.
- To relieve the pain of orchitis, which can be severe:
  - give ibuprofen, 400 mg orally, every eight hours;
  - provide support for the scrotum;
  - apply measures to cool the scrotum.

Plague

Plague is caused by the bacterium *Yersinia pestis*. It is a disease of wild rodents (rats, squirrels, and related animals) and infects humans only accidentally. The infection is spread among rodents by fleas; humans are usually infected by bites from rodent fleas or from handling dead rodents. The disease is widespread and epidemics have occurred recently in Africa and in India. Plague can have its main effects in the lymph nodes (bubonic plague), in the blood (septicaemic plague) or in the lungs (pneumonic plague). Bubonic plague is the commonest. Patients with pneumonic plague can transmit the disease to others via respiratory droplets.

► *Signs and symptoms*

- At onset:
  - fever
  - feeling unwell;
- soon after onset:
  - intense pain, severe tenderness, and swelling of lymph nodes (buboes), mainly in the groin;
- in septicaemic plague:
  - high fever and obvious illness.

COMPLICATIONS

- In some cases of bubonic or septicaemic plague, pneumonia with:
  - cough
  - breathlessness.

✔ *What to do*

- Give doxycycline, 100 mg orally, twice daily for 10 days.

- Isolate the patient, applying strict respiratory (droplet) precautions (see Chapter 26, *Nursing care and medical procedures*) until full recovery.
- If the patient has a cough or is breathless, give all face-to-face contacts of the patient doxycycline, 100 mg orally, twice daily for 10 days.
- Boil soiled linen and bed clothes for 10 minutes or destroy them.
- Do not lance the buboes: if they produce pus, which is highly infectious, cover them with a dry dressing, taking care to wear gloves, a mask, and protective clothing.
- If a case of suspected plague occurs on board ship, seek medical advice at once.
- After consultation with the port health authorities, send the patient to an onshore medical facility at the first opportunity.
- To ensure destruction of any fleas, treat the patient's quarters and those occupied by the rest of the crew with insecticide powder.

Note

- Plague is a disease subject to the International Health Regulations (see Chapter 32, *International Health Regulations*): the ship's master should notify the local health authorities at the next port of call that a case has occurred on board.
- Measures should be taken, as directed by the local health authority, to prevent spread of the disease.
- Dead rats found aboard ship should be picked up with tongs and placed in a plastic bag, which should be sealed with string, weighted, and thrown overboard; if the ship is in port, dead rats should be disposed of in the manner required by the port health authorities.

Rabies

Rabies is caused by a virus which attacks the brain. Once the disease has taken hold it is always fatal. The virus spreads through the bite of a rabid mammal (only mammals can be infected). It is not transmitted directly from person-to-person. In the less developed countries dog bites cause 90% of cases. Bats, foxes, and other wild carnivores are important vectors in some countries but mice, squirrels, guinea-pigs, and rabbits do not carry rabies. Bats often inflict very small bites, often at night, so that patients may not realize that they may have been exposed to the virus.

✔ *What to do*

- Immediately after a potentially infective bite, wash the wound thoroughly with soap and water.
- Swab with povidone–iodine solution.
- Seek medical advice as soon as possible: it may be necessary to evacuate the patient to a hospital for preventative treatment.
- Try to find out, and tell the doctor:
  - what animal was involved;
  - the circumstances of the bite: unprovoked attacks are more likely to transmit rabies than provoked attacks;
  - whether the animal can be captured for observation;

- the location of the bite: the incubation period of the disease is shorter if rabies is acquired from a bite to the head than to any other part of the body.

Rubella (German measles)

Rubella is caused by a virus transmitted by droplets from the mouth and nose. Patients are most infectious before they become ill. Once the rash appears they are less likely to transmit infection. Rubella is nearly always a mild illness in adults. The greatest risk from rubella is in women infected in the early stages of pregnancy: they can transmit the infection to the fetus, which, as a result, may be born deaf and with heart and eye defects.

Signs and symptoms

- At onset, mild fever, swelling of the lymph glands behind the ears and at the back of the neck but no other lymph nodes affected (this distribution is characteristic of rubella).
- A red rash of spots and blotches appearing first on the face, then spreading to the trunk.
- Joint pain and stiffness, possibly lasting for several weeks and occurring often in women but only occasionally in men.

✔ *What to do*

- Warn the patient to avoid all contact with pregnant women who have not been immunized against rubella.
- If the patient has been in close contact with a woman in early pregnancy in the previous two weeks, ask him to inform the woman that she should seek medical advice.

SARS (severe acute respiratory syndrome)

SARS was caused by a virus related to one that causes the common cold. There was a sudden outbreak with cases over a few months in early 2003, but at the time of writing, there had been no cases reported since 2004.

All of the cases occurred in people who had been in southern People's Republic of China or had contact with someone from southern China or were doctors or nurses caring for patients with SARS.

SARS began with fever (more than 38°C), followed after a few days by cough and breathlessness. The illness became rapidly more severe in nearly all cases and death occurred in 10% of cases.

Infection spread by droplets and by direct contact with respiratory secretions (the same as influenza).

PRECAUTIONS IN CASES OF POSSIBLE SARS

If another outbreak of SARS occurs, it should be considered if fever and cough or breathlessness occur in a person who has been in an area where SARS has occurred recently.

Seek radio medical advice at once. If the advice is to make for the next or nearest port notify medical authorities in that port immediately.

Meanwhile, have the patient stay in a single cabin and not leave it for any reason. As few attendants as possible should enter the sick bay, and they should wear masks, gowns, and gloves while attending the patient. They should remove these items (in the order gown, then gloves, then wash hands, then mask) before they leave the sick bay and dispose of them as hazardous infectious waste. They should wash their hands carefully before leaving and on returning. There is no need to isolate carers from other crew unless fever develops.

Sore throat

Sore throats are common and in most cases due to viral infections. Of these, glandular fever (see below) is the most important, though not the most common. In about 10–15% of cases of sore throat the cause is infection with Group A Streptococcus (GAS), also called *Streptococcus pyogenes*. Infection with this bacterium can produce abscesses around the tonsils ("quinsy") or, occasionally, provoke an attack of a joint and heart illness called rheumatic fever. There is no need to isolate a patient with GAS infection.

✔ *What to do*

- If the patient with a sore throat has three or more of the following symptoms, you can strongly suspect infection with GAS:
  - yellowish creamy material on the tonsils or back or sides of the throat;
  - tender, enlarged lymph nodes below the jaw;
  - fever, either reported by the patient or detected by taking the patient's temperature;
  - no cough.
- If you suspect GAS infection, give azithromycin, 500 mg orally, twice daily for five days.
- Note that antibiotic treatment will shorten the course of the illness and prevent rheumatic fever but only if the patient completes the full course of treatment even if symptoms subside after a day or two.
- If the patient has a sore throat but does not have symptoms suggestive of GAS infection give:
  - paracetamol, 1000 mg orally, every six hours; **OR**
  - liquorice tea, which will reduce the soreness in the throat.

Red flags

In rare cases, a sore throat can be part of a serious infection or can be due to abscesses in the tissues below, to either side of, or behind the throat: if a patient with a sore throat has in addition any of the following symptoms seek medical advice urgently:

- difficulty swallowing saliva
- drooling
- difficulty speaking
- difficulty breathing
- swelling of the neck not due to enlarged lymph nodes.

Tetanus (lockjaw)

Tetanus results from infection of a wound by the bacterium *Clostridium tetani*, which produces a toxin (tetanus toxin). The toxin travels to the brain and spinal cord and causes the symptoms of the disease (see below). The bacterium is usually present in soil and tetanus can occur when wounds, especially deep wounds, are contaminated with soil. The bacterium can also infect needle wounds of intravenous drug users.

Tetanus can be prevented by immunization with a vaccine prepared from inactivated tetanus toxin. To maintain protection, booster doses of the vaccine should be given every 10 years. All seafarers employed on a ship carrying horses, cattle, or animal hides must provide proof that they have completed initial (primary) immunization against tetanus plus the booster vaccine doses.

Signs and symptoms

- Onset a few days to weeks after the wound;
- first symptoms in most cases: spasm of the jaw muscles, leading to difficulty in opening the mouth and swallowing ("lockjaw");
- increasingly frequent, extremely painful muscle spasms, triggered by external stimuli such as touch, noise, or bright light, with the patient remaining fully conscious.
- spasms spreading to the chest, neck, and back;
- sweating;
- irritability;
- restlessness;
- rapid pulse.

What to do

- Carefully clean – but do not suture – wounds that may be contaminated with soil.
- Open out and wash thoroughly any puncture wounds that may contain contaminated material, such as a twig or soil.
- **If you suspect tetanus, seek medical advice and arrange for urgent evacuation to an appropriate onshore medical facility**.
- **While awaiting evacuation, nurse the patient in a darkened room**, with as few disturbances as possible.

Tuberculosis

Tuberculosis, which is caused by a bacterium, *Mycobacterium tuberculosis*. It remains a common disease throughout the world. It can affect any organ in the body but most cases involve the lungs. Only lung tuberculosis is infectious. Infection is spread by droplets coughed up by a person with active lung tuberculosis. The risk of infection is low if the period of contact is less than a few hours, so most infections are acquired from household or other close contacts.

Only about 10% of infected people develop tuberculosis disease. Infected people who do not develop the disease cannot transmit the infection. The disease is most likely to occur in very young children, in patients with illnesses such as diabetes, in people who are malnourished, and in people with HIV/AIDS. Tuberculosis may take years to develop into a severe illness.

Signs and symptoms

- Onset gradual and usually not sooner than a few months after infection.
- Cough, usually not so severe as to interfere with everyday activities, but present every day, often with a little sputum flecked with blood.
- In many cases, fever, especially in the evenings.
- In many cases, weight loss despite a good appetite.

Note

- Other important causes of a persistent cough are asthma, gastro-oesophageal reflux disease (see Chapter 16, *Gastrointestinal and liver diseases*), bronchiectasis, lung disease due to cigarette smoking, and lung cancer (which also causes a cough with blood or blood-streaked sputum).
- It is rarely possible to distinguish between these conditions without a chest X–ray.
- A person with active tuberculosis should be prevented from going to sea, since the entire crew would be at risk.
- Anyone with a cough lasting more than three weeks should see a doctor and have a chest X-ray to exclude tuberculosis.
- If a case of active tuberculosis is discovered on board, all members of the crew should be screened for tuberculosis by having an X-ray at the next port, and possibly a skin test or blood test that can detect infection.
- Crew members with tuberculosis infection and an abnormal chest X-ray will require treatment.
- Some crew members may have a normal chest X-ray despite being infected: medical advice should be sought as to whether or not these crew members should be treated.
- Several drugs are required to cure tuberculosis and the treatment must continue for several months.
- Medication for the treatment of tuberculosis should not be started at sea, because the right choice of drugs requires identification of the strain of bacterium present in a particular case.
- Most patients have been sick for several months before tuberculosis is diagnosed: a delay of a week or two before starting treatment would make little difference to the risk of spreading the infection, provided respiratory precautions are taken (see above, under *What to do – precautions against spread of infection*, and Table 23.2).

✔ What to do

- Have the patient sleep in a single-berth cabin and wear a mask outside of the cabin.
- You do not need to take special precautions in handling the patient's bedclothes, eating utensils, or clothing.
- Note that a patient loses the ability to transmit infection within a week or two of starting the correct treatment.

Typhoid and paratyphoid fever

Typhoid and paratyphoid fever are caused by two closely related bacteria of the *Salmonella* group. After an incubation period of two to three weeks, both infections produce much the same signs and symptoms and require much the same treatment. Further reference, therefore, to "typhoid" fever in this section of the guide, should be taken to cover both typhoid and paratyphoid fever.

Transmission of the infection occurs via food or, less often, water that is contaminated with *Salmonella*. Immunization does not prevent all cases of typhoid fever and does not prevent paratyphoid fever at all: it does, however, reduce the likelihood of an infection producing serious disease.

Signs and symptoms

- Fever, that typically rises steadily over the first week ("stepwise fever"), with a surprisingly slow pulse rate, given the high fever;
- abdominal pain;
- headache;
- feeling unwell;
- constipation (more common than diarrhoea);
- cough, in about a third of cases;
- in some cases, during the second week of illness, appearance of the classical rash, consisting of:
  - faint pale-pink spots ("rose spots") on the trunk and abdomen; note that because antibiotics are usually given in the first week of the illness, rose spots have become rare;
- in about 10% of untreated patients, during the third week of illness, symptoms due to perforation of the bowel and peritonitis:
  - blood in the stools;
  - dramatic worsening of abdominal pain and abdominal swelling.

What to do

- Give ciprofloxacin, 500 mg orally, twice daily for 10 days; **OR**:
  - azithromycin, 1000 mg orally, once daily for five days.
- For a patient who relapses and has fever again, give a second course of antibiotics.
- Make sure that contact precautions are taken, such as:
  - frequent, scrupulous hand-washing by the patient;
  - forbidding the patient to prepare or handle food;
  - forbidding a crew member responsible for food preparation and suspected of having typhoid to return as a food-handler before being cleared as a possible carrier of the typhoid organism (see *Note*, below).

Note

- A few patients become chronic carriers of typhoid organisms: they do not become ill but are likely to transmit the disease if they are food-handlers and may require repeated courses of antibiotics.

- Patients who have gallbladder disease are likely to become chronic carriers: removal of the gallbladder may be required to cure the carrier state.

Viral hepatitis (hepatitis A, B, and C)

Viral hepatitis is an infection of the liver by one of the hepatitis viruses. The three commonest viruses (A, B and C) are not related to one another, cause three different sets of signs and symptoms, and have in common only the fact that they cause hepatitis.

HEPATITIS A VIRUS INFECTION

Hepatitis A virus (HAV) infection is common throughout the world. When children are infected they rarely become ill but as living standards rise more people escape infection until adult life, when hepatitis with visible symptoms of illness is more likely to occur. The illness caused by HAV infection can be prevented by immunization. There is no specific treatment for HAV infection or illness.

HAV is spread only by faecal–oral transmission and is present in the patient's faeces long before the illness appears. Most transmission occurs in the patient's home and most patients have had direct contact with an infected person. Occasional cases are acquired from food, usually inadequately cooked shellfish.

Signs and symptoms

- Onset two to seven weeks after infection
- fatigue
- feeling unwell
- nausea
- loss of appetite
- fever
- pain in the upper right segment of the abdomen (over the liver)
- a week or so later, appearance of dark urine
- pale faeces
- jaundice (yellow colouring of skin and itching), peaking after a week or two then declining: onset of jaundice is associated with a lessening of fever and of feeling unwell.

COMPLICATIONS

- Severe liver failure in some patients who acquire HAV infection when already infected with the hepatitis B or hepatitis C virus.

✔ *What to do*

- Follow contact precautions.
- Make sure the patient does not prepare or handle any food that may be eaten by others.
- Have the patient use disposable plates and cutlery or plates and cutlery that only the patient uses.
- Have the patient wash the hands scrupulously and frequently: the virus can survive on unwashed fingers for several hours.

- Ensure that household bleach is used to disinfect surfaces potentially contaminated by HAV.
- Urge the patient to avoid alcohol during the illness but to eat a normal diet otherwise.
- If pain and fever are troublesome, give acetylsalicylic acid (Aspirin®), 600 mg orally, every four to six hours; note:
  - paracetamol should not be given to patients with viral hepatitis.
- Have the patient see a doctor at the next port.

HEPATITIS B VIRUS INFECTION

Hepatitis B virus (HBV) causes several illnesses affecting the liver and can also cause symptoms in other parts of the body. Chronic infection with HBV can cause cirrhosis and cancer of the liver (*Hepatocellular carcinoma*). HBV infection is spread by contact with the blood of an infected person and is preventable by immunization. There is no specific treatment for HBV infection or illness.

Note

- **In China, South-East Asia, and sub-Saharan Africa:**
  - 10–20% of the population has chronic HBV infection;
  - most people are infected at birth and do not develop hepatitis illness.
- **In Japan, the Mediterranean, the Middle East, and South America:**
  - 3–5% of the population is infected; most cases are acquired in childhood by contact with blood from an infected person's minor injuries.
- **In Australia, North America, and northern Europe:**
  - less than 2% of people are infected, most cases being acquired by sexual intercourse or intravenous drug use during adult life;
  - infection acquired by adults is most likely to cause hepatitis illness but seldom leads to chronic infection.

Signs and symptoms

- Onset following an incubation period of one to four months;
- loss of appetite;
- feeling unwell;
- discomfort in the right upper segment of the abdomen;
- jaundice (yellow colouring of the skin) in about a third of patients with acute HBV infection.

COMPLICATIONS

- Liver failure in a few cases, especially in patients whose liver is already damaged from another cause.
- liver failure causes:
  - darkening of the jaundice

- swelling of the abdomen
- skin bruising either without injury or after very minor injury
- irritability
- confusion.

✔ *What to do*

- Because only the blood is infectious, you do not need to isolate the patient.
- Warn the patient not to share razors, toothbrushes, or any other implement that could be contaminated with blood.
- Warn the patient not to have sexual intercourse until medically cleared.
- Have the patient see a doctor at the next port.
- Advise the patient not to drink alcohol but otherwise to eat a normal diet.

✘ *What not to do*

- DO NOT give paracetamol: it can cause liver failure in this condition.

HEPATITIS C VIRUS INFECTION

The hepatitis C virus (HCV) causes one of the commonest liver diseases in the more developed countries. Most cases are acquired by intravenous drug use or by other forms of exposure to the blood of an infected person. Close contact without exposure to blood cannot transmit the disease. The acute infection does not usually cause any illness but nearly all patients become chronically infected and have continuing liver inflammation without symptoms. Chronic HCV infection is a common cause of cirrhosis of the liver, but this usually develops many years after infection.

Whooping cough (pertussis)

Whooping cough is caused by the bacterium *Bordetella pertussis*. It is an important cause of illness and death in small children but also affects adults. Immunization against pertussis in childhood does not provide life-long immunity and many adults are susceptible to infection. The incubation period of pertussis is usually one to three weeks but it can be much longer.

Whooping cough is highly infectious and is spread by respiratory droplets but infection requires relatively close contact, usually at a distance of less than two metres. For this reason patients are often aware of contact with someone who has had a prolonged cough. Unfortunately, patients are most infectious at the beginning of the illness, when it is not possible to distinguish pertussis from viral bronchitis.

Signs and symptoms

- Cough, in most cases, dry and occurring mainly at night, in paroxysms (bouts), with many coughs in rapid succession followed, in half of the cases, by vomiting.
- In children, cough paroxysms followed by a noisy, whistling intake of breath (the "whoop").
- Cough lasting for several weeks, in most cases, and up to three months, in some cases.
- No fever.

✔ *What to do*

- If you suspect whooping cough, isolate the patient and apply precautions against droplet transmission (see above, under *What to do – precautions against spread of infection*, and Table 23.2).
- For a patient who has had a cough occurring in paroxysms for more than one week, give azithromycin, 500 mg orally, then 250 mg orally, every day for the next four days; note:
    - this treatment reduces the infectivity of a patient but does not relieve the cough, for which there is no specific treatment.

Worms

PINWORM (OR "THREADWORM")

Pinworm *(Enterobius vermicularis)* most often affects children but the infection can spread to adults. It occurs in all parts of the world. The adult worm lives in the human bowel. At night the females migrate out of the infected person's rectum to lay their eggs around the anus. These eggs are then transferred to the fingers of the infected person, who ingests them or passes them to another person. Infection can also be transmitted through contaminated bedclothes or food.

► *Signs and symptoms*

- No symptoms in most cases;
- in some cases, itching around the anus;
- in some cases, adult female worms, which are white and about 10 mm long, can be seen around the anus or in faeces.

✔ *What to do*

- If you suspect pinworm, give a single dose of mebendazole, 100 mg orally, both to the patient and to all the patient's close contacts.

ROUNDWORM AND WHIPWORM

Roundworm (*Ascaris lumbricoides*) and whipworm (*Trichiura trichiuriasis*) infections are common in tropical areas with poor sanitation. They are acquired by eating food or, less often, by drinking water contaminated with the worms' eggs. The two worms are considered together here because their geographical ranges are similar and they often occur simultaneously.

A roundworm is a large worm, about 5 mm across and up to 30 cm long. When its eggs are eaten by a person, they hatch and form larvae. The larvae penetrate the bowel wall to reach the bloodstream, which they use to travel to the lungs. The larvae mature within the lungs for a few days, then pass up the airways to reach the throat, where they are swallowed. Back in the bowel, they become adults. Roundworms live for months or even a year or two. When they die, they are passed in the stool, which is often the first indication of infection.

A whipworm is about 4 cm long and lives in the large bowel (colon). A person acquires infection by eating food contaminated by whipworm eggs, which hatch in the bowel and attach themselves to the wall of the colon. Eggs are then passed in the faeces.

Signs and symptoms

- No symptoms in most cases.

What to do

- If worms are visible in the faeces, give mebendazole, 100 mg orally, twice daily for three days.

HOOKWORM

Hookworm infections occur in areas with plentiful rainfall and poor sanitation. Infected people pass the worm's eggs in the faeces. If the faeces reach moist soil, the eggs hatch and form larvae, which can penetrate the skin of humans walking barefoot on contaminated soil. Only a few larvae – and therefore only brief exposure to contaminated soil – are needed to cause infection.

From the skin, the larvae enter the bloodstream, which takes them to the lungs and upper respiratory tract. They pass up the bronchi to the throat, where they are swallowed and then pass into the bowel. There they mature into adult worms, attach to the bowel wall, and feed on blood. They may live for many years, so that infection can be present in people who have not travelled in the recent past to an area where infection is common.

Signs and symptoms

- An itchy rash ("ground itch"), when the worms enter the skin of a person walking on contaminated soil.
- In many cases, when the worms first return to the bowel from the lungs:
  - diarrhoea
  - vomiting
  - abdominal pain.
- Severe anaemia caused by blood loss, especially in undernourished children and women in poor communities: each worm consumes about 0.5 ml of blood a day.

What to do

- If you suspect hookworm, give mebendazole, 100 mg orally, twice daily for three days.

TAPEWORM

BEEF AND PORK TAPEWORM

The cattle tapeworm (*Taenia saginata*) and pig tapeworm (*Taenia solium*) infect the animals through food or water contaminated by human faeces that harbour the worms' eggs. Infection is, therefore, commonest where animals and humans live in close proximity and sanitation is poor. The eggs eaten by cattle or pigs hatch in the animals' bowel. The worms reach the animal's muscles via the bloodstream, where they form cysts a few millimetres in diameter. Humans acquire the infection by eating undercooked meat.

Adult tapeworms are large, often 10 metres long, and most infected humans have only one or a few worms. The head of the worm clings to the upper bowel wall by suckers and hooks. The rest of the worm consists of a chain of segments (proglottids) containing eggs. The proglottids, which are about a centimetre across, can move under their own power. They enter the bowel and pass out in the faeces, where they may be noticed by the patient. Otherwise the worms usually cause no symptoms.

Note

- Beef tapeworm eggs passed in human faeces cannot infect other humans, only cattle.
- Pig tapeworm eggs can infect humans, causing a disease called cysticercosis.
- In cysticercosis, worm larvae migrate out of the bowel to reach muscle or the brain, where they form cysts, as in the pig: cysts in the brain can cause epilepsy.

FISH TAPEWORM

Infection with the fish tapeworm (*Diphyllobothrium latum*) occurs most often in northern Europe and Japan. As with other tapeworms, the adult worms live in the human bowel and eggs are passed in the faeces. When the eggs reach fresh water they hatch and release embryos which are eaten by water fleas, which are in turn eaten by crabs and fish. Larvae develop in the crabs and fish and infect humans who eat the crab or fish raw or undercooked.

Signs and symptoms

- No symptoms in most cases.
- Very rarely, a proglottid visible in faeces.

What to do

- Since the dose of anti-worm drug has to be adjusted to the species of worm and since retesting is required after treatment to be sure that all the worms have been killed, have a patient who has passed a proglottid see a doctor at the next port.
- To prevent tapeworm infection:
  - make sure all meat is inspected: tapeworm cysts are visible to the naked eye;
  - make sure meat is adequately cooked or frozen;
  - prevent crew members who pass a proglottid from handling food and urge them to be meticulous about hand-washing in order to minimize the risk of cysticercosis;
  - warn crew members not to eat raw or undercooked fish or crab, especially fresh-water varieties.

TRICHINELLOSIS (OR TRICHINOSIS)

Trichinellosis is an infection by a worm of the *Trichinella* species. It is acquired by eating undercooked pork in which the worm has deposited infective cysts. In some areas of the world, the meat of predators, such as bears, contains *Trichinella* larvae and can thus infect humans. Two to seven days after a person eats the contaminated meat, the larvae are released from the cysts by gastric juices. These larvae pass into the small intestine and become adults. After mating, adult female worms lay eggs, which develop into larvae that travel through the bloodstream to reach muscles. In the muscles, the worms curl into a ball and become enclosed in a capsule (cyst).

Signs and symptoms

- In some cases, when adult worms are in the bowel:
  - abdominal pain
  - vomiting
  - diarrhoea;
- a week or two after infection, when the larvae produced in the bowel enter the blood and travel to muscles:
  - severe pain
  - tenderness and weakness of many muscles
  - eyes red and swollen
  - in many cases, high fever.

✔ What to do

- If you suspect trichinellosis, seek medical advice.
- Give mebendazole, 300 mg orally, three times daily for three days, then 500 mg orally, three times daily for 10 days; **AND**:
  - prednisone, 50 mg orally, daily for 10 days.
- To prevent trichinellosis:
  - make sure that pork is adequately cooked or that it has been frozen for a minimum of three weeks;
  - make sure that meat from wild animals, such as wild boar, bear, and walrus, is thoroughly cooked.

Yellow fever

Yellow fever is caused by a virus carried by a mosquito. More than 90% of cases occur in Africa, where the disease is endemic from coast to coast between the south of the Sahara and Zimbabwe. In Africa the vector is the *Aedes* mosquito, which lives in and around human houses, so that in Africa yellow fever occurs in cities and towns, where epidemics can develop ("urban yellow fever"). Yellow fever is also present in parts of Central and South America, but is spread by a mosquito that lives in trees, so most cases occur in people who enter heavily forested areas ("jungle yellow fever"). All seafarers operating in these areas should be immunized against yellow fever. Many countries require immunization of travellers to, or through, yellow fever zones (see www.who.int/ith/ for a current list of these countries).

Signs and symptoms

- Onset three to six days after infection, with:
  - fever, often very high, but with a surprisingly slow pulse rate
  - feeling unwell
  - headache
  - pain in the back and legs
  - irritability;
- three to four days later, recovery in mild cases; **OR**
- one to two days later, in about 15% of patients, onset of a "period of intoxication", with:

- return of fever
- vomiting
- pain in the upper abdomen
- jaundice
- a tendency to bleed from the bowel, urinary tract, and gums
- low urine output;

- after a few days, about 75% of patients recover and about 25% die.

Note

- There is no specific treatment for yellow fever.
- Because the incubation period is relatively short, most cases occur in areas lacking modern hospital facilities.
- If there is a suspected case of yellow fever on board ship, medical advice should be obtained.
- The ship's master should notify the local health authorities at the next port of call and take such measures for prevention of spread of the disease as the authorities require.

Endnotes

1. Based on Garner JS. Guideline for isolation precautions in hospitals. The Hospital Infection Control Practices Advisory Committee. *Infection control and hospital epidemiolology*, 1996, 17:53–80.
2. Based on *Guidelines for the treatment of malaria*, Geneva, World Health Organization, 2006.

Dental problems

A tooth has a central core, or pulp, which contains nerves and blood vessels. The central core is surrounded by dentine, a hard bone-like substance, which itself is surrounded by a smooth layer of enamel: the enamel forms the surface of the tooth and is harder than bone. Each tooth has a crown, the part of the tooth which projects above the gum, and roots, which are embedded in the jaws. The neck of the tooth is where the crown and roots join up.

SOME COMMON DENTAL PROBLEMS

Tooth decay (caries)

- Bacteria form a film, or plaque, on the surface of teeth that are not cleaned regularly.
- The bacteria produce acids from sugar in the plaque.
- The acids dissolve the enamel surface of the tooth.
- There are no symptoms until the enamel is so damaged that the bacteria can reach and infect the pulp.

Pulpitis and peri-apical abscess

- Bacteria can be present in an infected tooth or in a tooth from which a filling has been lost or is cracked.
- The bacteria reach the pulp through a gap in the enamel caused by caries (see above).
- The resulting toothache may be constant or may come and go but is usually made worse by cold drinks and when the patient lies down.
- Pus can form an abscess around the tooth (peri-apical abscess or gumboil).

Periodontal disease (gum inflammation)

- The gums are reddened and bleed easily, when the patient brushes the teeth, for example.
- The gums may withdraw to expose the necks of the teeth.
- Discoloured plaque is clearly visible around the base of the teeth.
- Pus may be present between the gums and the teeth.
- There is usually no pain.

Pericoronitis

- Pericoronitis is a form of toothache caused by infection under the gum flaps around partly emerged wisdom teeth (fourth molars), causing, over the affected tooth:
  - redness
  - swelling
  - pain and tenderness.

✔ ***What to do in a case of toothache***

- Check for red flags (see below).
- If there is a lost filling or obvious defect in the enamel, apply oil of cloves to the tooth surface.

- If there is a large defect in the tooth, apply a temporary dressing as for a lost filling (see below, *Lost fillings*).
- Give amoxycillin/clavulanate, 875/125 mg orally, twice daily for seven days.
- To relieve pain, begin by giving paracetamol, 1000 mg orally.
- If a stronger analgesic is needed, as is often the case, replace paracetamol with tramadol, 50 mg orally, twice daily.
- Have the patient rinse out the mouth with warm saline solution (a quarter teaspoonful of table salt in 200 ml of warm water) for five minutes of each waking hour.
- Note that once an abscess forms, pain often subsides and is relieved dramatically when the abscess bursts.
- Have the patient continue to rinse out the mouth with saline solution until a dentist can be seen at the next port.

Red flags

Spread of infection can occur into the tissues around the jaws, and then backwards or upwards towards the neck or the brain. If any of the following are present seek medical advice urgently:

- difficulty opening the mouth
- difficulty swallowing
- drooling
- difficulty breathing
- swelling in the neck
- pain much beyond the area of the infected tooth.

Lost fillings and broken teeth

Recurrent decay around a filling or a fractured filling or tooth can cause a filling to be dislodged from a tooth or for the tooth to break around a filling.

✔ *What to do*

- If there is no pain or sensitivity to cold, no treatment is required but have the patient see a dentist at the next port of call.
- If the tooth is painful or sensitive to cold, give amoxycillin/clavulanate, 875/125 mg orally, twice daily for seven days and put a temporary dressing into the cavity, as follows:
    - isolate the tooth by placing a 5×5 cm piece of gauze on each side of it;
    - use a cotton bud or pellet to dry the cavity;
    - place a drop of oil of cloves on cotton wool, gently press the cotton wool into the cavity and leave it in place;
    - remove the isolating gauze;
    - repeat this procedure two or three times daily, as necessary;

A bleeding socket

Bleeding normally occurs after extraction of a tooth. However, prolonged or profuse bleeding from a tooth socket calls for treatment.

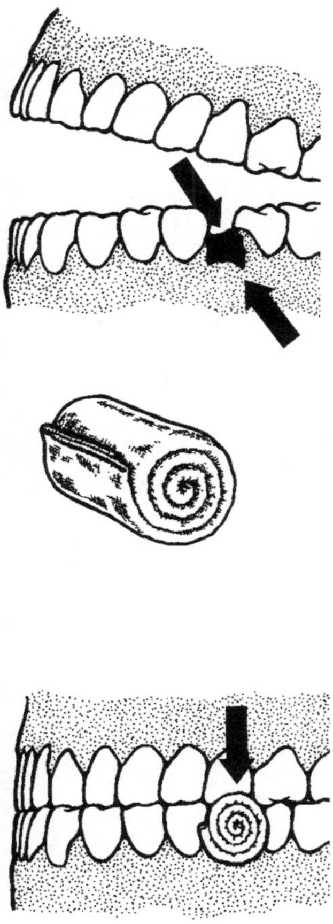

Figure 24.1 How to control bleeding following removal of a tooth.

✔ *What to do*

- Clear excessive blood and saliva from the mouth.
- Place a piece of gauze, 5×5 cm, over the extraction site, after folding it to a size that fits the extraction site, and have the patient bite on it to apply pressure (Figure 24.1).
- Leave the pad undisturbed for 7–10 minutes, then replace it with a new piece of gauze, as necessary.
- Once bleeding has stopped, leave the area undisturbed.
- If bleeding is difficult to control, pack a piece of gauze, 5×5 cm, twisted into a thin cone shape or rolled, into the site and place a second gauze pressure pack over it.
- Have the patient apply biting pressure for 30 minutes to an hour, or longer, if necessary.
- Ask the patient not to rinse the mouth for 24 hours and to eat only soft food for two days.

Lost teeth

If a crew member loses a tooth after a blow to the face or jaws **and** you are in port, it may be possible to save the tooth. Rapid action is needed: the likelihood of saving the tooth is diminished if the tooth is replaced after 15 minutes and is nil after an hour.

✔ *What to do*

- Handle the tooth by the crown **only**.
- Rinse the tooth in tap water: **DO NOT** brush the tooth.
- Put the tooth back in its socket.
- Have the patient keep the tooth in place with a finger or by biting on it.
- Have the patient go to a dentist **immediately**.

External assistance

MEDICAL ADVICE

Medical advice from doctors stationed in ports throughout the world is available 24 hours a day to all ships at sea, and should be sought whenever the caregiver is uncertain about the best course of action. The advice is given by direct radio-telephonic contact, satellite communications, fax, or Internet. Advice may, on occasion, be obtained from another ship in the vicinity with a doctor on board.

Clearly, it is preferable for the exchange of information to take place in a language common to both parties. If this is not possible, using a translator fluent in both languages is preferable to one party attempting to convey medical information, or trying to understand advice, in an unfamiliar language. Coded messages are a frequent source of misunderstanding and should be avoided as far as possible.

✔ *What to do*

- Provide the doctor with **all** possible information about the patient, using the form provided below:
  - complete the form before calling for assistance, except in emergencies;
  - when giving the doctor details of a patient's symptoms or past illnesses miss nothing out, however long it takes;
  - do not leave out points you may judge to be unimportant.
- Make sure you understand clearly and can record, preferably with the help of an electronic recording device, **all** the advice and instructions given by the doctor.
- Repeat back to the doctor any advice given, to make sure you have fully understood it.
- As soon as possible after the call, note the details of the exchange in the patient's records and in the ship's records.
- Since the doctor may not be aware of the contents of your ship's medical chest, have ready a complete list of the drugs and appliances available on board.

Forms to be used in communicating to a doctor information about a patient's illness (part A) or injury (part B)

(A) IN THE CASE OF ILLNESS

1 Routine information about the ship

1.1 Name of ship
1.2 Call sign
1.3 Date and time (GMT)
1.4 Course, speed, position, and cargo
1.5.1 Port of destination ...., which is......hours/days away
1.5.2 Nearest port ...., which is......hours/days away
1.5.3 Alternative port ...., which is......hours/days away
1.6 Local weather (if relevant)

2 *Routine information about the patient*

2.1 Surname
2.2 Other names
2.3 Rank
2.4 Job on board (specify kind of work, not just the trade)
2.5 Age and sex

3 *Details of illness*
- 3.1 When did the illness first begin?
- 3.2 Has the illness occurred before? If so, when?
- 3.3 How did the illness begin (suddenly, slowly, etc.)?
- 3.4 What did the patient *first* complain of?
- 3.5 List *all* the patient's complaints and symptoms.
- 3.6 Describe the course of the *present* illness from the start of the illness to the present time.
- 3.7 Give details of *past* illnesses/injuries/operations.
- 3.8 List serious illnesses of parents, brothers, and sisters, if known (family history).
- 3.9 List social pursuits and previous occupations, including hobbies (social and occupational history).
- 3.10 List *all* medicines/tablets/drugs that the patient was taking *before the present illness began* and indicate the dose(s) and how often taken (see 6.1).
- 3.11 Does the patient smoke? If so, how much and how often?
- 3.12 Does the patient drink alcohol? If so, how much (on how many days a week, on average, and how many drinks a day, on average)?
- 3.13 Does the patient take any herbal or folk medicines? If so, how are they taken?
- 3.14 Does the patient use recreational drugs? If so, how are they taken?

4 *Results of examination of patient*
- 4.1 Note temperature, pulse, blood pressure, and respiration.
- 4.2 Describe the general appearance of the patient (healthy, obviously ill, pale, etc.).
- 4.3 Describe the appearance of affected parts of the body (consider faxing or e-mailing a digital photograph).
- 4.4 Describe your observations about the affected parts of the body (swelling, tenderness, lack of movement, etc.).
- 4.5.1 What tests have you done (urine, blood, other) and what were the results?
- 4.5.2 Give the results, if available, of any previous blood tests, X-rays, or other investigations.

5 *Diagnosis*
- 5.1 What is your diagnosis?

6 *Treatment*
- 6.1 List **ALL** given or frequency of administration (see 3.10).
- 6.2 Describe how the patient responded to the treatment.

7 *Problems*
- 7.1 What problems are you worrying about now?
- 7.2 What do you need advice about?

8 *Other comments*

9 *Comments by the doctor*

(B) IN THE CASE OF INJURY

1 *Routine information about the ship*
- 1.1 Name of ship
- 1.2 Call sign
- 1.3 Date and time (GMT)
- 1.4 Course, speed, position, and cargo
- 1.5.1 Port of destination ...., which is......hours/days away
- 1.5.2 Nearest port ...., which is......hours/days away
- 1.5.3 Alternative port ...., which is......hours/days away
- 1.6 Local weather (if relevant)

2 *Routine information about the patient*
- 2.1 Surname
- 2.2 Other names
- 2.3 Rank
- 2.4 Job on board (specify kind of work, not just the trade)

2.5 Age and sex

3 *History of the injury or injuries*

3.1 ***Exactly*** how did the injury or injuries occur?

3.2 Did the patient lose any blood? If so, how much?

3.3 When did the injury or injuries occur?

3.4 How long before the accident did the patient last eat or drink?

3.5 What does the patient complain of? (List the complaints in order of importance or severity.)

3.6 List all past illnesses/injuries/operations.

3.7 List **ALL** medicines/tablets/drugs that the patient was taking **before the present injury or injuries** occurred, indicating doses and frequency of administration.

3.8 Has the patient been taking any alcohol?

3.9 Do you think the patient might have taken narcotic drugs, amphetamine, etc?

3.10 Does the patient remember everything that happened? If not, how long before the accident is his or her last clear memory?

3.11 Did the patient lose consciousness, even for a very short time? If so, for how long and when in relation to the injury?

4 *Results of examination of patient*

4.1 Note temperature, pulse, blood pressure, and respiration.

4.2 Describe the general condition of the patient.

4.3 List what you believe to be the patient's injuries in order of importance and severity.

4.5.1 What tests have you done (urine, blood, other) and what were the results?

4.5.2 Give the results, if available, of any previous blood tests, X-rays, or other investigations.

5 *Treatment*

5.1 Describe first aid and other treatment you have administered since the injury or injuries occurred.

5.2 List **ALL** the medicines/tablets/drugs that the patient has taken or been given, and indicate the dose(s), the number of times given, and frequency of administration.

5.3 How has the patient responded to the treatment?

6 *Problems*

6.1 What problems are worrying you now?

6.2 What do you need advice about?

7 *Other comments*

8 *Comments by the doctor*

EVACUATION BY HELICOPTER

Evacuation by helicopter should be requested only for a patient in a serious condition: apart from the expense of this service, the helicopter crew often risk their lives to render assistance to ships at sea and their services should be used only in an emergency.

The following guidelines for medical evacuation by helicopter are reproduced from the *International aeronautical and maritime search and rescue manual*, Vol. III. London/ Montreal, the International Maritime Organization and the International Civil Aviation Organization, 2006.

- **Requesting helicopter assistance:**
  - arrange a rendez-vous position as soon as possible if the vessel is beyond helicopter range and must divert;

- give as much medical information as possible, particularly about the patient's mobility;
- advise immediately of any changes in the condition of the patient.

- **Preparation of patient before the helicopter arrives**:
  - move the patient as close to the helicopter pick-up area as the patient's condition permits;
  - ensure the patient is tagged to show details of any medication which has been administered;
  - prepare the patient's seaman's papers, passport, medical record, and other necessary documents in a package ready for transfer with the patient;
  - ensure that personnel are prepared as necessary to move the patient to the special stretcher (lowered by the helicopter) as quickly as possible;
  - the patient should be strapped in the stretcher face-up, in a lifejacket if the patient's condition permits.
- **The following information should be exchanged between the helicopter and the vessel to prepare for helicopter operations**:
  - position of the ship;
  - course and speed to the rendez-vous position;
  - local weather situation;
  - how to identify the ship from the air (such as flags, orange smoke signals, spotlights, or daylight signalling lamps).
- **Shipboard safety checklist for the officer in charge**:
  - ***General***:
    - Have all loose objects within and adjacent to the operating area been secured or removed?
    - Have all aerials and standing or running gear above the operating area been secured or removed?
    - Has a pennant or windsock been hoisted where it can be clearly seen by the helicopter pilot?
    - Has the officer of the watch been consulted about the ship's readiness?
    - Does the leader of the deck party have a portable radio transceiver (walkie-talkie) for communicating with the bridge?
    - Are the fire pumps running and is there adequate pressure on deck?
    - Are fire hoses ready (hoses should be near to but clear of the operating area)?
    - Are foam hoses, monitors, and portable foam equipment ready?
    - Are dry powder fire extinguishers available and ready for use?
    - Is the deck party complete, correctly dressed, and in position?
    - Are the fire hoses and foam nozzles pointing away from the operating area in case of inadvertent discharge?
    - Has a rescue party been detailed?
    - Is a person-overboard rescue boat ready for lowering?
    - Are the following items of equipment to hand:

- large axe
- crowbar
- wire cutters
- red emergency signal/torch
- marshalling batons (at night)
- first-aid equipment?

› Has the correct lighting (including special navigation lights) been switched on prior to night operations and not directed towards the helicopter?
› Is the deck party ready, wearing brightly coloured waistcoats and protective helmets, and are all passengers clear of the operating area?
› Has the hook handler been equipped with helmet, strong rubber gloves and rubber-soled shoes to avoid the danger of static discharge?
› Is access to and egress from the operating area clear?
› Has the radar been secured or placed in stand-by mode just before the helicopter arrives?

- ***Landing on deck***:

› Is the deck party aware that a landing is to be made?
› Is the operating area free of heavy spray or seas on deck?
› Have side rails and, where necessary, awnings, stanchions, and other obstructions been lowered or removed?
› Where applicable, have portable pipes been removed and have the remaining apex ends been blanked off?
› Are rope messengers to hand for securing the helicopter, if necessary? (Note: only the helicopter pilot may decide whether or not to secure the helicopter.)
› Have all personnel been warned to keep clear of rotors and exhausts?

SHIP-TO-SHIP TRANSFER OF DOCTOR OR PATIENT

This operation demands high standards of seamanship that are beyond the scope of this guide. A few reminders may be appropriate, however, for yachtsmen or small craft operators carrying a doctor to, or a patient from, a large vessel.

✔ *What to do*

- For your own safety, make sure you are seen by the crew of the larger ship and that your actions are communicated to that ship's master.
- Act promptly on the master's instructions.
- Use your daylight signalling apparatus or VHF radio as soon as possible since:
  - a large tanker or other ship under way at sea may require 30 minutes or more to put its main propulsion machinery on stand-by;
  - loaded, large tankers require several miles to stop headway and are difficult to manoeuvre close to small craft.

- Take care in approaching light (unloaded) ships of any type and high-sided passenger ships, since they will make considerable leeway when stopped.
- Keep clear of the larger ship's overhang of bows or stern, especially if there is any sea running.
- Beware of the larger ship's permanent side fendering.
- Note the general rule that the ship with the higher freeboard should provide illumination and facilities for boarding and should indicate the best position.
- As soon as the operation is completed use full power to get your craft clear: a dangerous suction effect may hold you alongside.

REFERRAL INFORMATION TO ACCOMPANY EVACUATED PATIENTS

A letter or form should always be sent with any patient who is going to see a doctor. The patient will be a stranger to the doctor and there might even be a language difficulty. The letter should include routine particulars about the crew member (name, date of birth) and about the ship (name of ship, port, name of agent/owner). The medical content of the letter should be set out in a systematic way, informing the receiving doctor of everything known about the patient that may be relevant, including *copies* of any information from doctors who have seen the patient in previous ports.

Nursing care and medical procedures

This chapter deals with the nursing care of ill patients on board ship until they recover or are sent to a hospital.

Good nursing contributes to the recovery from an illness and cheerful, helpful, and intelligent nursing can encourage the patient to take a positive attitude towards a health problem. For this reason, the person chosen to attend a patient should be selected with care and the ship's master or a senior officer should keep a check on how the designated attendant is coping with the task.

NURSING CARE

Preparing sick-quarters

- To provide the patient with a peaceful environment and at the same time reduce the risk of spreading a possible infection, have the patient put in the ship's hospital or in a relatively isolated cabin.
- To lessen accumulation of dust and facilitate cleaning, remove superfluous fittings and all pictures and carpets from the sick-quarters.
- Have the deck washed daily and scrubbed twice a week.
- Have fittings dusted daily with a wet cloth and then polished with a dry duster.
- Ensure that the sick-quarters have adequate ventilation and do not undergo sudden or marked changes of temperature: the ideal temperature for the sick-room is that at which the patient is comfortable; this may be warmer than is comfortable for the attendant because nursing procedures often require the patient to be uncovered.
- If possible, admit direct sunlight into the cabin, and also fresh air if the weather is warm and the portholes are suitably situated.

First steps on a patient's arrival

- If necessary, assist the patient to undress and get into bed.
- Undress an unconscious or helpless patient.
  - For a patient with a severe leg injury, you may have to cut off the trousers by cutting down the outside seam of the injured leg first.
  - For a patient with an arm injury, remove the shirt sleeve from the sound arm first, slip the shirt over the head, and then withdraw the injured arm carefully from its sleeve.
- Ensure that the clothing the patient wears in bed does not have to be removed for procedures such as blood pressure measurement and does not conceal wounds, injured parts, or the sites of injections or of access to a vein for intravenous administrations:
  - long-sleeved garments should be avoided.
- Although in the tropics blankets are unnecessary, provide the patient with a sheet that is spread over the patient's body or folded once lengthwise and wrapped around the midriff.

- If the patient has a chest condition that causes coughing and spitting, provide a sputum pot or suitable jar or a tin fitted with a cover or piece of lint to distinguish it from a drinking receptacle:
  - if the sputum pot is not of the disposable variety, add a little disinfectant and have the pot thoroughly cleaned out twice daily with boiling water and a disinfectant.
- Leave a urine bottle for the patient on a chair, stool, or locker, and cover it with a cloth.
- Remove food, plates, cups, knives, forks, and spoons from the sick-quarters immediately after a meal, UNLESS:
  - the patient is infectious, in which case wash these items in the cabin in a basin or bucket and stack them neatly away, covered with a cloth.
- Protect the patient from long and tiring visits from well-meaning shipmates:
  - for a patient who is ill or feverish, limit visits to 15 minutes.

Basic principles of nursing care

- Ensure that the patient is comfortable in bed.
- For each patient, keep an individual, separate, written, record, or log, of the illness and all relevant information about the illness, with the patient's name clearly written on the cover **and** on every page:
  - remember that the patient must be allowed to consult this medical record;
  - for **all** entries in the record, note the date, time, and identity of the person making the entry;
  - make sure that entries in the record are in strict chronological order and leave as little blank space as possible between them;
  - note the patient's progress at least once a day, recording:
    - trends in vital signs (see below, *Monitoring vital signs*);
    - changes in symptoms;
    - medication given;
    - food and fluid consumed;
    - mood and behaviour;
    - why medication was started or stopped, if that is the case;
    - any medical advice given, with the date and time of the communication and the identity of the doctor consulted;
  - if you enter incorrect information or information relating to another patient in the record, simply cross out the erroneous entry so that it remains legible and add below it "Written in error", affixing your signature and the date.
- Give top priority to accurate medication records.
- Keep a special medications chart for each patient, with his name clearly written on every page.
- It will save time if you keep in each chart a list of the crew members authorized to make entries in the charts and administer medications, with their usual signature and initials, so that entries and records of drug administration need only be initialled.
- Use the medication chart to record:

  - the administration of every dose of every drug, using the generic name (not the trade name) of the drug and recording the date and time it is given and the identity of the person giving it;
  - the consumption of any personal medications, with the approved (i.e. generic) names, or herbal or traditional medicines;
  - any allergies the patient may have to any medication.
- Check the patient's vital signs – temperature, pulse, respiration, and level of consciousness – every day, morning and evening, or more often if the results are not in the normal range (see below, *Monitoring vital signs*):
  - check every four hours in a case of serious illness and record the results each time.
- On arrival of the patient in the sick bay, test a specimen of urine and record the result: do this test every second day if the patient is seriously ill and every few days if the patient is mildly-to-moderately ill.
- Arrange for water to be readily available, unless fluids must be restricted.
- Note whether the patient is on a normal diet or has to comply with dietary restrictions.
- Ensure that the patient knows to ask for a urine bottle or a bedpan – some patients do not ask unless told to.
- Ask and record each day whether or not the patient has had a bowel movement.
- Check fluid intake and fluid loss by questioning the patient about drinking and passing urine:
  - in certain illnesses it is a good idea to keep an intake-loss fluid chart but this is time-consuming and difficult to do accurately: recording body weight every day or every second day is often more accurate.
- If there is blood loss, measure or estimate it and record the amounts.
- Check that the patient is eating and record the status of the patient's appetite.
- Tidy the bedclothes at least twice a day or more often if necessary for the patient's comfort; take care to remove crumbs and creases.
- To prevent boredom, provide suitable reading and hobby material, and, if possible, a radio.
- Provide the patient with the means to summon help, such as a bell, telephone, or intercom.
- Fit bunk boards for seriously ill patients and at night or in heavy weather for all patients.
- Release retaining catches of swinging beds when the ship is rolling.

Caring for the bed-bound patient

THE BED

- Make sure the bed is made up and the linen changed at regular intervals; note:
  - bed-making and changing an occupied bed should not be attempted single-handed.
- Remember that creases in sheets can be uncomfortable and cause bedsores.
- If the patient is gravely ill, incontinent, or likely to sweat excessively, use a waterproof sheet covered by a draw-sheet across the bottom sheet.

- If the patient has a fracture or if the weight of the bedding causes discomfort, have the bedding supported by a bed cradle (or cradles); note:
  - a bed cradle can be improvised by removing two facing sides from a topless wooden box and then inverting it over the affected part of the patient with the bedding resting on top of the box.
- If the patient cannot get out of bed:
  - change the bed linen by rolling the patient gently to one side of the bed and untucking the used linen on the unoccupied side, rolling it up and placing it against the patient;
  - tuck the clean linen under the mattress with its outer edge rolled up and placed beside the roll of used linen;
  - gently roll the patient onto the clean side of the bed;
  - for a sitting patient use the same technique, but from the bottom to the top of the bed linen instead of side-to-side

BED BATHS

- Ensure that a patient confined to bed is washed all over at least every other day and once a day in hot weather or if the patient is feverish.
- Wash and dry one part of the body at a time, beginning with the face, so that the patient is not uncovered throughout the whole procedure.
- When the patient is dry, dust the pressure areas and skin creases with talcum power.

FEEDING THE BED-BOUND PATIENT

- Encourage the patient to drink a lot in order to prevent dehydration.
- Find out what the patient would like to eat or drink: people who are ill or injured may not feel like eating or may be unable to enjoy food.
- Ensure that food is presented as attractively as possible.
- Follow strictly any special diets prescribed for the patient.
- Remember that in a patient who is not fully conscious food can be inhaled into the lungs and cause an obstruction to the airway resulting in an infection or even death.
- In a patient who is not fully conscious or has just recovered from a period of reduced consciousness, do not give food or oral medication without checking the patient's ability to swallow.
- To check a patient's ability to swallow:
  - give the patient a mouthful of clean plain water to swallow;
  - if the patient does not cough or splutter, you can give food and oral medication;
  - if the patient does aspirate a small amount of water no harm will be done but give the patient intravenous fluids and re-test for swallowing ability after 24 hours.

MOUTH CARE OF THE BED-BOUND PATIENT

- Make sure that plenty of fluid and facilities for brushing teeth and dentures are available at least twice a day.
- Remove the dentures of a very ill or unconscious patient.

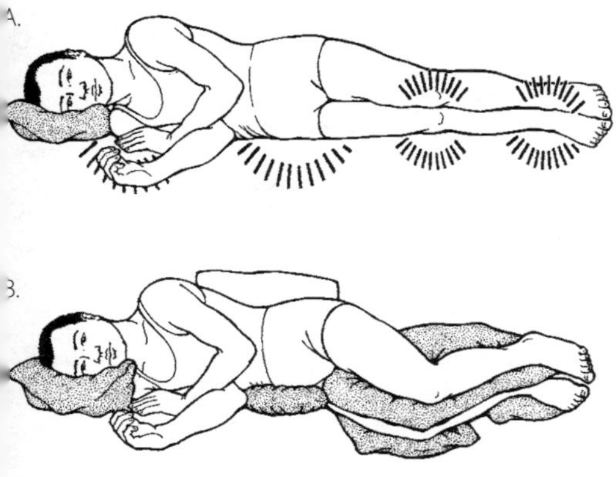

gure 26.1 Sites of the body where pressure sores ay occur (A), and how to use pillows and ring ds to prevent them (B).

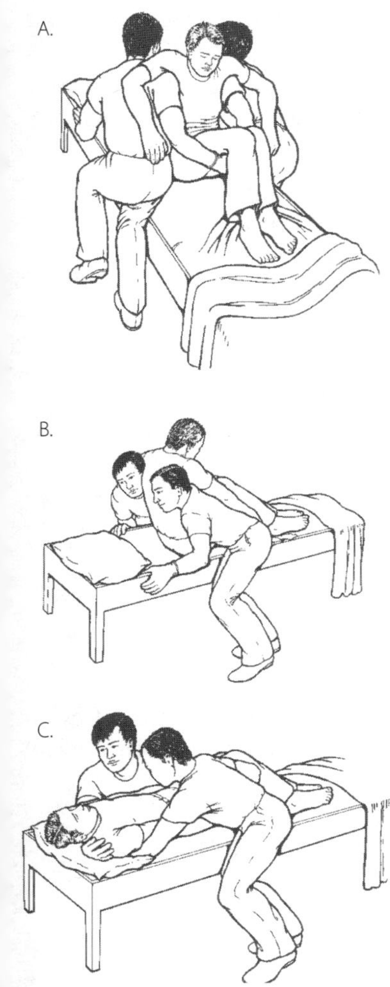

Figure 26.2 How to move a patient in bed.

- Swab the inside of the cheeks, gums, teeth, and also the tongue with cotton wool, cotton buds, or other suitable materials soaked in water.
- If the patient's lips are dry, apply petroleum jelly thinly and repeat as often as necessary.

BEDSORES

- Bedsores are ulcers caused when pressure of the patient's body weight on the bed blocks blood flow to the skin and deeper tissues, which then die (necrosis).
- Bedsores are commonest over bony prominences, such as the heels, buttocks, and vertebrae (Figure 26.1).
- Healthy people do not get bedsores, even when they are sick, as long as they can move around and relieve the pressure on the tissues.
- Unconscious patients are most at risk of bedsores but anyone with severely reduced mobility is at high risk of bedsores, especially if the person is incontinent (whether of urine or faeces) or malnourished.
- To prevent bedsores:
  - change the patient's posture at least every two hours day and night, systematically rotating the patient's posture (e.g. from back, to left side, to right side, to back); to turn a patient:
    - make sure that at least two attendants are available (Figure 26.2);
    - lift the patient a few centimetres from the bed (never drag a patient across the sheets) and roll the body over slowly and gently.
  - Have the bed equipped with a foam mattress rather than a spring mattress.
  - Keep the bed sheets taut and smooth.
  - Keep the patient's skin clean and dry, especially if there is incontinence or heavy sweating.
  - For a patient with reduced mobility avoid the half-sitting position: slipping down across the sheets creates shearing forces on the tissues over bony prominences and increases the risk of bedsores.
  - Use pillows, rubber rings, and other padding to relieve pressure.

BREATHING DIFFICULTIES IN A BED-BOUND PATIENT

- To reduce the discomfort of a bedridden patient with difficulty breathing, place the patient in a half-seated position (Figure 26.3), either lying back or leaning forward, with forearms and elbows supported with pillows on a bedside table.
- To prevent distress in a patient with heart failure who is likely to suffer breathlessness if made to lie flat, allow the patient to sleep sitting up.
- Allow a patient with lung disease, who may be less breathless lying down, to find the most comfortable position in bed; note:
  - if the patient has difficulty breathing when sitting up but not when lying down, there may be a foreign body blocking the airway.

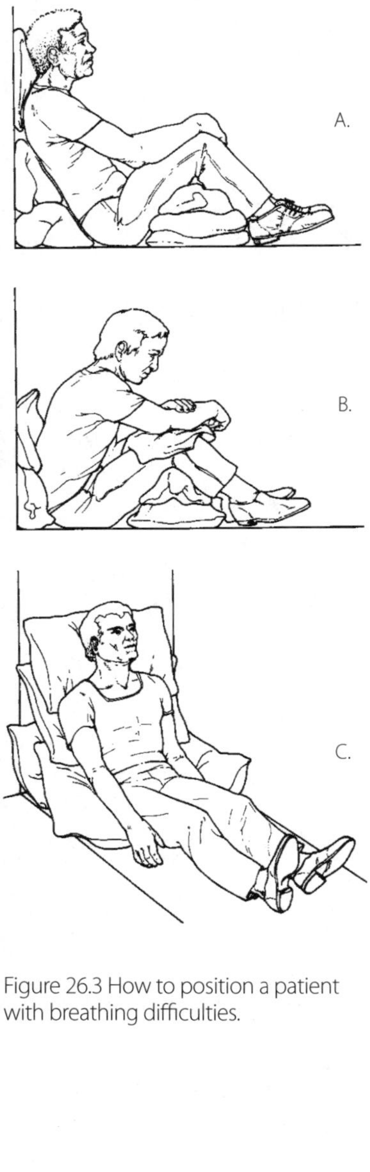

Figure 26.3 How to position a patient with breathing difficulties.

Monitoring the vital signs

The vital signs indicate how well the body is performing its essential functions. The main vital signs are:

- body temperature
- pulse rate and rhythm
- respiration rate
- blood pressure
- level of consciousness.

How to take the body temperature

- Use a temperature chart or, if temperature charts are not on board, write down your findings, noting the hour at which they were recorded (Figure 26.4).
- Take temperature readings twice a day, always at the same time of day, say, 07:00 and 19:00 (7 a.m. and 7 p.m.) or more frequently if justified by the severity of the symptoms; note:
  - it is rarely necessary to record the temperature more frequently than once every four hours; exceptions in which more frequent temperature recordings are required are:
    - cases of severe head injury (see Chapter 4, *Head injuries*);
    - acute abdominal conditions (see Chapter 7, *Abdominal and chest injuries*, and Chapter 16, *Gastrointestinal and liver diseases*);
    - heat stroke (see Chapter 10, *Heat stroke and other heat disorders*).
- Use a clinical thermometer to take body temperature, except in cases of hypothermia, for which you should use a low-reading thermometer.
- Shake down the mercury in the clinical thermometer to about 35°C.
- Place the thermometer under the patient's tongue and keep it there for at least one minute, asking the patient to keep the lips closed and not to speak.
- After one minute, read the thermometer, then put it back in the patient's mouth for a further minute.
- Check the reading:
  - if it is the same as the first reading, record the temperature on the chart;
  - if it is different, repeat the procedure.
- Disinfect the thermometer.
- If a rectal temperature reading is necessary, as for example in a case of hypothermia, use a rectal thermometer, which has a short, blunt tip to prevent injury to the rectum:
  - lubricate the thermometer with petroleum jelly;
  - with the patient lying on one side, push the thermometer gently into the rectum for a distance of about 5 cm and leave it there for two minutes;
  - record the temperature;
  - disinfect the thermometer.

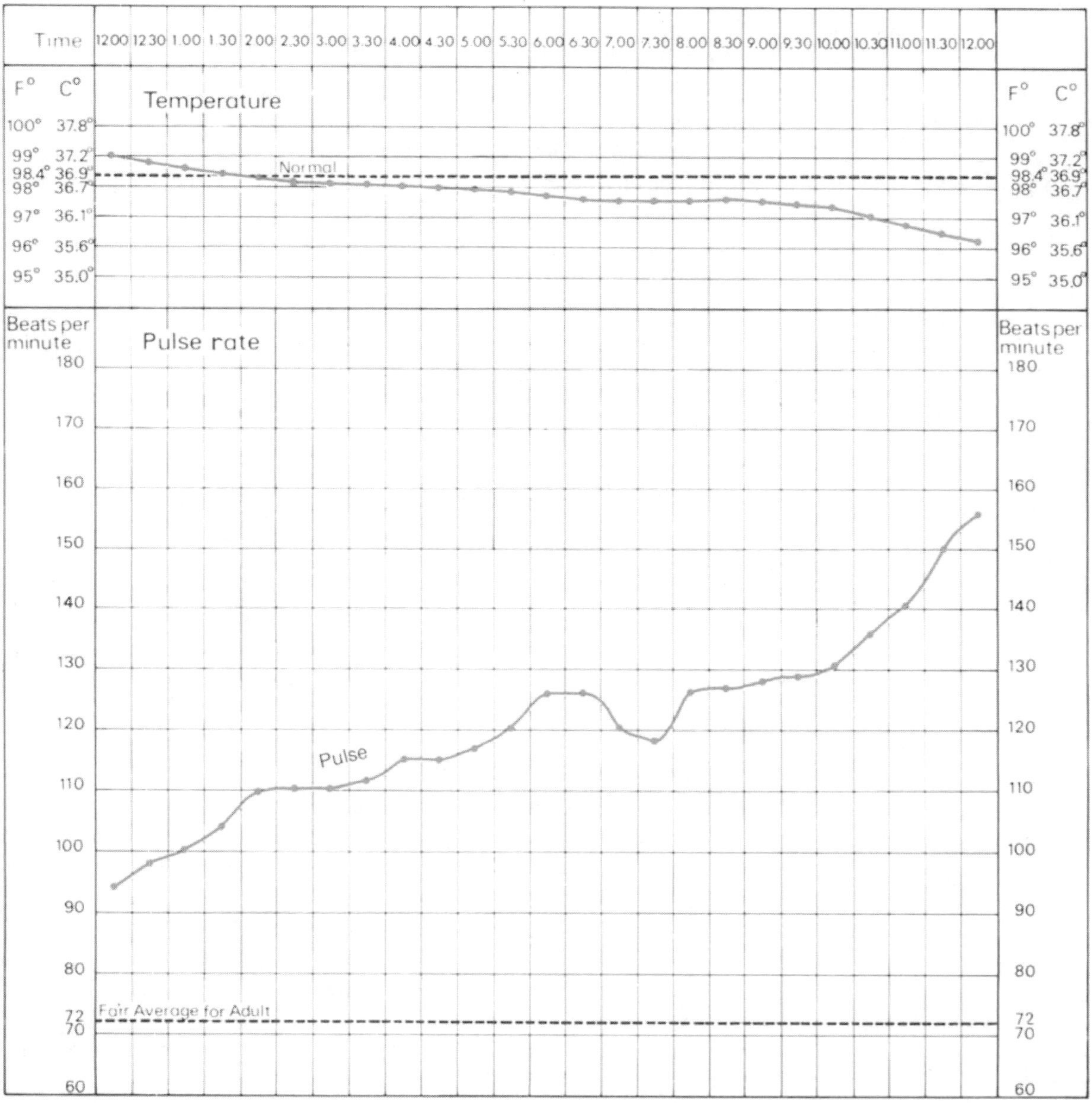

Figure 26.4 A temperature chart showing a falling temperature and a rising pulse rate.

- If the patient is unconscious, restless, or drunk, take the temperature by placing the thermometer in the armpit and holding the arm against the side of the body for five minutes before reading the thermometer.
- If body temperature rises above 40 °C, see section on *Heat stroke*, in Chapter 10, *Heat stroke and other heat disorders*.

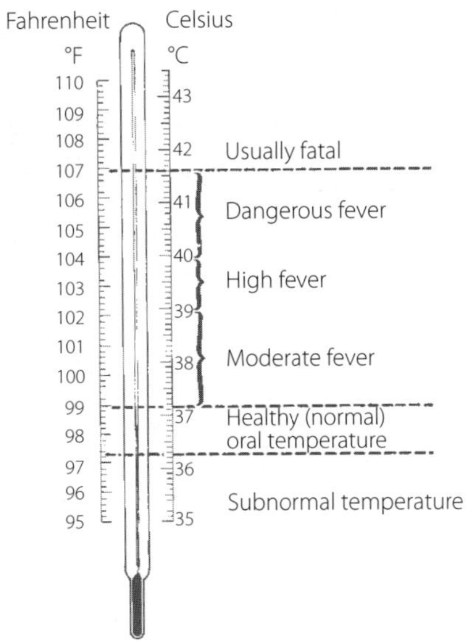

Figure 26.5 A thermometer with the normal ranges of temperature.

Note

- The normal body temperature, measured in the mouth, is about 37°C.
- Temperatures outside the range 36.3–37.2°C are abnormal (Figure 26.5).
- Temperatures taken in the armpit (or groin) are 0.5°C lower and in the rectum 0.5°C higher than temperatures taken in the mouth.
- Body temperature is slightly lower in the morning and slightly higher at the end of the day.
- Body temperature is normal in some, even severe, cases of infection.
- An increased body temperature means fever:
  - fever is most often caused by infection;
  - a wide range of other illnesses can also cause fever;
  - the pattern of fever, i.e. how it fluctuates, is important;
  - in many illnesses caused by bacterial infection, such as pneumonia and abscesses:
    - fever rises sharply each day towards the evening;
    - as body temperature rises, the patient feels cold and shivery, and as the temperature peaks, the patient becomes hot to the touch but may not necessarily feel hot or uncomfortable;
    - as the temperature starts to fall, the patient may feel uncomfortably hot and sweat profusely, requiring a rapid change of clothing and sheets.
  - in other febrile illnesses the temperature remains high and does not vary greatly: the patient does not experience alternating chills and sweats, and often feels relatively comfortable.

How to take the pulse rate

- To determine the pulse rate (the number of heart beats per minute), you can feel the pulse at the wrist or, particularly for patients who have a rapid pulse rate (120 beats per minute or more), you can listen to the heart beat over the left nipple on the chest; note that the pulse rate:
  - varies with age, sex, and physical activity (see Table 26.1);
  - becomes more rapid with exercise and excitement;
  - becomes less rapid in sleep, in physically fit people, and when a person is relaxed;
  - usually increases with rising body temperature – about 10 beats per minute for every 0.5°C increase above 38°C.
- To take the pulse rate at the wrist:
  - ask the patient to relax the forearm and hand;
  - place your fingers over the radial artery on the thumb side of the patient's wrist;
  - move your fingers until you feel the pulse beat and exert enough – but not too much – pressure until you feel the pulse distinctly;
  - count the beats for one minute and record the result.
- Note and record whether the pulse beat is regular or irregular, i.e. whether

Table 26.1 Normal pulse rates.

Age and sex	Pulse rate (beats per minute)
Age 2–5 years	about 100
Age 5–10 years	about 90
Male adults	65–80
Female adults	75–85

able 26.2 Normal respiratory rates.

Age and sex	Number of breaths per minute
Age 2–5 years	24–28
6 years–adult age	progressively less
Male adult	16–18
Female adult	18–20

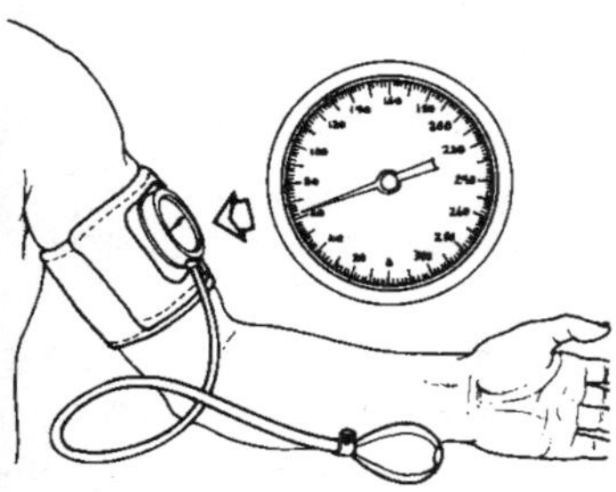

Figure 26.6 An aneroid sphygmomanometer – for measuring blood pressure.

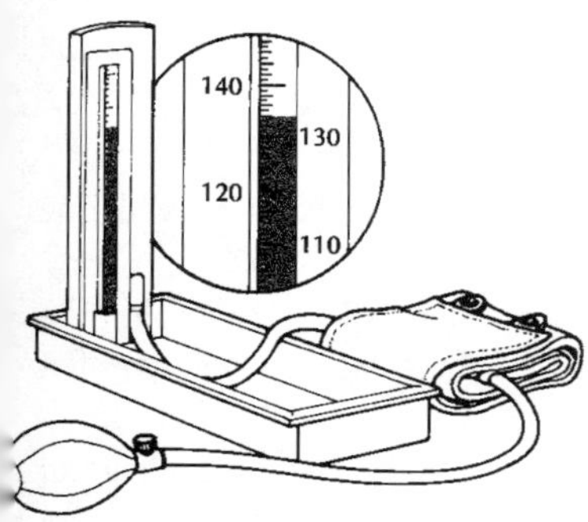

igure 26.7 A mercury sphygmomanometer – for measuring blood ressure.

there are the same number of beats in every 15-second period and whether each beat has about the same force.

- If the pulse beat is irregular, count the pulse at the wrist and also listen over the heart for a full minute in each case; note:
  - the rates may appear to be different between the wrist and the heart: that is because you are able to hear weak heart beats but you may not be able to feel a weak pulse at the wrist.

How to take the respiratory (breathing) rate

- To determine the respiratory rate, namely, the number of times per minute that the patient breathes in:
  - watch the patient and count the inspirations for a full minute but do so unobtrusively (while you are taking the pulse at the wrist, for example): if the patient is aware of what you are doing, the respiratory rate is likely to be irregular;
  - note that the respiratory rate:
    - is a good indicator of the severity of many chest illnesses and chest injuries: in general, a rate of over 40 breaths per minute in an adult suggests serious damage to the respiratory system;
    - varies with age, sex, and physical activity (see Table 26.2);
    - increases with exercise, excitement, and emotion;
    - decreases in sleep and when the body is at rest.

How to take the blood pressure

- Use a sphygmomanometer and a stethoscope for blood pressure readings in an artery in the arm.
- Ensure that the instrument used for measuring blood pressure is carefully maintained and checked regularly:
  - you cannot assume that an aneroid sphygmomanometer (with a dial showing the reading; Figure 26.6) will give accurate measurements unless it has been checked against a mercury sphygmomanometer (one with the height of a column of mercury in a glass tube indicating the pressure level; Figure 26.7).
- Note:
  - blood pressure is expressed in millimetres of mercury (mmHg);
  - two levels of pressure are recorded: systolic pressure, as the heart beats or contracts, and diastolic pressure, as the heart relaxes;
  - a blood pressure recording of 120/80 means the systolic pressure is 120 mmHg and the diastolic pressure 80 mmHg.
- Remember that in a healthy person blood pressure varies in response to many factors, including:
  - emotion
  - physical activity
  - alcohol consumption
  - smoking.

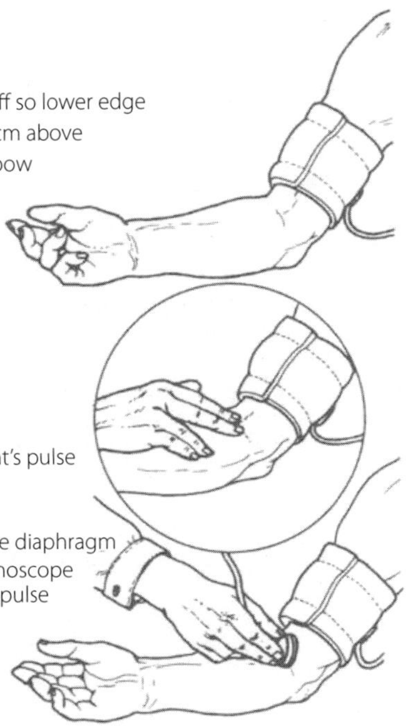

Figure 26.8 How to measure a patient's blood pressure.

- Blood pressure falls with:
  - vigorous exercise;
  - prolonged bed rest (for two or three days);
  - blood loss (such as from an injury or internal bleeding).
- Note:
  - shock is a dangerous drop in blood pressure;
  - when blood pressure is low because of shock the pulse rate is rapid;
  - low blood pressure with a normal pulse rate is usually not significant.
- Blood pressure rises with:
  - alcohol consumption;
  - smoking;
  - talking while your blood pressure is being taken.
- To take a blood pressure reading, have the patient lie down or sit, with an arm (either arm) supported at about the level of the heart.
- Check that the valve on the inflation bulb, or pump, is fully closed (turned clockwise).
- Place the sphygmomanometer cuff around the patient's arm, above the elbow (Figure 26.8); note:
  - it is very important that the bladder, or compression bag, inside the cuff is centred over the artery and that the cuff fits snugly;
  - the bladder must cover 80% of the arm's circumference and its width must be half the arm's circumference;
  - if the patient's arm is fat or very muscular the cuff is likely to be too small and you risk over-estimating the blood pressure.
- Find the arterial pulse, located on the front (in the crook) of the elbow, below the inner edge of the biceps muscle.
- Keeping your fingers on this arterial pulse, inflate the cuff by pumping on the rubber bulb until you can no longer feel the pulse.
- Note the pressure and deflate the cuff.
- Place the earpieces of the stethoscope in your ears (the earpieces should be directed slightly forward) and position the disc of the stethoscope over the spot where you felt the pulse.
- Ask the patient to keep his elbow straight.
- Hold the disc of the stethoscope snugly in position over the pulse with one hand, while inflating the cuff with the other.
- Inflate the cuff until the mercury column or the needle on the dial of the aneroid apparatus is about 30 points above the pressure where you felt the arterial pulse disappear.
- Loosen the valve on the inflation bulb slightly and allow the pressure to drop slowly (no faster than 2–3 mmHg per second), listening carefully for the sound of the pulse as a definite beat.
- When you hear the first sound or beat, record the reading on the mercury scale or dial: this is the systolic pressure.

Table 26.3 The Glasgow Coma Scale.

Eye opening	
■ Spontaneously	= 4 points
■ In response to a verbal command	= 3 points
■ In response to pain	= 2 points
■ No eye opening	= 1 point
Best verbal response	
■ Oriented	= 5 points
■ Confused	= 4 points
■ Inappropriate words (e.g. swearing)	= 3 points
■ Incomprehensible words	= 2 points
■ No speech	= 1 point
Best motor response	
■ Obeys commands	= 6 points
■ Moves a hand to site of painful stimulus	= 5 points
■ Pulls away from painful stimulus	= 4 points
■ Flexes limbs when painful stimulus applied	= 3 points
■ Straightens limbs when painful stimulus applied	= 2 points
■ No motor response	= 1 point

he score can range from 3 (the worst) ɔ 15 (the best). A painful stimulus is est produced by vigorous pinching f the trapezius muscle (the muscle hat shrugs the shoulders and that runs etween the back of the neck and the ɔp of the shoulder).

- If you miss the beginning of the beat or if you suspect that the pressure reading may be wrong, begin again.
- Do not keep pressure in the cuff high and do not repeatedly pump the cuff to above systolic pressure: this is painful and will cause the blood pressure to rise.
- After you have recorded the systolic pressure, continue to deflate the cuff slowly until the sound becomes abruptly softer and then disappears.
- When you hear the sound disappear, note the reading on the mercury scale or dial: this is the diastolic pressure.
- Open the valve completely and allow the cuff to deflate.
- Troubleshooting:
  - you cannot hear the sounds appearing and disappearing at all:
    - the valve may be opened too far, causing the pressure in the cuff to drop too rapidly;
    - the cuff may be wrongly placed or loose;
    - the stethoscope may not be snugly on the patient's skin: this is likely to happen if the patient's elbow is bent;
    - the blood pressure may actually be too low, as in shock, to be measured with the stethoscope:
    - check that you can measure the systolic pressure by feeling (palpating) for disappearance of the pulse as the cuff is inflated;
    - if you cannot, the problem is probably in the placement of the cuff;
    - in difficult or emergency situations it is easier and therefore usually more reliable to palpate than use a stethoscope;
  - you can measure the systolic pressure but the sounds do not disappear until the pressure is zero:
    - in pregnancy and in a few other conditions this is normal.

How to assess level of consciousness

- Use the Glasgow Coma Scale (Table 26.3) to determine and track changes in a patient with disturbed consciousness and also to inform a medical consultant about the patient's level of consciousness; note:
  - a large part of the brain must be affected to produce alterations in consciousness;
  - neurological diseases are not common causes of alterations of consciousness; the only exception is epilepsy;
  - if brain disease or injury is responsible, it is usually very severe and the outlook is poor;
  - common causes are:
    - sudden, marked falls in blood pressure (see *Sudden loss of consciousness (syncope)* in Chapter 13, *Paralysis, strange behaviour, unconsciousness*);
    - things that circulate in the blood and so affect large parts of the brain – drugs and alcohol;
    - low blood sugar (hypoglycaemia).

Bodily functions

URINARY AND INTESTINAL EXCRETION

- If the toilet or a suitable commode is available, encourage the use of these facilities if the patient's condition permits.
- Remember that some people will have difficulty using toilet facilities with an observer present but an attendant should remain within hearing distance.
- Remind patients who do not have a bowel movement regularly that there is no need for a bowel movement every day: even after a week without a bowel movement there is no risk to health, especially as food intake is often restricted in ill patients and bowel movements will inevitably become less frequent.
- Be ready to help very ill patients in using the bedpan.
- Empty all recipients immediately after use and make sure they are thoroughly cleaned and disinfected.
- Inspect voided matter – faeces, urine, vomit, or sputum – and record the amount, colour, consistency, and smell.
- To manage incontinence (urinary or faecal):
  - have an understanding, reassuring attitude to the patient;
  - assemble everything needed to restore the patient to a clean, dry condition:
    - gloves and, if necessary, a rubber or plastic apron
    - soap and warm water
    - toilet paper
    - cotton wool
    - towels
    - talcum powder
    - clean bed linen
    - a change of clothing/pyjamas
    - a plastic bag for soiled tissues
    - a plastic bag for dirty linen/clothing.
- Clean up with toilet paper.
- Wash soiled areas with cotton wool, soap, and water.
- Wash the patient and dry thoroughly by patting, not rubbing, to avoid damaging soiled skin.
- Apply plenty of talcum powder.
- Remake the bed with clean linen.
- If the patient can stand up and walk, suggest a bath or shower.
- In male patients with urinary incontinence, consider setting up an improvised system, as follows (Figure 26.9):
  - make a small cut in the teat of a condom;
  - stretch the teat over the end of a suitable length of flexible tubing and secure it firmly;

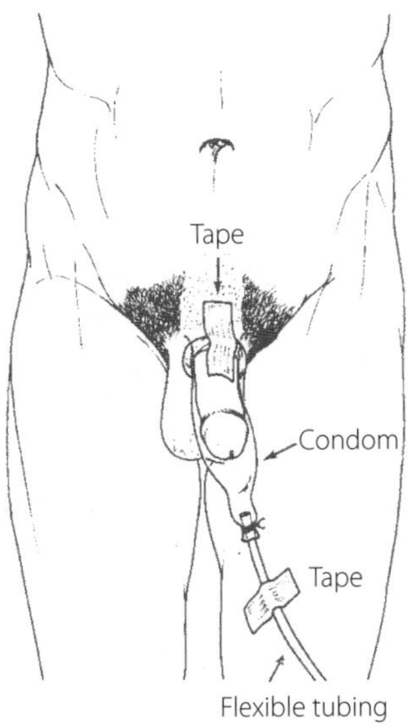

Figure 26.9 A simple device for use in urinary in continence.

- insert the patient's penis into the open end of the condom; to prevent the tube from chafing the penis, make sure that there are at least three to four centimetres between the tip of the penis and the junction between the teat and the tube;
- to keep the condom correctly positioned, shave the patient's pubic hair and use lengths of sticky tape attached to the skin of the abdomen;
- avoid using encircling bands round the penis;
- to prevent tension on the tubing, fix it to the patient or the bed;
- have the free end of the tubing drain into a suitable container, which should be emptied at appropriate intervals.

FLUID BALANCE

Note

- The body has self-regulating mechanisms that maintain a balance between fluid intake and fluid loss; two main mechanisms are:
  - the sensation of thirst;
  - the capacity of the kidneys to reduce or increase the amount of water lost in the urine.
- Maintaining fluid intake is mainly a problem for patients who are unable to drink (because they are unconscious, for example).
- Maintaining the right fluid output is only a problem for patients with severe kidney and heart disease.
- An indication that fluid intake is too low is:
  - the patient is thirsty; **AND**
  - the patient's urine concentration is high:
    - › the specific gravity of the urine (i.e. the difference in its density compared with that of water, as measured by a dipstick) is 1.010 or more; **AND**
    - › the urine is a dark amber colour; **BUT**
    - › patients with head injuries or stroke sometimes produce concentrated urine without having a low fluid intake.
- Another indication that fluid intake is too low is:
  - dryness of the mouth; **BUT**
  - this could be caused by breathing through the mouth.
- Therefore, if the patient is thirsty **and** is producing concentrated urine, increase fluid intake.
- An indication that the intake of fluid is too high is oedema, or swelling of the tissues with fluid; note:
  - oedema usually appears first around the ankles; **BUT**
  - in a patient confined to bed oedema may occur in the lower back instead;
  - oedema is not necessarily a reason to restrict fluid intake, because it is due in most cases to kidney or heart disease and will not go away until the underlying cause goes away.

- Therefore, if the patient has oedema seek medical advice; you may be advised to:
  - give a diuretic drug to increase urine output;
  - restrict fluid intake – but do not do this without medical advice.
- Note that in a previously healthy person and in most cases of illness on board ship drinking too little fluid is more likely to cause problems than drinking too much: patients should be encouraged to drink enough to keep their urine plentiful and pale.
- To monitor fluid intake and fluid loss:
  - a hospital-type fluid balance chart is not necessary for patients who can say when they are thirsty;
  - in patients who are unconscious or have severe kidney disease, a simplified fluid chart can be used (see Table 26.4).

Table 26.4 Sample chart record of fluid intake and output.

Date and time	Type of fluid	In	Out		
		Mouth	Urine SG	Vomit	Other
12/8/06					
11:00	clear soup	1 cup			
11:15				large	diarrhoea
12:00			500 1.008	small	
12:30	milk	half cup			
13:00				small	diarrhoea
14:00	ORS solution	half cup			
17:00	ORS solution	1 cup			
20:00	ORS solution	1 cup			
20:15			200 1.010		
23:00	ORS solution	1 cup			

ORS = Oral rehydration salt.

SG = Specific gravity of urine.

If the specific gravity of the urine cannot be measured, urine colour should be noted. This patient is drinking fluid and is passing urine. The specific gravity of the urine is a little high: the patient should be encouraged to increase fluid intake.

Examining faeces, urine, sputum, and vomited matter (see also Table 16.1 in Chapter 16, *Gastrointestinal and liver diseases*)

FAECES

- You should check faeces for blood, pus, slime (mucus), unusual colour, or worms:
  - blood in the faeces:
    - black, tarry faeces, either formed or fluid but always of an extremely offensive, penetrating odour, indicate bleeding from the stomach or from high up in the intestines;
    - bright-red blood, alone or mixed with faeces, suggests an abnormal condition (but rarely cancer) of the lower bowel, rectum, or anus;
    - a streak of blood on the surface of faeces or on toilet paper is usually a sign of haemorrhoids (piles);
  - pus or mucus in the faeces:
    - pus is found in faeces in severe dysentery or ulceration of the intestines or when an internal abscess has discharged into the intestine;
    - slimy faeces, from excess mucus, are found mainly in acute and chronic inflammation of the large bowel, in which case the mucus is often streaked with blood;
  - colour of the faeces:
    - pale, putty-coloured faeces is a sign of diminished bile content caused by a disease of the liver, pancreas, or gallbladder.

URINE

- Always test the urine if:
  - the patient is ill enough to be confined to bed; OR
  - the symptoms suggest an abdominal problem; OR
  - the symptoms (such as pain on urinating) suggest a disease of the urinary system; OR
  - there is a genital problem.
- Make sure the urine specimen for testing is uncontaminated:
  - in males, if there is a discharge from the penis or from behind the foreskin, and in females, if there is a vaginal discharge, wash the genitalia with soap and water and dry with a paper towel or tissue before asking the patient to pass urine;
  - wash urine glasses or other collecting vessels with detergent solution or soap and water and rinse them at least three times in fresh water to remove all traces of detergent or soap;
  - examine and test the urine immediately after it has been passed.
- Holding the urine glass towards a source of light, note:

- the colour:
  - normal urine varies from pale-straw to dark amber;
  - in jaundice (but also sometimes in a healthy person), the urine may be the colour of strong tea or even slightly greenish;
- whether the urine is:
  - crystal clear;
  - slightly cloudy;
  - hazy (turbid);
- whether there are threads floating in the urine or at the bottom of the glass: they are usually associated with infections of the bladder or urethra.

- Look for deposits that may appear as the urine cools and note their colour and appearance.
- Note any odour from the urine, such as that of acetone or ammonia.
- Look for frothing of the urine, which suggests the presence of protein.
- Look for blood in the urine, which may come from anywhere in the kidneys and urinary tract;
  - only a very small amount of blood is needed to make urine visibly blood-stained;
  - if you see blood clots, the bleeding is probably coming from a site in the urinary tract below the kidneys.
- Test urine for protein, blood, glucose, ketone, pH (acidity or alkalinity), and bilirubin using the test strips in the ship's medical stores (see Chapter 33, *The ship's medicine chest*): follow the test strip manufacturer's instructions carefully.

Note

- Urine normally contains no sugar (glucose) or protein.
- Protein may sometimes be present in the urine of healthy young people after strenuous exercise, but in this case it will not be found in urine passed immediately on rising in the morning.
- If there is no protein in this specimen, the presence of protein in other specimens taken during the day is unlikely to be significant.
- A similar situation can arise with sugar, but there is no test available for use on board ship that can clarify whether the sugar found in the urine is normal or due to diabetes.

SPUTUM

- Sputum may be:
  - **clear and slimy** in cigarette-induced lung disease (chronic bronchitis or emphysema);
  - **sticky and hard to cough up** or sometimes in the form of branching plugs of mucus in asthma;
  - **copious** (more than half a tea-cup per day), thick and yellow or green in bronchiectasis;
  - **rust-coloured** (from small amounts of blood) in pneumonia;

- **blood-streaked** or as pure blood (without sputum) in tuberculosis or lung cancer;
- **foul-smelling** (like faeces) in lung abscess.

VOMITED MATTER

- In a case of suspected poisoning, collect vomited matter in a suitable receptacle, cover with an airtight lid, label, and store in a refrigerator ready for later analysis.
- Vomit containing:
  - **undigested food** that tastes sweet to the patient because the food did not reach the stomach suggests an obstruction in the oesophagus;
  - **partly digested food** suggests obstruction at the outlet of the stomach;
  - **bile**, which is greenish-yellow in colour and will taste bitter to the patient, suggests obstruction below the entry of the bile duct;
  - **blood**, which may be dark in colour and resemble coffee grounds, suggests:
    - gastric or duodenal ulcer; **OR**
    - a tear in the oesophagus caused by repeated vomiting of any cause; **OR**
    - cirrhosis of the liver;
  - **faecal matter**, in the form of watery brown fluid with the odour of faeces, suggests advanced intestinal obstruction.

Mentally disturbed patients

- Have a constant watch kept on a patient who appears to be of unsound mind; note:
  - violence on board ship is far more likely to be due to alcohol intoxication or abuse of stimulant drugs, such as amphetamine than to mental illness;
  - self-harm, including suicide, is more common in mental illness than is harm to others;
  - harsh restraint or imprisonment is rarely necessary.
- Look for these warning signs of violence in a mentally disturbed patient:
  - a recent history of violent acts;
  - specific threats of violence;
  - a belief that a particular person or group is threatening the patient;
  - known drug abuse or intoxication;
  - shouting, pacing, or other evidence of inability to remain still;
  - having a weapon (see below, under *What to do when threatened by a violent patient*).
- Look for these warning signs of possible suicide in a mentally disturbed patient:
  - a recent suicide attempt;
  - hearing voices telling the patient to commit suicide;
  - having a well-thought out plan likely to result in a successful suicide attempt.
- If you believe suicide is likely, do not allow the patient out on deck while the ship is at sea, unless accompanied by two people; see also Chapter 13, *Paralysis, strange behaviour, unconsciousness*.

✔ What to do when threatened by a violent patient

- Gather as many crew members as possible, preferably five or six.
- Have each crew member stand behind a thick mattress held upright.
- Have the group keep close together and rush the patient in a coordinated, rapid, and decisive push so as to overwhelm the patient with little risk of injury.
- Immobilize the patient on a berth or stretcher by tying one folded bed sheet across the chest and another across the legs.
- To prevent the patient from standing or sitting up, keep the patient's heels off the ground or bed surface by placing an object under the calves; note:
  - a Neil-Robertson stretcher is a useful instrument of restraint in these circumstances.
- If the master considers it necessary to isolate the patient for the protection of the crew, have the patient housed in a single-berth cabin, with ports firmly screwed home and no potentially harmful object within reach, such as:
  - a mirror
  - glass
  - an unperforated plastic bag
  - an unprotected light bulb.
- Remove razors and matches from the patient's possession.
- If running water is available in the cabin, have the flow controlled from outside the cabin.
- Have the cabin door firmly secured from the outside.
- Allow only the attendant to enter the cabin, unarmed, but with a second person standing by in case assistance is required.

✘ What not to do when threatened by a violent patient

- DO NOT ask about, or attempt to search for, a weapon until you are in a position to apply overwhelming force: the patient could perceive your attempt as threatening and attack you.
- DO NOT forget that the simplest way to reduce the risk of violence is by isolating the patient.

The unconscious patient

- Make sure that an unconscious patient:
  - has a clear airway;
  - is placed in the recovery position;
  - is never left alone.
- Maintain a clear airway, keeping the patient in the unconscious position (see Chapter 1, *First aid*, and below, *How to insert an airway in an unconscious patient*).
- Never leave an unconscious patient unattended: he/she may move, vomit, have a fit, or fall out of the bunk.

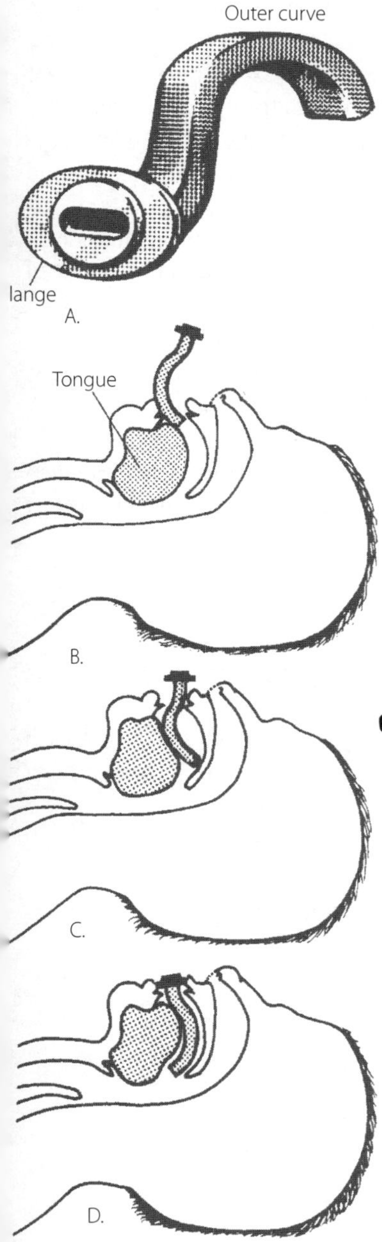

igure 26.10 How to insert an airway
n an unconscious patient.

How to insert a guedel airway in an unconscious patient

- Insert an airway if the patient is breathing without assistance but is doing so with difficulty: the airway ensures a clear passage between the lips and the back of the throat.
- Remove any dentures and suck or swab out any blood or vomit that is in the mouth.
- With the patient's head pushed fully backwards, wet the airway and slide it gently into the mouth with its outer curve towards the tongue (Figure 26.10).
- If the patient gags, retches, or vomits, stop and try again later.
- Continue to insert the airway until its flange reaches the lips.
- Rotate the airway through 180° so that its outer curve is turned upwards towards the roof of the mouth.
- Bring the jaw upwards and push the airway in until the flange at the end of the airway is in front of the teeth (or gums) and behind the lips.
- If necessary tape one or both lips so that the end of the airway is not covered.
- Check that the patient's breath is coming through the airway.
- Continue to push the patient's jaws upwards with the head bent fully back: the airway will be held in place by the teeth or gums.
- The patient will probably spit out the airway as consciousness returns: make sure the airway is retained until the patient is fully conscious.

✔ What to do – general principles in managing an unconscious patient

- Make sure that a semi-conscious patient cannot suffer further injury, such as by falling on the floor or hitting against a hard edge or surface:
  - a cot with sides is probably the safest place for a semi-conscious patient but make sure there are no pillows or other padding where the patient might lie face down.
- To prevent bedsores, turn the patient from one side to the other at least once every two hours:
  - in turning a patient, keep the head in a straight line with the neck and prevent the head from bending forwards with the chin sagging;
  - have an attendant hold the patient's head in the correct alignment during turning, in order to keep a clear airway and prevent spinal injury if there is a fracture of a neck vertebra;
  - if you suspect a neck or spine injury, do not turn the patient, especially if evacuation will occur within 24–48 hours;
  - check breathing and make sure that the airway is securely in place as soon as you have turned the patient.
- Make sure the patient's joints are neither fully straight nor fully bent but, ideally, midway between the two extremes.
- Place pillows under and between the bent knees and between the feet and ankles.
- Use a bed cage (a large stiff cardboard box will do) to keep the bedclothes from pressing on the feet and ankles.

- Check that elbows, wrists, and fingers are in a relaxed mid-position after turning.
- Never pull, strain, or stretch any joint.
- Make sure that the eyelids are closed and remain closed at all times, to prevent damage to the eyeball: if necessary use light tape to keep the eyelids closed.
- Irrigate the eyes every two hours by opening the lids slightly and pouring some saline solution gently into the corner of each eye so that it runs across the eye and drains from the opposite corner:
  - use 0.9% sodium chloride solution (normal saline) for intravenous infusion or make a saline solution by dissolving one level teaspoonful of salt in half a litre of boiled water that has been allowed to cool.
- Over the first 12 hours of unconsciousness do not worry about fluid intake.
- After 12 hours of unconsciousness, seek medical advice and give fluid intravenously, particularly in hot climates and/or if the patient is obviously sweating.
- Set up an input–output fluid chart (see Table 26.4).
- To collect the urine of a male patient, use an incontinence container with a condom over the penis (see above, under *Bodily functions*) and for a female patient, a bladder catheter.
- Moisten the patient's mouth, cheeks, tongue, and teeth every 20 minutes with a small swab moistened with water.
- Carry out mouth care every time the patient is turned.
- After 48 hours of unconsciousness, move the patient's joints at least once a day:
  - move all the joints in all the limbs very gently in such a way as to put each joint through a full range of movement, provided there is no fracture or other contraindication to this exercise;
  - ensure that exercising the arms does not interfere with breathing;
  - take your time, moving each joint fully before going on to the next.
  - begin on the side of the patient that is most accessible, working in this order:
    - fingers
    - wrist
    - elbow
    - shoulder
    - toes
    - foot
    - ankle
    - knee
    - hip;
  - turn the patient with the help of another person and move the joints on the other side.
- Remember that unconscious patients may be relaxed and floppy, so do not let go of a limb until you have placed it safely back on the bed.
- Hold the limbs firmly but not tightly and do everything slowly, with the utmost gentleness.

MEDICAL PROCEDURES

Applying cold

Cold may be applied:

- in order to constrict the blood vessels and prevent or reduce haemorrhage in any part of the body that is injured and may bleed;
- in patients with certain infections, such as an infected appendix or an abscessed tooth, in order to prevent swelling and further damage.

Note

- Prolonged application of cold may cause cells to die.
- If the skin turns pale or blue when cold is applied, the procedure should be stopped for 15 minutes and then resumed.

COLD EYE COMPRESSES

Cold compresses are often applied to an inflamed eye to diminish blood flow to the eye, thereby reducing its bloodshot appearance and the pain caused by swelling.

How to apply a cold eye compress

- Assemble sterile compresses or eye pads.
- Place several large pieces of ice in a basin and add tap water.
- Dip a compress into the cold water, wring it out, and place it over the eye.
- Prepare the next compress in the same way.
- Remove the compress already on the eye and replace it with the fresh compress.
- Apply cold compresses for 15–30 minutes.

How to apply an ice bag

- Fill a plastic bag about half full of ice.
- Expel the air in the bag before closing it (air increases the melting speed of the ice and decreases the flexibility of the bag).
- Test the bag for leakage.
- Cover the bag with a soft absorbent material such as a towel (do not apply a plastic bag filled with ice directly to the skin).
- Apply the bag to the affected part (if the bag has a metal top, keep it turned away from the patient's body).
- Apply the bag for 30 minutes and take it off for an hour, then reapply it.
- Remove the bag if the patient complains of numbness or if the affected part becomes white or blue.
- Refill the bag with ice to replace melted ice.

COOLING A PATIENT WITH A VERY HIGH TEMPERATURE

Cold baths are usually given to patients with a temperature of over 40°C. Such high temperatures usually occur with heat stroke (see Chapter 10, *Heat stroke and other heat disorders*) or after haemorrhage into the brain, although they may rarely occur in an infection. Cold baths can be given in a bath tub with cold or ice water, but if the patient is very ill or bedridden the procedure must be performed as a sponge bath.

How to give a cold sponge bath to a bedridden patient

- Assemble the following items:
  - a thermometer
  - a large basin with cold water
  - two washcloths or a sponge
  - a large waterproof sheet
  - two cotton blankets
  - two towels
  - an electric fan (if possible).
- Remove the patient's clothes.
- To protect the bedding, place the waterproof sheet, covered with a cotton blanket, under the patient.
- Check the patient's pulse rate and temperature (see above) and record them.
- Sponge the patient's body systematically, in this order:
  - chest
  - abdomen
  - front part of legs
  - back
  - buttocks
  - back of legs
  - arms.
- Stop if the patient's pulse becomes weak or the lips turn blue.
- Continue for 20 minutes.
- Add ice to the water to keep it cold.
- If a fan is available, use it to blow air on the patient, increase evaporation of water, and thereby speed cooling of the patient's body.
- Take the patient's rectal temperature frequently, leaving the thermometer in position for five minutes.
- When you have lowered the patient's temperature to at least 39°C, dry the skin and powder with talcum powder.
- If the patient complains of being cold and starts to shiver, and if body temperature has fallen sufficiently, cover the patient with a thin sheet.
- Use another thermometer to take the temperature orally every 30 minutes until it drops to below 39 °C for at least an hour: then take the temperature every hour until fever has disappeared.

Applying heat

Heat can reduce the pain and stiffness caused by inflammation of joints and muscle, and may lessen the need for drugs to reduce pain.

How to apply heat with a hot water bottle

- Assemble the following items:
  - an electric kettle
  - hot water
  - a hot water bottle.
- Fill the hot water bottle (half or three-quarters full) with water at about 50°C.
- Expel the air from the bottle until the water comes to the top.
- Check for leakage of the bottle.
- Cover the bottle with a towel.
- Apply the bottle to the affected area of the body.
- After 15 minutes, check the patient's skin for excessive redness or a possible burn.
- Refill the bottle at least every hour to keep the water at the desired temperature.

Note

- A heating-pad can be used to supply dry heat.
- Care must be taken to ensure that the temperature of the pad is not increased accidentally.
- To avoid possible injury to the patient, electrical wiring and connections should be checked for flaws.
- The affected area of the body should be checked at least every hour to avoid burning of the patient's skin.

Catheterizing the urinary bladder

Catheterization is the insertion of a catheter (tube) through the urethra into the bladder to remove urine. A patient who has been consuming a normal amount of fluid but has not urinated **at all** in 24 hours **and** feels the need to pass urine probably needs catheterization.

The most common cause of failure to pass urine is obstruction to the outflow of urine from the bladder. This problem is much more common in men than in women and is usually due to an enlarged prostate gland. Rarer causes are obstruction to both ureters (the tubes that lead from the kidney to the bladder) and a few disorders of the kidney: in both circumstances the bladder is empty and the patient will not feel the need to pass urine. Often, a full bladder can be felt in the lower abdomen as a soft, dome-shaped mass rising up from behind the pubic bone; when tapped with the fingers, the bladder gives a dull rather than hollow resonating sound (unlike the bowel, which gives a resonating sound).

Bladder catheterization is also required in unconscious female patients and in unconscious male patients in whom a condom urine collection device (see description above, under *Bodily functions of bed-bound patients*) cannot be kept in place.

When performed in a hospital by skilled personnel, bladder catheterization is relatively safe. When not properly performed, there is danger of infection or perforation of the urethra. For this reason:

- catheterization should be done only by a person with appropriate training;
- aboard ship, catheterization should be carried out only in a patient with urinary tract obstruction.

✔ What to do before catherizing for suspected urinary tract obstruction

- Attempt to induce urine flow by:
  - providing privacy and having the patient hear the sound of running water;
  - letting the patient stand, sit, or kneel;
  - applying a hot water bottle to the lower abdominal area or having the patient pour warm water (at a temperature of about 38–40 °C) over the bladder area;
  - having the patient lie in a hot bath, relax, and try to pass urine; **BUT**
    - if there is severe discomfort, give morphine, 15 mg intramuscularly, before the patient goes into the bath;
    - give the patient nothing to drink.
- If, in spite of these measures, the patient has still not passed urine and catheterization is considered necessary, seek medical advice.

How to perform bladder catherization in a male patient

- Tell the patient that he will feel only slight discomfort: allaying his fears may help him to relax his muscles and make it easier to pass the catheter into the bladder.
- Assemble the following items:
  - a sterile disposable catheterization tray containing:
    - a #14 French (5 mm) straight catheter
    - sterile gloves
    - small forceps
    - cotton balls
    - lubricant
    - antiseptic solution
    - an underpad
    - a drape
    - a specimen container
    - a label;
  - if a disposable catheterization tray is not available, sterilize the rubber catheter and the forceps by boiling.
- Before opening the catheterization tray, prepare the patient, as follows:
  - fold the top covers to the foot of the bed and cover the patient with a sheet or light blanket;
  - have the patient lie on his back with knees bent;
  - expose his penis, keeping the rest of the body covered.
- Scrub your hands thoroughly, especially under the fingernails.
- Open the catheter and catheter tray, following the instructions on the wrapper.
- Put on sterile gloves.
- Stand at the patient's right side and hold his penis with your left hand.

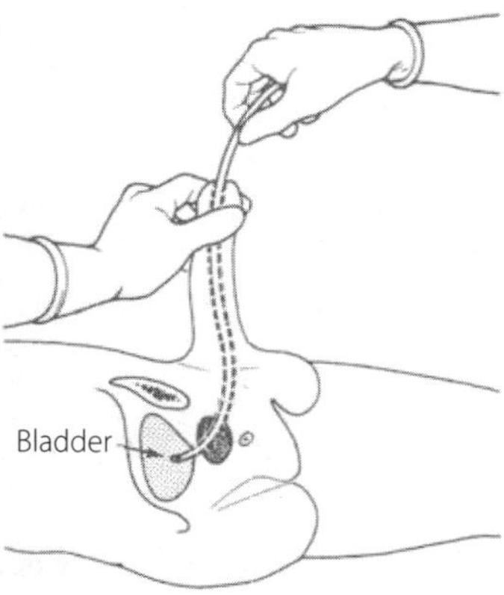

Figure 26.11 How to insert a urinary catheter in a male patient.

- With your right hand, swab the end of the penis, using the cotton balls and antiseptic solution.
- Pick up the catheter, without touching the tip.
- Apply lubricant thoroughly to a 15 cm length of catheter.
- With your left hand, hold the penis straight and at right angles to the abdomen and insert the catheter with your right hand (Figure 26.11).
- Use gentle but steady pressure to insert the catheter: you may feel slight resistance as the catheter approaches the bladder's sphincter muscle but gentle pressure should push the catheter past the muscle.
- If you cannot insert the catheter with gentle pressure and you feel firm resistance, **stop** and seek medical advice: **never force the catheter: you may seriously damage the bladder or urethra.**
- Position the basin under the outside tip of the catheter.
- Continue to insert the catheter until urine begins to flow (which it will usually do when you have inserted 15–20 cm of catheter).
- When urine flow stops, withdraw the catheter.
- Record the date, time of day, and the amount and colour of urine withdrawn.
- Dipstick test the urine and record the result.

How to perform bladder catherization in a female patient

- Assemble the necessary equipment as for a male patient (above), adding a floor lamp to illuminate the area of the urethral orifice (the external opening of the urethra).
- Before opening the catheterization tray, prepare the patient, as follows:
  - fold the top covers to the foot of the bed and cover the patient with a sheet or light blanket;
  - drape her thighs and legs with the right and left corners of the sheet and tuck the free edges under her feet;
  - have the patient lie on her back, still covered by the drape, with knees bent, thighs apart, and feet flat on the mattress;
  - place the lamp on the far side of the bed and adjust the light to shine on the perineal area.
- Scrub your hands thoroughly, especially under the fingernails.
- Open the catheter and catheter tray, following the instructions on the wrapper.
- Fold back the drape sheet to expose the patient's vulva.
- Encourage the patient to relax and to breathe regularly.
- Put on sterile gloves.
- Place four cotton balls in a sterile container and pour antiseptic solution over them.
- Squeeze the lubricant on to a gauze sponge.
- Fold about three inches of the sterile towel over your gloved hands to avoid contamination of the gloves as you place the towel between the patient's thighs with the top edge of the towel just under her buttocks.
- With your gloved left hand, separate the labia to expose the urethral orifice, which should be visible as a small opening about half a centimetre above the vagina (Figure 26.12).

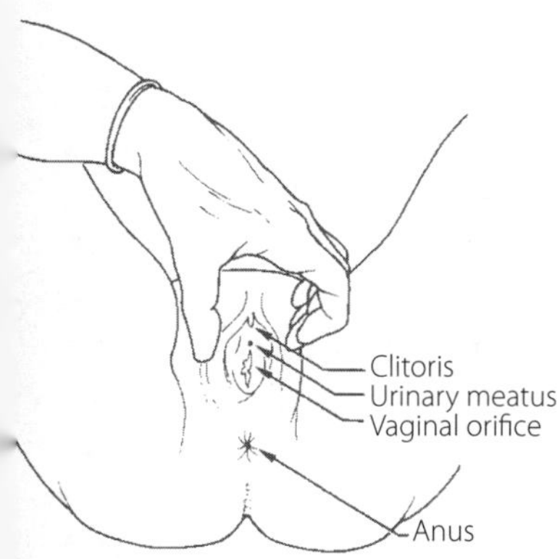

ure 26.12 Where to insert a urinary theter in a female patient.

- Keep your left hand in position holding the labia apart until the catheter has been inserted.
- **Remember: your gloved left hand is now no longer sterile.**
- With your gloved right hand, pick up a cotton ball saturated with antiseptic solution and, without going over the same area twice, clean the vestibule (the part of the vulva between the small labia) from above downwards, including the urethral orifice.
- Repeat the cleaning procedure with the remaining cotton balls: try not to touch the urethral orifice with the right hand.
- Discard used cotton balls.
- With your gloved right hand, pick up the sterile basin and place it on the sterile towel, close to the buttocks and below the labia.
- With your gloved right hand, pick up the catheter, holding it about 8 cm from the tip.
- Lubricate the catheter by passing it gently over the gauze sponge containing the lubricant.
- Insert the catheter into the urethral orifice to a distance of about 5 cm or until urine starts flowing: if there is resistance **do not use force and do not insert the catheter more than 5 cm**.
- When the flow of urine stops, pinch the catheter and gently withdraw it.
- Leave the patient dry, covered, and comfortable.
- Record the date, time of day, and the amount and colour of the urine obtained.

Surgical dressings

The proper procedure for changing a dressing allows removal of the old dressing without contaminating the wound or the fingers of the person removing it and the application of a new dressing.

How to change a surgical dressing

- Assemble the necessary equipment (two sets are needed: one to remove the old dressing and clean the wound; another to put a new dressing on the wound):
  - sterile dressings: size, number, and types will depend on the nature of the wound
  - forceps
  - a waxed paper bag
  - surgical tape.
- Wash your hands thoroughly.
- Put on gloves.
- Undo materials securing the dressing.
- Lift off the dressing, touching only the outside portion and using forceps if the dressing is soiled.
- Drop the soiled dressing into a waxed paper bag.
- Open the gauze-dressing pack.
- Using sterile forceps, remove the gauze dressing from its wrapper and place it on the wound, taking care not to touch the portion of the dressing that is going to be in contact with the wound.

- Tape the dressing in place.
- Staple the paper bag to close it and place it in a refuse container for bodily waste.

Administering medicines - basic principles

- Always give medicine on time.
- Read the label three times before administering medication.
- Check that the patient is not already taking the medication under a different name.
- If the patient is fully conscious, ask:
  - "What is your name?"
  - "What medicines do you think you are taking?"
- Before giving any new medication for the first time, check in the patient's medical record to see if any allergies have been recorded and ask the patient directly:
  - "Do you have any allergies that you know of?"
  - "Have you ever been told you are allergic to [*drug name*] or that you should not take [*drug name*]?"
- When the medicine has been taken by the patient, record the date, time of day, name of the medicine, amount given, and route of administration.
- If a medicine has to be given more than once a day, space the doses at a reasonable interval; for example;
  - three times a day: at 08:00, 16:00, 00:00.
- Distinguish carefully between medicines to be given four times daily (e.g. at 08:00, 12:00, 16:00, 20:00) from those to be given every six hours (e.g. at 08:00, 14:00, 20:00, 02:00).
- For medicines that have to be taken before a meal, give them half an hour before the meal.

Routes of administration

ORAL

- Giving a medicine by mouth is the easiest and generally the safest route of administration.
- Tablets and capsules are swallowed more easily if placed on the tongue and washed down with water:
  - tablets are more easily swallowed if the patient tilts the head back;
  - capsules usually float in water and are more easily swallowed if the patient tilts the head forward rather than back.

SUBLINGUAL

- Placing a medicine under the tongue is the best route of administration for substances that may be destroyed by digestive juices, such as isosorbide dinitrate tablets for a heart attack.

RECTAL

- Medicines administered rectally, in liquid form or as suppositories, tend to be absorbed erratically: this route is rarely desirable.

SUBCUTANEOUS (see below, *How to give a subcutaneous injection*)

- The most usual sites for injecting medicines under the skin are:
  - the lower abdomen;
  - the lateral surfaces (outer sides) of the thighs;
  - the outer surface of the upper arm.

INTRAMUSCULAR (see below, *How to give an intramuscular injection*)

- The intramuscular route can be used when a medicine is likely to irritate the subcutaneous tissue (just under the skin) or in some cases when a prolonged action is desired, such as for treatment with procaine benzylpenicillin.

INTRAVENOUS (see below, *How to give an intravenous injection*)

- To avoid serious risks, intravenous administration of a medicine should only be carried out by a person with appropriate training.

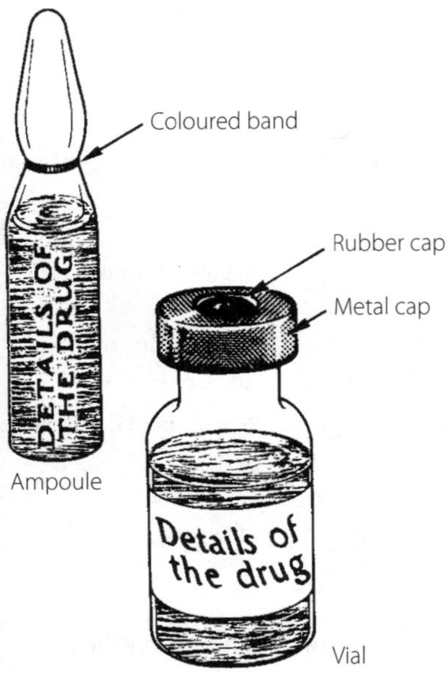

Figure 26.13 Vials and ampoules of medicines for injection.

Injections

- **SYRINGES AND NEEDLES MUST BE USED ONCE ONLY**;
- if disposable syringes are not available, sterilize glass syringes and needles by boiling:
  - medicines for injection are supplied either in rubber-capped vials or in glass ampoules (Figure 26.13);
  - the use of multi-dose vials carries a risk of contamination: a new needle and syringe **MUST ALWAYS BE USED** when drawing medicines from a multi-dose vial;
  - check that the name and strength of the medicine is marked on the vial or ampoule;
  - if you cannot see or decipher the name of the medicine, discard the vial or ampoule;
  - glass ampoules may have a coloured band around the neck indicating the level at which the top of the ampoule will break off cleanly;
  - the rubber cap of a vial is held on by a metal cap with a small tear-off seal: do not remove this seal until the drug is required.

AFTER YOU HAVE GIVEN AN INJECTION

- Place the needle, together with the syringe, directly into a proper sharps disposal bin.
- **NEVER, UNDER ANY CIRCUMSTANCES, REPLACE THE NEEDLE GUARD ON THE NEEDLE OR ATTEMPT TO BREAK THE NEEDLE AND SYRINGE.**

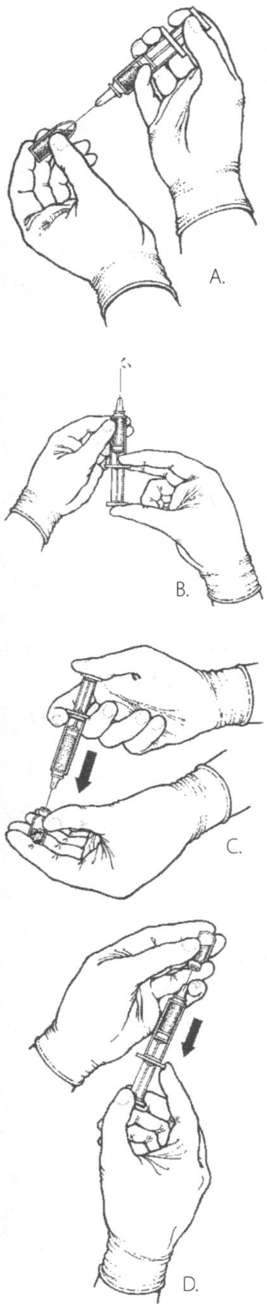

Figure 26.14 How to draw up liquid from a glass ampoule into a syringe (A), expel air, and a bead of medication (B), inject sterile water into a vial (C), and withdraw the dissolved drug from the vial (D).

- If you accidentally pierce your skin with a needle used for an injection, see Chapter 23, *Infectious diseases*, under *Needle-stick injuries*.

How to give a subcutaneous injection

- Assemble the following items:
  - a disposable syringe
  - a 19- or 21-gauge needle for drawing the medicine into the syringe
  - a disposable 23- or 25-gauge needle for injecting the medicine
  - alcohol swabs
  - the medicine.
- If the medicine is in a multiple-dose vial, clean the rubber diaphragm on the vial with alcohol.
- If the medicine is in an ampoule, tap the ampoule gently with a finger to ensure that all the liquid is below the neck of the ampoule, then break off the top with a sharp snap:
  - if you are not experienced in this procedure, hold the top of the ampoule with a cloth or swab to avoid being cut by the edge of the glass.
- Remove the guard from the needle without touching the needle.
- If the medicine is in a vial, inject into the vial an amount of air equal to the amount of medicine to be withdrawn: this will make it easier to withdraw the medicine (Figure 26.14).
- Withdraw the correct amount of medicine.
- Point the needle upwards and push the plunger to expel any air in the syringe.
- Select a site for the injection and disinfect the skin with an alcohol swab.
- Grasp between your thumb and forefinger a fold of skin large enough to offer plenty of space between the site of injection and your fingers (Figure 26.15).
- Insert the needle firmly and quickly at an angle of about 45°.
- Once the needle is under the skin, draw back the syringe plunger.
- If no blood appears in the syringe, inject the medicine and withdraw the needle.
- If blood appears, repeat the procedure at a new site, using sterile equipment.
- Place the needle, together with the syringe, directly into a proper sharps disposal bin.
- **NEVER, UNDER ANY CIRCUMSTANCES, REPLACE THE NEEDLE GUARD ON THE NEEDLE OR ATTEMPT TO BREAK THE NEEDLE AND SYRINGE.**
- If you accidentally pierce your skin with a needle used for an injection, see Chapter 23, *Infectious diseases*, under *Needle-stick injuries*.

How to give an intramuscular injection

- Assemble the following items:
  - a disposable syringe
  - a disposable 19- or 21-gauge needle
  - alcohol swabs
  - the medicine.
- If the medicine is in a multidose vial, clean the rubber diaphragm on the vial with an alcohol swab.

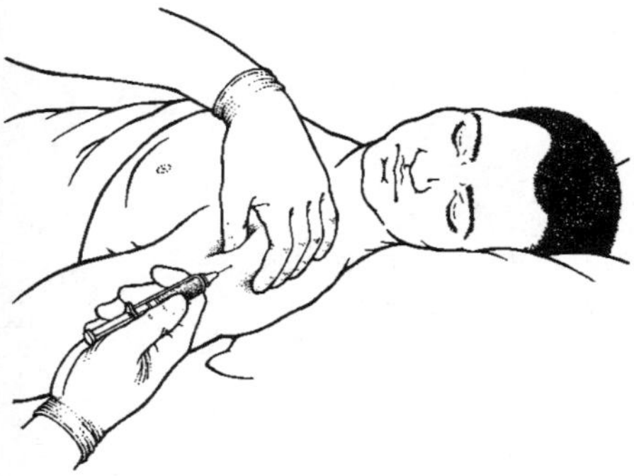

Figure 26.15 How to give a subcutaneous injection.

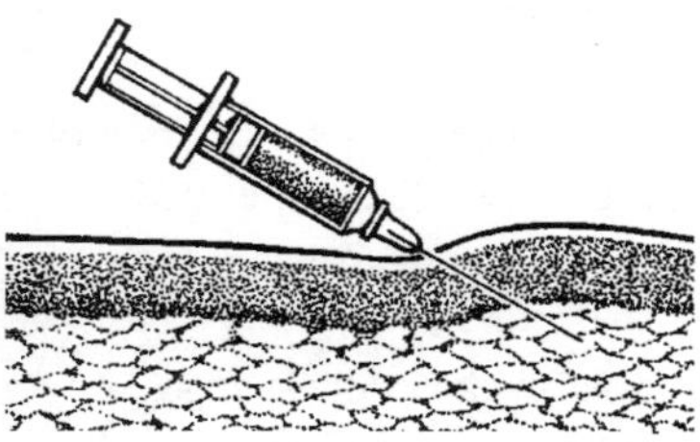

Figure 26.16 The correct depth of the needle for a subcutaneous injection.

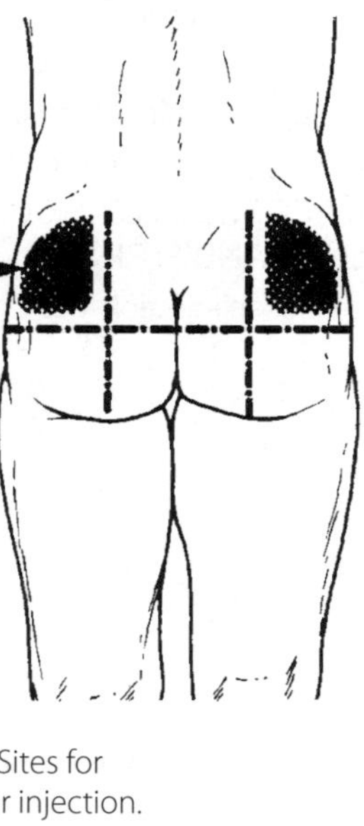

Figure 26.17 Sites for intramuscular injection.

- If the medicine is in an ampoule, break off the top of the ampoule.
- Remove the guard from the needle without touching the needle.
- If the medicine is in a vial, inject into the vial an amount of air equal to the amount of medicine to be withdrawn in order make withdrawal easy.
- Withdraw the correct amount of medicine.
- Expel any air from the syringe.
- Select a site for the injection: the preferred sites are the outer upper quadrant of either buttock or the outer thigh muscle (Figure 26.17): **DO NOT USE OTHER PARTS OF THE BUTTOCK.**
- In infants use **only** the outer thigh muscle.
- Swab the skin at the injection site with alcohol swabs.
- Stretch the skin with thumb and forefinger and insert the needle at a right angle to the skin to a depth of about 2 cm so as to penetrate the subcutaneous fat and enter the muscle (Figure 26.18).
- Draw back the syringe plunger.
- If no blood appears, inject the medicine and withdraw the needle.
- If blood appears, repeat the procedure at another site, using new sterile equipment.
- Place the needle together with the syringe directly into a proper sharps disposal bin.
- **NEVER, UNDER ANY CIRCUMSTANCES, REPLACE THE NEEDLE GUARD ON THE NEEDLE OR ATTEMPT TO BREAK THE NEEDLE AND SYRINGE.**
- If you accidentally pierce your skin with a needle used for an injection, see Chapter 23, *Infectious diseases*, under *Needle-stick injuries*.

How to perform an intravenous fluid infusion

- Assemble the following items:
  - latex gloves
  - a sterile, disposable intravenous administration set
  - a 19- or 21-gauge intravenous cannula:
    - there are different types of cannula but most are of steel or plastic;
    - plastic cannulas have a steel guide needle inside them to pierce the skin: you must remove the guide needle before giving the infusion;
    - the correct way of removing a guide needle differs between different manufacturers: check carefully the instructions given by the manufacturer of your cannula;
    - plastic cannulas are suitable for prolonged infusions but **MUST BE CHANGED AT LEAST EVERY SECOND DAY**;
  - a tourniquet
  - adhesive tape (1 cm in width)
  - dextrose (glucose), 5% solution, or sodium chloride, 0.9% solution, in a sterile glass bottle or plastic container; note:
    - glass bottles of infusion solution have a rubber diaphragm through which the spike of the administration set is pushed;
    - glass bottles require a second needle to be inserted through the rubber diaphragm to allow air into the bottle to replace the fluid that runs out;

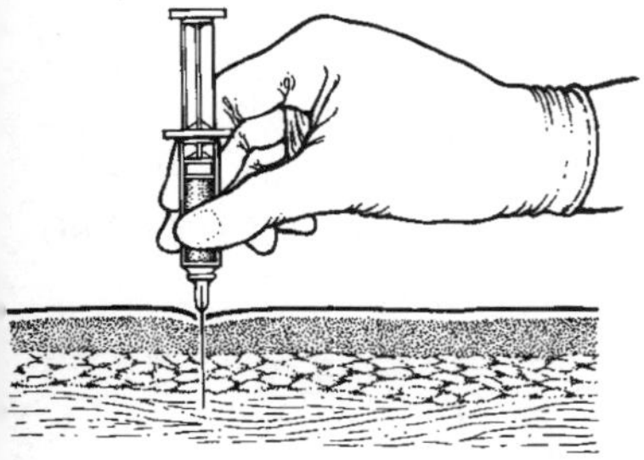

Figure 26.18 How to give an intramuscular injection.

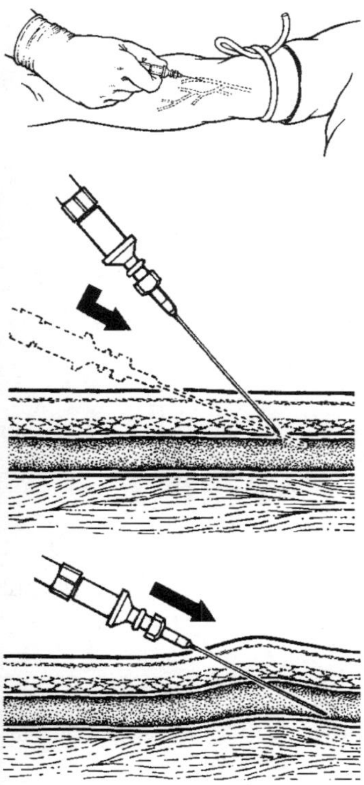

Figure 26.19 How to give an intravenous infusion.

    - › plastic containers have a teat at one end for the spike of the administration set: the sheath covering the teat must be removed before inserting the spike;
  - alcohol swabs
  - several paper towels.
- Remove the protective covering from the rubber diaphragm or teat of the bottle of solution.
- Remove the administration set from the package.
- Remove the protective cover from the spike and insert the spike into the diaphragm of the bottle.
- Remove the protective cover from the end of the administration set.
- Invert the bottle so that the solution flows into the drip-chamber and through the tubing: **DO NOT REMOVE THE COVER FROM THE PATIENT END OF THE TUBING.**
- When the tubing is completely full of solution, close the slide clamp.
- Place the fluid container stand in a convenient position near the bed.
- Cut three 5-cm lengths of tape.
- Choose a site for the infusion:
  - the back of the forearms and the back of the hands are the best sites;
  - the large vein usually visible just above the thumb side of the wrist is ideal;
  - a site where a vein divides is ideal because the vein is less mobile at this point and therefore easier to pierce;
  - avoid the front of the forearms and elbows, if possible;
  - never place the cannula across a joint.
- Put on the gloves.
- Apply the tourniquet about 5 cm above the site of the infusion and direct the ends away from the injection site.
- Ask the patient to open and close the fist vigorously so as to enlarge the veins.
- Disinfect the skin thoroughly with an alcohol swab at and around the injection site.
- Use your thumb to apply tension to the skin and to the soft tissue about 5 cm below the intended injection site.
- Hold the needle parallel to the skin, with the bevel up and in line with the vein, directly alongside the wall of the vein at a point about 2 mm away from the point at which you intend to puncture the vein.
- If you are able to use a point where the vein divides, hold the needle parallel to the skin in the line of the vein about 2 mm below the dividing point.
- Insert the needle through the skin (this requires a firm push), wait a moment, then insert it into the vein (this requires only a light push): you will feel resistance that suddenly gives way as the needle pierces the vein wall (Figure 26.19).
- When blood passes through the needle gently push the needle 1–2 cm further into the vein.
- Release the tourniquet.
- Remove the inner needle if you are using a plastic cannula.
- Blood may flow out of the cannula, so be ready to attach the infusion set quickly.
- Use paper towels to prevent blood dripping onto the bed.

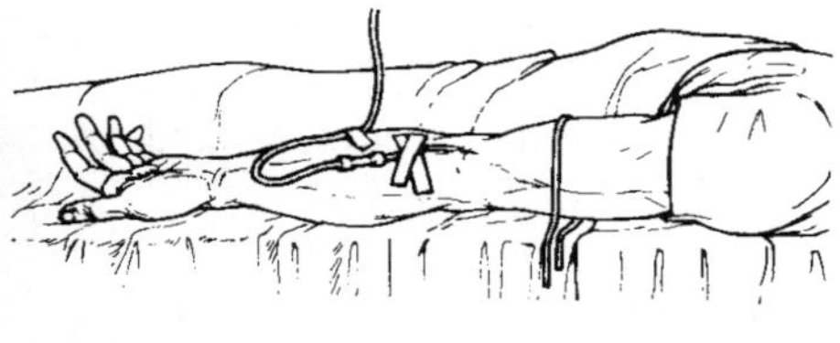

Figure 26.20 How to secure an intravenous catheter.

- Remove the cap on the infusion tubing, attach it to the cannula, and open the clamp on the infusion tube: check that fluid flows freely.
- Tape the needle securely in place (Figure 26.20).
- Place the guide needle directly into a proper sharps disposal bin.
- **NEVER, UNDER ANY CIRCUMSTANCES, REPLACE THE NEEDLE GUARD ON THE NEEDLE.**
- If you accidentally pierce your skin with a needle used for an injection, see Chapter 23, *Infectious diseases*, under *Needle-stick injuries*.
- Regulate the flow rate (drops per minute) carefully:
  - check often to make sure that the flow rate does not change or that the flow does not stop before all the solution is administered;
  - the flow rate will vary with the administration set but will be indicated on the packaging:
    - for example, if your set delivers 15 drops per ml and you wish to administer 1000 ml of solution over five hours, the flow rate should be about 50 drops per minute.
- Check the infusion site every day for redness, tenderness, warmth, or tissue swelling around the cannula: **if any of these signs is present, stop the intravenous infusion and start the procedure again in another vein, using another sterile needle.**

How to give an intravenous injection

- Assemble the following items:
  - latex gloves
  - alcohol swabs
  - cotton swabs or cotton-wool balls
  - a disposable syringe
  - a disposable needle to draw up the medicine
  - a disposable 19- or 21-gauge needle for the injection
  - the medicine.
- Note that some medicines have to be injected slowly, often over several minutes: check this point carefully before you begin the injection.
- Put the gloves on.
- Choose a site for the injection:
  - the large vein on the lateral (thumb) side of the elbow is the best site but the patient must keep the elbow straight during the injection; **OR**
  - choose a vein lower down the forearm;
  - **do not** use the vein in the medial (inner side) of the elbow unless you have no alternative: you may damage the nearby median nerve and brachial artery if you have not positioned the needle correctly.
- Draw up the medicine, as for an intramuscular injection.
- Apply the tourniquet to the upper arm above the chosen injection site.
- Swab the skin with alcohol.

- Bring the needle to the vein, with the bevel up, holding it alongside and almost parallel to the vein and to the skin.
- Gently press the point of the needle down so that the skin billows up a little around it, then push the point forward into the vein.
- Advance the needle and syringe gently along the vein for 1 cm or so, then place your left thumb (if you are right-handed) over the syringe to keep the needle steady in the vein.
- Gently draw back the syringe plunger and check that the blood is flowing easily into the syringe.
- Remove the tourniquet.
- Inject the medicine.
- Withdraw the needle and place a cotton swab or cotton-wool ball over the injection site, asking the patient or an attendant to press down firmly on the swab or cotton-wool ball: bleeding should be minimal and should stop completely within a few minutes.
- Place the needle and syringe directly into a sharps disposal bin.
- **NEVER, UNDER ANY CIRCUMSTANCES, REPLACE THE NEEDLE GUARD ON THE NEEDLE OR ATTEMPT TO BREAK THE NEEDLE AND SYRINGE.**
- If you accidentally pierce your skin with a needle used for an injection, see Chapter 23, *Infectious diseases*, under *Needle-stick injuries*.

Eye medication

The eye is susceptible to infection and injury. Solutions and ointments introduced into the conjunctival sac (the inside of the eyelids) should be sterile, as should the equipment used to introduce them.

Medicines chosen for their action on the eye or eyelids should not be applied directly to the sensitive cornea (the clear membrane covering the eye) but rather should be instilled into the lower conjunctival sac.

How to instill eye drops into the eye

- Note that sterile eye drops are supplied either in a glass or plastic bottle fitted with a sterile dropper or in a plastic bottle fitted with a device that dispenses drops when held upside down and squeezed.
- Remember to use only a sterile medicine prepared specially for the eyes.
- Wash your hands.
- If discharge is coming from the patient's eyes:
  - have ready sterile cotton balls moistened with sterile 0.9% sodium chloride solution;
  - clean the discharge with the cotton balls, wiping the eyelids from the inner to the outer side and using a new cotton ball for each stroke;
  - **never use dry cotton on the eye.**
- Have the patient look up.
- Drop the prescribed number of drops into the pocket formed by the lower eyelid: make sure the dropping device does not touch any part of the eye.

- Instruct the patient to close the eyes slowly and rotate the eyeballs to spread the medicine evenly.

How to apply eye ointment

- Before applying an ointment, clean off any discharge from the eyelids and eyelashes (as described above, *How to instil eye drops into the eye*).
- Hold the tube of eye ointment horizontally so as to control the quantity of ointment leaving the tube and to reduce the risk of touching the eyeball or the conjunctiva with the tip of the tube.
- Have the patient look up.
- Place a thumb near the margin of the lower lid, immediately below the eyelashes (see Figure 5.2 in Chapter 5, *Eye injuries and diseases*).
- Press down on the bony part of the cheek.
- Expose the conjunctival sac by pulling the lower eyelid down and away from the eyeball.
- Squeeze out about 1–1.5 cm of ointment and distribute it in the lower conjunctival sac,
- Instruct the patient to close the eyelids and move the eyes, in order to spread the ointment under the lid and over the surface of the eyeball.

How to perform conjunctival irrigation

- Use potable water in a clean container.
- Wipe off any discharge from the eye (as described above, *How to instil eye drops into the eye*).
- Separate the eyelids.
- Gently pour the water, using enough to produce a continuous flow of solution from the inner to the outer corner of the eye (see Figure 5.3 in Chapter 5, *Eye injuries and diseases*).
- Wipe the patient's cheeks with a towel or absorbent tissue.

Ear medication

How to instill ear drops into the ears

- Have the patient lie on one side with the affected ear uppermost.
- Straighten the ear canal by gently pulling the ear lobe upwards and backwards (in an adult) or downwards and backwards (in an infant or small child).
- Hold the tip of the dropper or inverted dropper-bottle at the opening of the ear taking care not to introduce the dropper or dropper-bottle into the ear canal.
- Instil a few drops of the medicine into the ear.
- Ask the patient to keep quite still for a few minutes to allow the medicine to remain in contact with the surfaces of the canal and to prevent leakage of drops from the ear.

INFECTION CONTROL (see *Table 26.5*)

Sterile conditions are difficult to achieve and maintain on board ship, and are rarely necessary. Hand-washing is the best way of reducing the risk of infection.

Table 26.5 Disinfection and sterilization guidelines.

Item	Means of disinfection or sterilization	Exposure time
Smooth, hard-surface objects (non-food-handling area)	■ 2% cetrimide solution, or 3% aqueous phenolic solution	30 minutes
Food-handling area: cutlery, dishes, plates, glasses	■ sodium hypochlorite, 100 mg/litre (100 parts per million) chlorine	30 minutes
	■ boiling	20 minutes
Instruments[a]	■ 3% aqueous phenolic solution ■ boiling	30 minutes 20 minutes
Thermometers[a]	■ 3% aqueous phenolic solution ■ 2% cetrimide solution (rinse thoroughly before use)	30 minutes 30 minutes
Items entering skin or mucous membranes[b]	■ autoclaving (sterilization by steam under pressure)	30 minutes at 121 °C
Environmental surfaces: walls, floors, etc.	3% aqueous phenolic solution or 2% cetrimide solution	

[a] Must be cleansed with soap and water before disinfection.

[b] All items that enter the skin or are in direct contact with mucous membranes (i.e. injection needles, urinary catheters, suction catheters, etc.) should be single-use, disposable items.

Note

- Most wound infections are caused by organisms on the patient's skin that are introduced into the wound at the time of the injury: the most careful, aseptic wound care will not prevent infection from this source.
- Infections caused by organisms introduced by dressings or from an attendant's skin do occur occasionally but will be rare if careful hand-washing is carried out.

✔ *What to do*

- Make sure that people coming into contact with the patient wash their hands before and after every contact with the patient and with the equipment and supplies used for the patient's care.
- Provide the patient with all that is needed for hand-washing after using the urinal or bedpan.
- Provide the patient with cotton handkerchiefs and insist that the mouth and nose be covered and the head turned away from others whenever the patient coughs or sneezes.
- Have the disposable articles that have been taken from an infected patient's room sealed in a bag with strong adhesive tape and then put that bag in a second, sealed bag.
- Store all potentially infectious articles and all articles contaminated by body fluids safely until they can be autoclaved (exposed in an autoclave device to steam under high pressure) or burned.

Death at sea

When nothing can be done to save a patient's life, everything should be done to alleviate the patient's suffering and loneliness in the final moments of life.

SIGNS OF DEATH

- Early signs of death:
  - the heart has stopped:
    - there is no pulse and no heart sounds can be heard with a stethoscope;
  - breathing has stopped:
    - with your ear over the patient's nose and mouth, you feel no air and see no chest or abdominal movement;
    - no breath sounds can be heard with a stethoscope;
  - there is no activity in the brain:
    - the pupils are very large, and do not become smaller when you shine a bright light directly into them;
  - the patient looks dead:
    - eyes dull;
    - skin pale.
- A person who is suffering from extreme cold (hypothermia) may look dead but still be alive (see Chapter 28, *Medical care for survivors at sea*).
- A person who has been struck by lightning may have large unresponsive pupils and still be alive (see Chapter 9, *Burns, chemical splashes, smoke inhalation, and electrocution*).
- If you are not confident declaring a patient dead from the early signs, wait for rigor mortis to appear (see below).
- Later signs of death:
  - stiffness of the muscles (rigor mortis) sets in three to four hours after death:
    - most easily felt in the jaw, elbow, and knee;
  - reddish or purplish patches resembling bruises (post-mortem lividity *or* staining) appear on the lower parts of the body (back, and back of the limbs, if the body has been placed or left face upwards after death);
  - the cornea takes on a milky appearance about 15 hours after death;
  - changes due to decomposition can be seen two to three days after death, usually first appearing in the abdomen, which may turn a greenish colour: this is a certain sign of death:
    - discoloration spreads to the rest of the abdomen and trunk, then upwards to the neck and head and downwards into the limbs.

✔ *What to do*

- If the dead person was ill on board, consult any records that were made of the nature and course of the illness and the treatment given.
- If the person was injured, investigate and record the circumstances of the injury or injuries.

- If the circumstances of death were unusual, sudden, or unknown, or if there is **any** possibility of criminal intent, a post-mortem examination is indispensable. You may be suspected of concealing a crime if a person is buried at sea under these circumstances:
    - to preserve the body for examination put it in a body bag and then in a refrigerator or cold-store;
    - failing this, place the body in a bath in which you have put a large amount of ice.
- Only if the ship is not near a port and the body cannot be kept on board because it poses a risk of infection should you proceed to burial at sea:
    - seek medical advice to confirm that it is dangerous to keep the body on board and record this advice in the log;
    - examine the body thoroughly (see below, *Examining a dead body*);
    - if the patient's identity is not known, look for signs that might assist in subsequent identification.
- Strip the body of all clothing, without tearing or cutting any clothes:
    - note if there is blood on the clothing.
- List each item of clothing briefly and note any initials or names on the garments.
- Remove and clean any dentures and place them with the other articles to be kept for future examination.
- List any papers, wallet, money, etc., that you find.
- Dry any wet articles and put them into a plastic bag, which you should seal, label, and keep in a safe place for delivery to the police or to other authorities at the next port.
- Have a witness present while you do this and have them sign all the records you make of your findings.

EXAMINING A DEAD BODY

- Record the exact time and date of the examination.
- Use universal body fluid precautions (gloves, eye protection, gown, if necessary).
- If the circumstances of death were unusual, photograph the body where it was found from several angles. When the body is moved, take more photographs of the scene to show any blood on the deck or any other evidence.
- Photograph the unclothed body, particularly any wounds, scars, and injuries.
- Photograph the face from the front and the side.
- Record the dead person's:
    - skin colour
    - approximate age
    - height
    - body size and shape (fat, thin, wasted, muscular, etc.)
    - hair length and colour

- eyebrow thickness
- complexion (sunburned, pale, etc)
- eye colour
- shape of the nose
- state of the teeth (sound, decayed, missing)
- birthmarks, moles, tattoos (photograph them if possible), scars (including vaccination scars), wounds, bruises (noting type, position, length, width, depth, and so on – photograph them if possible).

- Note down:
  - if facial hair is present;
  - if the patient was circumcised or not;
  - if there is any skin blackening around an entrance to a bullet wound and look for an exit wound (always larger than the entry wound);
  - the extent of discoloration from putrefaction:
    - late signs of putrefaction appear as swelling or bloating due to gas in the tissues;
    - the abdomen is swollen;
    - the skin becomes moist and peels;
    - bags of reddish or greenish fluid may form on the surface;
    - there is a foul odour;
    - froth or fluid may appear at the nose, mouth, and anus;
    - the tongue may protrude.
- Look for:
  - a bullet that may be lodged under the skin and note its position;
  - blood in the area where the body was found – this could help distinguish bleeding injuries caused while the patient was still alive from non-bleeding injuries caused after death;
  - broken bones;
  - signs of disease, such as boils, ulcers, or skin rashes.

DISPOSAL OF THE BODY

Wherever possible, the body should be kept for post-mortem examination or burial ashore. Care should be taken to observe the laws and regulations of both the flag state of your ship and of the country in whose waters you are sailing.

✔ *What to do to preserve the body*

- Thoroughly wash and dry the body all over:
  - do not wash the body if there is any possibility that a forensic post-mortem examination may be needed (seek medical advice if in doubt);
  - take care to observe as far as possible the requirements of the deceased person's religion.

- Comb the hair.
- Straighten the arms and legs, and interlock the fingers over the thighs.
- Tie the ankles together to keep the feet perpendicular.
- Use forceps to place a large plug of cotton wool well up into the rectum.
- Pass a catheter tube to empty the bladder completely:
  - if this is not possible, tie a string or ribbon around the base of the penis.
- Insert a plug of cotton wool into each nostril.
- Put the body into a body bag and keep it in a refrigerator or cold store set aside for the purpose or, if the ship is near a port, put the body into a bath in which you have put a large amount of ice.

BURIAL AT SEA

Burial at sea should be considered a last resort; always take the body to the next port if you can. The body may be buried at sea if there is no suspicion of foul play and it is not possible to keep the body safely on board, or if the next-of-kin have so requested (be wary of agreeing to requests of this type if you cannot be sure of the cause of death).

For burial at sea, the body has traditionally been sewn into a wide sheet of canvas about 4.5 metres in length. The canvas is weighted by fire bars sewn onto it on either side of the legs below the knees. These items may not be available on a modern ship. In seeking substitutes, note that the shroud needs to be made of very strong material and the weights must be heavy enough to ensure rapid sinking and permanent submersion of the body. There should be three or four slits or openings in the material to allow decomposition gases to escape and prevent flotation due to trapped air. Burial should not take place in soundings in any part of the world.

Efforts to observe the customs of the deceased person's religion should be made. If you are unsure of the requirements in a particular case seek advice.

To prepare the body for burial at sea:

- lay the body on a flat surface;
- straighten the legs and arms;
- interlock the fingers over the thighs;
- brush the hair clear of the forehead;
- wash the face;
- secure the jaw by passing a bandage under the chin and over the top of the head, where it may be tied or clipped;
- place the body on an improvised platform resting on the ship's side-rail and a suitable trestle or other support and cover it with a ship's flag;
- secure the body to the inboard edge of the platform;
- screw wooden blocks under the platform and rest them against the ship's side-rail in order to prevent the platform from sliding outboard when the inboard end is raised to allow the body to slide from under the flag into the sea;
- if the ship is small and there is a heavy sea, fasten guide-rails on the platform;

- brief the seamen assigned to the disposal that on receiving a discreet signal they should raise the inboard end of the platform to allow the body to slide from under the flag into the sea;
- the ship's master will notify the family that the remains were committed to the sea, indicating the longitude and latitude of the burial and, if the next-of-kin wish it, sending the flag used in the burial to the family with the personal effects of the deceased.

Medical care for survivors at sea

Following the abandonment of a vessel at sea, survivors on a survival craft or rescue vessel are likely to require medical treatment. Since there will be little or no time to consult a manual during or shortly after ditching of the ship, training of crew in the principles and procedures needed to provide such medical treatment is essential. This training should include regular lifeboat drills and regular briefing of crew and passengers in procedures to be followed after abandoning ship.

ABANDONING SHIP

The following advice, adapted from a pamphlet published by the International Maritime Organization[1], is aimed at increasing the chances of survival in cold water following a disaster at sea. The pamphlet should be available on board ship and should be used for training the crew in coping with this crisis situation.

1. Put on as many layers of warm clothing as possible, including foot protection, making sure to cover head, face, neck, hands, and feet. Fasten, close, and/or button up clothing to prevent cold water flushing through the clothing.
2. If an immersion suit is available, put it on over the warm clothing.
3. If the immersion suit does not have inherent flotation, put on a lifejacket and be sure to secure it correctly before immersion. In cold water you will lose full use of your fingers immediately.
4. If there is time to access the medicine chest and if it is possible to do so safely, take ondansetron, 4 mg orally before or immediately after boarding the survival craft. Vomiting will interfere with your survival chances because it removes body fluid, makes you more prone to hypothermia and impairs your will to survive.
5. Avoid entering the water if possible, e.g. board davit-launched survival craft on the embarkation deck or by the marine escape system. If davit-launched survival craft, a marine escape system, or other means of dry-shod embarkation are not available, use over-side ladders or, if necessary, lower yourself by means of a rope or fire hose.
6. Stay out of the water as long as possible! Try to minimize the shock of sudden cold immersion. A sudden plunge into cold water can cause rapid death or an uncontrollable rise in breathing rate may result in an intake of water into the lungs. If jumping into the water is unavoidable, you should try to keep your elbows to your side and cover your nose and mouth with one hand while holding the wrist or elbow firmly with the other hand. Avoid jumping onto the life-raft canopy or jumping into the water astern of a life raft, in case the ship has some remaining headway.
7. Once in the water, whether accidentally or by ship abandonment, orient yourself and try to locate the ship, lifeboats, life rafts, other survivors, or other floating objects. If you were unable to prepare yourself before entering the water, button up clothing now. In cold water, you may experience violent shivering and pain. These are natural body reflexes that are not dangerous. You do, however, need to take action as quickly as possible before you lose full use of your hands: button up clothing, turn on signal lights, locate whistle, etc.
8. While afloat in the water, do not attempt to swim unless it is to reach a nearby craft, a fellow survivor, or a floating object on which you can lean or climb. Unnecessary swimming will 'pump' out any warm water between your body and the layers of clothing,

thereby increasing the rate of body heat loss. In addition, unnecessary movements of your arms and legs send warm blood from the inner core to the extremities (arms and legs) and thus to the outer parts of the body. This can result in very rapid heat loss. Stay calm and take up a good position to prevent drowning.

9. The body position you assume in the water is also very important in conserving heat. Try to float as still as possible – with your legs together, elbows close to your side, and arms folded across the front of your life jacket. This position minimizes the exposure of the body surface to the cold water. Try to keep your head and neck out of the water.
10. Try to board a lifeboat, raft, or other floating platform or object as soon as possible in order to shorten the immersion time. Remember: you lose body heat many times faster in water than in air. Since the effectiveness of your insulation has been seriously reduced by water soaking, you must now try to shield yourself from wind to avoid a wind-chill effect. If you manage to climb aboard a lifeboat, shielding can be accomplished with the aid of a canvas cover, a tarpaulin, or an unused garment. Huddling close to the other occupants of the lifeboat or raft will also conserve body heat.
11. Keep a positive attitude of mind about your survival and rescue. This will improve your chances of extending your survival time until rescue comes. Your will to live does make a difference!

SURVIVING IN A SURVIVAL CRAFT

Surviving in a survival craft (lifeboat or life raft) is one of the most strenuous ordeals an individual can face. It involves combat against all the elemental forces at sea, one's own physical limitations, and – most of all – panic and despair.

- A healthy uninjured person can be confident of surviving three days at sea in a lifeboat or raft, and survival for more than a month is common.
- The single most important factor in survival is the **will to live.**
- The second most important factor is the morale of the group:
  - keeping active by fulfilling specific tasks – nursing care, supply tally, rescue watch, and so on – can occupy the mind and keep hopes high.
- Lone survivors should make every effort to conserve energy and resources:
  - keeping the mind active with mental exercises may prevent hallucinations.
- Mental derangement may appear at any time before or after the rescue.
- Panic is contagious and can destroy chances of survival on the open sea.

✔ *What to do*

- Before other survivors are picked up or as soon as immediate rescue operations have been completed, establish a firm chain of command based on previous positions of authority on board ship.
- The person in command of a survival craft has responsibility for the physical safety, health, and morale of the occupants of the survival craft and for deciding such issues, as:
  - how long artificial respiration should be continued on an unconscious victim;
  - how food, water, and medical supplies are distributed;
  - when to signal for help.

- In transferring a survivor to the survival craft, apply the first-aid instructions given in Chapter 1, *First aid*.
- Rapidly triage survivors according to their physical condition, grouping:
  - those whose injuries require immediate treatment;
  - those with injuries whose condition will not be worsened by delaying treatment;
  - those for whom no treatment will prevent death (the only survivors likely to be in this group will be older persons with extensive burns).
- Treat immediately survivors rescued from drowning (see below, under *Near-drowning* and in more detail, Chapter 1, *First aid*, under *Basic life support*).
- If a medical kit (see Table 28.1) is not available, provide life-saving treatment by:
  - controlling haemorrhage with direct pressure;
  - giving mouth-to-mouth artificial respiration when needed;
  - applying chest compressions if the survivor has no pulse or heartbeat;
  - treating a survivor in shock by placing the head lower than the rest of the body and keeping the body warm;
  - treating fractures by strapping the extremity to the opposite side;
  - relieving pain by reassurance.
- To counter anxiety:
  - reassure survivors;
  - assign small tasks to keep survivors occupied.
- To treat acute agitation promptly:
  - use forced restraint, if necessary; OR
  - if a medical kit is available, morphine sulfate, 10 mg intramuscularly, repeated every four hours as needed.
- When survivors are rescued by a large vessel, triage immediately as above, but add a category for survivors who require evacuation to a hospital.
- **Evacuate all submersion victims to a hospital for follow-up care, even if only minimal treatment is required.**

Near-drowning

There are three main elements to near-drowning, present to a variable degree in each case:

- inhaling water, which can cause lung damage that can become progressively worse over a period of up to eight hours after rescue;
- lack of oxygen caused by vocal cord spasm preventing the passage of either air or water;
- hypothermia.

✔ *What to do*

- The effects of inhaling water cannot be treated effectively without the facilities of a hospital: seek medical advice with a view to evacuation even if the patient appears well.
- If the patient is unconscious, check for pulse and breathing: if they are absent immediately apply mouth-to-mouth artificial respiration and, if needed, chest compressions (see Chapter 1, *First aid*).

Table 28.1 Recommended medical survival kit[a] for lifeboats aboard merchant vessels. These supplies are intended for 20–30 survivors for a period of one week.

Description of item	Container	No. of units	Usage, class
Medicines			
Paracetamol tablets, 500 mg, 100s	Bottle	1	Minor aches or pains, fever
Morphine sulfate injection, 10 mg/ml, 1-ml disposable cartridge,[b] 10s	Package	1	Analgesic, sedative (controlled substance)
Sodium chloride tablets, 1 g, 100s	Bottle	1	Heat cramps
Sunscreen preparation	Package	40	Protection against sunburn
Amoxycillin/clavulanate tablets, 875/125 mg	Bottle	2	Broad-spectrum antibiotic
Surgical supplies			
Bandage, elastic, 10-cm roll, 12s	Box	1	
Bandage, gauze, roll, sterile, 10 cm×10 m, 12s	Box	1	
Bandage, absorbent, adhesive, 2 cm×8 cm, 100s	Box	1	
Pad, sterile, 10 cm×10 cm, 100s	Box	2	
Lister bandage scissors	Item	1	
Soap	Cake	20	
Sunglasses	Item	20	
Syringe, hypodermic cartridge holder[b]	Item	2	
Tape, adhesive, surgical, 5 cm×5 m roll, 6s	Box	1	
Low-reading clinical thermometer	Item	2	

[a] To be available in the event of forced abandonment of a vessel sailing in infrequently used waterways.

[b] The disposable cartridge holding the medication and the syringe holder should be purchased from the same supplier to ensure that the cartridge will fit the syringe. Injectable doses of morphine sulfate may be stored in these kits. However, the ship's compartment in which morphine sulfate is stored should be locked securely at all times and checked at frequent intervals by the master. The master and officer concerned should be the only persons on board with the key or lock combination.

- In checking if the patient's heart has stopped, be aware that the pulse may be irregular; it may also be difficult to feel because of the extreme slowing of the heart caused by hypothermia.
- Continue resuscitation efforts for 30 minutes, then stop if:
  - there is no carotid or femoral pulse; **AND**
  - the patient's Glasgow coma scale score is less than 5 at 30 minutes (for the Glasgow coma scale, see Table 26.3 in Chapter 26, *Nursing care and medical procedures*).

✗ *What not to do*

- Do not try to drain water from the lungs of a nearly drowned person.

Generalized hypothermia due to cold water immersion

Generalized hypothermia is the leading cause of death among shipwreck survivors. In a cold environment, the body will automatically increase its heat production efforts in order to compensate for heat loss. However, if the rate of heat loss exceeds the rate of heat production, body temperature falls and hypothermia will result.

Note

- Forced immersion is the main threat to life after hitting the water.
- Anyone immersed in cold water anywhere will lose heat and the heat loss will lower internal body (core) temperature.
- Loss of body heat is one of the greatest hazards to survival in the sea.
- Some degree of hypothermia occurs in most survivors extracted from cold water.
- The degree of hypothermia depends on the duration of immersion and the water temperature (and so on latitude and season), the person's activity in the water, and body insulation (the amount of fat and clothing on the individual).
- Most ordinary clinical thermometers do not measure temperatures below 34 °C: a special low-reading thermometer must be used if hypothermia is suspected.
- The severity of hypothermia is defined as follows:
  - mild hypothermia – core temperature above 32 °C;
  - moderate hypothermia – core temperature between 32 °C and 28 °C;
  - severe hypothermia – core temperature below 28 °C.
- Mild hypothermia causes:
  - an increase in pulse and breathing rates
  - poor muscular co-ordination
  - slurred speech
  - impaired judgement
  - shivering.
- Moderate hypothermia causes:
  - a slowing of pulse and breathing rates
  - drowsiness
  - confusion
  - in many cases, "paradoxical undressing", or a false sense of warmth, and cessation of shivering
  - death – in many cases, even with hospital care.
- Severe hypothermia causes:
  - coma
  - shock
  - lung failure

- kidney failure
- death – in most cases, even with hospital care.

✔ *What to do*

- For survivors who, although shivering dramatically, are rational and capable of recounting their experiences:
  - have their wet clothes replaced with dry clothes or blankets;
  - check quickly for injuries;
  - forbid the use of alcohol.
- In more serious cases, in which the survivor is not shivering but is semi-conscious, unconscious, or apparently dead, apply immediate first aid.
- If the survivor is not breathing:
  - ensure that the airway is clear and start mouth-to-mouth or mouth-to-nose artificial respiration immediately;
  - continue basic life support for at least 30 minutes.
- If the survivor is breathing but unconscious:
  - place in the recovery position to ensure that breathing is not obstructed by the tongue or by vomit;
  - check for other causes of unconsciousness, such as head injury;
  - avoid all unnecessary manhandling, such as removing wet clothes or massaging the limbs.
- To prevent further loss of heat from evaporation or exposure to the wind, immediately wrap the survivor in blankets, keeping the body horizontal with the head slightly lower than the rest of the body.
- A patient with mild hypothermia who is shivering will recover if further heat loss is prevented.
- A patient with moderate or severe hypothermia, especially if he is not shivering, requires external rewarming:
  - place a waterproof sheet on a bunk, and lay the patient on the sheet;
  - cover him with two or three blankets;
  - put four towels (or other large pieces of cloth) into a bowl of hot water (about 40 °C), then put the dripping wet towels into four plastic bags;
  - put the plastic bags on the patient's armpits and each groin;
  - after 10 minutes replace with fresh wet hot towels;
  - continue until the patient's temperature is over 32 °C.

✗ *What not to do*

- Do not try to warm a survivor in hypothermia by using an external source of radiant heat, such as a fire or electric radiator: this will divert blood from the core of the body to the skin, causing the body temperature to fall further.

Cold exposure injuries

Cold injuries to parts of the body – most commonly the face and extremities – are caused by exposure of tissues and small surface blood vessels to abnormally low temperatures. Cold exposure injuries are common in patients in hypothermia.

The extent of a cold injury depends on:

- temperature
- duration of exposure
- wind velocity
- humidity
- presence or absence of protective clothing
- whether or not skin comes into direct contact with cold metal or frozen cloth.

Frostnip

Frostnip, the mildest form of cold injury, is caused by exposure to temperatures above freezing (0–16 °C) in conditions of relatively high humidity.

Signs and symptoms

- Tingling
- itching
- burning sensation, possibly aggravated by warmth
- no blistering or skin discolouration.

Frostbite

Frostbite, involving the death of skin, is a more severe injury than frostnip.

Signs and symptoms

- In cases of superficial frostbite:
  - only skin involved
  - skin pale and swollen
  - blisters filled with clear fluid.
- In cases of deep frostbite:
  - involvement of skin and deeper tissues, such as muscle
  - ulcers, in some cases:
    - especially when skin is separated from metal or frozen fabric with which it has been in direct contact
  - blisters filled with blood
  - in severe cases, presence of gangrene.

What to do

- Test for skin sensation:
  - normal ability to feel a light touch indicates that the small nerve fibres immediately under the skin surface are alive;
  - loss of sensation suggests that injury has extended through the full thickness of the skin.
- Warm the injured part in water at 40 °C (not warmer) for 15 to 30 minutes, using a basin for hands and feet and warm compresses for face and ears.
- To relieve pain, which may be severe, give tramadol, 100 mg orally, every 8 hours or, if needed, morphine, 10–15 mg intramuscularly, every three to four hours.

- If the skin has blisters, leave them alone as long as possible:
  - if the blisters burst:
    - cut the dead skin away with sterile scissors;
    - swab the area with povidone–iodine solution;
    - cover with a sterile dressing.

✗ *What not to do*

- **Never** rewarm frostbitten tissue with direct heat from a fire.

Immersion foot (trench foot)

Immersion foot is caused by exposure of the lower extremities to water at above freezing temperatures but usually below 10 °C, for more than 12 hours. It typically occurs in shipwrecked sailors surviving, but remaining for the most part inactive, on lifeboats or rafts, and living on a poor diet, with wet and constricting clothing, and in adverse weather conditions.

► *Signs and symptoms*

- Swelling of the feet and lower legs
- numbness
- tingling
- itching
- pain
- cramps
- skin discoloration
- in the absence of trauma, usually no tissue destruction.

✔ *What to do – preventing immersion foot*

- Survivors should make every effort to keep their feet warm and dry.
- Several times a day, survivors should loosen shoe laces, raise the feet, and perform toe and ankle exercises.
- When possible, survivors should remove shoes and wrap spare clothing around the feet to keep them warm.
- Survivors should refrain from smoking.
- After rescue, avoid rapid rewarming of the affected limbs.
- Remove wet footwear.
- Allow the skin to dry in warm air.
- Avoid damaging skin or breaking blisters.

✗ *What not to do*

- Do not rub the skin.
- Do not massage affected limbs.

Other medical problems aboard survival craft

Seasickness

Seasickness (motion sickness) is an acute illness characterized by loss of appetite, nausea, dizziness, and vomiting. Preventive measures may be effective but few medications are effective once motion sickness has developed.

✔ *What to do – preventing seasickness*

- Give an anti-seasickness drug. Two widely used drugs are:
  - **scopolamine**, in the form of transdermal patches:
    - apply every 72 hours to the skin behind the ear;
    - wash the hands carefully after applying the patch to avoid any drug inadvertently entering the eye;
    - this treatment is effective but causes sedation, so **crew members using scopolamine cannot take watch, and are likely to make errors of judgement in emergencies**;
    - patches have to be applied at least two to three hours (preferably 12 hours) before they are needed;
  - **ondansetron**, 4–8 mg every 12 hours, orally, beginning 30 minutes before it is needed:
    - the tablets disintegrate on the tongue and are easy to swallow;
    - the drug treats only the nausea and vomiting of motion sickness, not the loss of appetite and dizziness;
    - the drug is non-sedating.

Sunburn

Sunburn is one of the main hazards facing a survivor on the open sea, regardless of latitude. It may vary from a first- to a third-degree burn, depending on the degree of exposure and the protection available to the victim.

✔ *What to do – preventing sunburn*

- Keep fully clothed at all times.
- Stay under a canopy, if possible.
- Wear sunglasses during daylight hours.
- Apply a sunscreen, preferably a physical agent such as zinc cream, to all exposed parts of the body.

Dehydration and malnutrition

If rescue is delayed, maintaining both hydration and nutrition aboard a survival craft is difficult. The need for water is more urgent and more vital than the need for food. Survival craft carry a limited quantity of potable water, but they may be equipped with desalting kits or a solar still which provides additional drinking-water.

✔ *What to do – preventing dehydration*

- Try to store rainwater.
- Ensure that each survivor drinks a minimum of half a litre of water daily.
- Increase the water ration:
  - for survivors who have a demanding thirst from having spent a considerable time in the water or from having swallowed seawater;
  - in tropical climates, to compensate for loss of water due to sweating.

Heat exposure (see also Chapter 10, *Heat stroke and other heat disorders*)

Special problems are created aboard survival craft by exposure to tropical heat. In certain circumstances, fluid loss by sweating alone can be extremely high. The body will adjust to some extent to exceptional heat but full acclimatization rarely occurs. Dehydration can be prevented by minimizing physical activity during daylight hours and by making the best use of clothing as a canopy. A survivor suffering from dehydration should be given an increased water ration, if supplies permit (see previous section, *Deydration and malnutrition*).

See Chapter 10, *Heat stroke and other heat disorders* for *Heat exhaustion*, which is caused by loss of body water and salt; for *Stoker's cramps*, which are painful spasms of the muscles of the extremities, back, or abdomen due to salt depletion, and for *Heat stroke*.

Contamination with oil

✔ *What to do*

- Once the survivor is warm and comfortable, clean the oil off the skin (except around the mouth and eyes).
- Take survivors who have recovered from hypothermia to a warm shower room or bathroom and have them take off all their clothes.
- Wipe their skin with a soft cloth and strong paper towels to remove as much of the oil as possible.
- Take care in wiping injured or burned areas (or avoid doing so).
- If available, use a strong warm shower to remove the oil.
- Use shampoo to remove oil from the hair and to help remove oil from the body.
- Use good toilet soap to clean the skin.
- Wash off the rest of the oil.
- Avoid using solvents, scouring compounds, kerosene, and other cleaners not designed for skin-cleaning: prefer jellied cleansing agents designed for skin cleaning.

FOOD AND WATER FOR RESCUED SURVIVORS

Malnutrition results from several weeks of minimal food intake. It should be suspected if there is marked loss of normal fat under the skin, and of muscle: this is most easily appreciated around the buttocks and upper arm. Note that rapid refeeding of a severely malnourished survivor and rapid rehydration of a survivor who has been dehydrated for a long time can be dangerous.

✔ *What to do*

- For a survivor who has had inadequate water intake for **less** than 48 hours:
  - allow as much fluid as desired;
  - give oral rehydration solution.
- For a survivor who has had inadequate water intake for **more** than 48 hours:
  - avoid rapid rehydration;
  - if possible, calculate the fluid deficit by subtracting the daily fluid intake of the survivor from three litres and multiplying the result by the number of days on reduced intake (for example, if a survivor has had one litre each day for five days the deficit is 3 – 1=2 then 2 x 5 = 10 litres);
  - if fluid intake is not known, assume the deficit is two and a half litres for each day (i.e. in a survivor rescued after five days and whose fluid intake is uncertain, assume a deficit of 12 litres);
  - over a five-day period, give the daily amount of fluid needed to replace the fluid deficit plus the three litres normally needed, up to a maximum of five litres per day (for example, if the total fluid deficit is 15 litres, give 2 + 3 = 5 l a day for five days).
- For a survivor who does not appear severely malnourished (see above), or has had inadequate food for a week or less, allow food as desired.
- For a survivor who does appear severely malnourished (see above), or who has had little or no food intake for several weeks:
  - on the first day, if the survivor is of average height and weighs about 50 kg, give half the food ration provided for a crew member engaged in ordinary shipboard work;
  - increase or reduce the allowance in proportion if the survivor is larger or smaller;
  - increase this amount each day by two pieces of fruit **or** two slices of bread **or** one serving of vegetables **or** half a serving of meat;
  - give a multivitamin pill, if available.

MEDICAL RESOURCES ON A LIFEBOAT

Lifeboats, life rafts, life floats, and buoyant apparatus should carry certain provisions. Every lifeboat on an ocean-going, seagoing, or coastal ship or on a self-propelled vessel should be equipped with a first-aid kit. Ships sailing on infrequently used waterways or in colder climates should, in addition, carry a more complete survival kit (see Table 28.1) that is kept at temperatures above freezing but not above room temperature, protected by waterproof packaging, and ready to be placed aboard lifeboats or life rafts when needed.

Endnote

1. *A pocket guide to cold water survival,* 3rd ed. London, International Maritime Organization, 2006.

Environmental control and hygiene

Environmental controls are concerned with the climatic, physical, and biological factors that act on an individual and on the community.

A seafarer's health and survival depend mainly on:

- personal efforts to maintain optimum physical and mental efficiency;
- the organization of the physical facilities and the supplies needed to maintain optimum efficiency;
- the efforts of other personnel, ashore and afloat, to create and maintain conditions conducive to health.

A give-and-take attitude is particularly important in maintaining good environmental sanitation on board ship. Proper sanitation is impossible unless each crew member cooperates. The ship's master should ensure good sanitary conditions on board through periodic inspections, and compliance with the guidance given in the most recent edition of the *Guide to Ship Sanitation*.

VENTILATION

Adequate ventilation in living spaces and food stores is important for the health of all on board ship. This is often achieved by a recirculating air-conditioning system. As it is obviously undesirable that the air from a room occupied by a person with an infectious disease should be recirculated, purpose-built ships' hospitals have separate ventilation systems. However, when a person with an infection has to occupy a cabin, steps should be taken to prevent contaminated air from recirculating. For example, a porthole or external door not subject to an inflow of air should be opened, wherever possible, to remove the contaminated air.

For effective ventilation, there must be:

- an adequate flow of clean air with sufficient oxygen content;
- controlled humidity to prevent sweating and mould growth;
- controlled temperatures to make the atmosphere comfortable.

Modern vessels use ventilation and forced air to create conditions suitable for working on board.

Old ships still in service may have cowl ventilators, which are not very effective in the tropics. However, judicious use of all openings and efficient electric fans can achieve some measure of comfort.

Ships built for service in temperate climates need to improve their air supply system if they are to be used for tropical runs.

A common hazard aboard ship is the accumulation of gases in holds, bunkers, paint lockers, tanks, and other confined areas (see Chapter 11, *Poisoning*). Such gases may be poisonous or they may displace oxygen, and crew members entering an enclosed space may become ill or die of asphyxia.

Among common toxic gases are carbon monoxide, carbon dioxide, ammonia, chlorine, hydrogen sulphide, and petroleum gases. These and other gases are found in varying combinations in:

- shipboard fires;
- empty oil, chemical, and storage tanks;

- bilges:
  - skin tanks
  - certain cargo holds, such as those containing products of plant origin, such as:
    - linseed cakes
    - resin
    - tobacco.

Poisonous gases or fumes may be formed from:

- decomposing residues in emptied tanks that have contained:
  - chemicals
  - petroleum
  - whale-oil
  - cargoes of hides that have become moist and have fermented;
- enclosed freshly painted compartments or tanks.

Mechanical refrigeration systems are potentially dangerous owing to the risk of leakage into enclosed spaces of ammonia, Freon, or other refrigerants. Cyanide or other gases used to fumigate ships present a serious hazard during fumigation and also after fumigation until the fumigated areas have been properly aired.

In all cases, safety depends on proper ventilation and proper individual precautions. When compartments or tanks must be entered for cleaning or other purposes, the deck officer and/or chief engineer must ensure that the area has been ventilated thoroughly, that all explosive gases have been vented, and that the oxygen supply is adequate. In addition, the first person to enter the area must wear a lifeline to be used in the event of malaise or illness and the work crew should be checked continuously during the first half-hour after entering the area. Proper canister-type oxygen gas masks should be available if a rescue operation becomes necessary. Frequent training demonstrations and emergency drills in the use of rescue and mask equipment should be organized for all ship's personnel.

LIGHTING

Without good lighting on board ship:

- fatigue and eyestrain develop rapidly
- work performance is reduced
- the risk of accidents increases
- morale deteriorates.

Good lighting is particularly important in:

- the engine room
- galley (ship's kitchen)
- chartroom
- companion-ways
- ladder-wells
- pantry
- scullery
- head.

FOOD HYGIENE

The ship's master should monitor the health of crew handling food and make regular and unscheduled inspections of areas used for the storage, preparation, and serving of food and of any self-dispensing food units aboard ship.

Food-handlers

The ship's master must ensure that all food-handlers aboard have proper health certification.

Applicants for food-handling work should undergo a pre-recruitment medical examination and a professional assessment should be made of their clinical history. Only those who are free from infection, with or without symptoms, should be hired. Food-handlers must report any conditions likely to present a risk of food contamination.

Persons carrying an organism that can spread through food or water should not be employed in food preparation or food-handling. See Chapter 26, *Nursing care and medical procedures* for guidance on isolation.

Food-handlers should be kept under regular surveillance for such infections.

Staff should be excluded from food-handling until given medical clearance to return to work if they:

- have wounds or sores that cannot be covered by a waterproof dressing;
- are suffering from a gastrointestinal infection;
- are suffering from any other condition likely to cause the contamination of food or of surfaces coming into contact with food.

Physical examinations for food service personnel are carried out in major ports by the medical department of the shipping company, the city health department, or any other suitable facility designated by the company, union, or country.

All food-handlers should receive basic instruction in hygiene and its application to:

- their work;
- company regulations and procedures;
- health requirements;
- use of equipment;
- use of protective clothing;
- the code of practice in:
  - handling food
  - reporting of sickness
  - personal hygiene
  - general standards of hygiene in working areas.

All food-handlers must:

- pay scrupulous attention to cleanliness of body and clothing;
- wear clothing designed for food service areas and do so only for food-handling work;
- have this clothing laundered regularly and wear it only during working hours.

Food service facilities

The surfaces of all decks, bulkheads, and deckheads close to the area where food is processed, served, and stored should be:

- corrosion-free
- smooth
- easy to clean.

All surfaces coming into contact with food should be of material that is:

- corrosion-resistant
- non-toxic
- non-absorbent
- smooth
- durable
- easy to clean.

Cooking utensils and equipment should be kept in a place where they can be used safely and efficiently and should not be made of potentially toxic metals, such as:

- cadmium
- lead
- zinc
- antimony.

Proper plumbing equipment in food service areas is mandatory. Only potable water should be piped into such areas, although non-potable water may be piped to garbage-grinder eductors. Food service equipment and areas should be adequately drained and the drains protected from backflow of waste matter.

The chief steward and the chief engineer must make regular sanitary inspections to ensure that these recommendations are implemented.

Food storage

NON-REFRIGERATED ITEMS

Non-refrigerated foods comprise bulk items and broken or lot items. The bulk items are boxed, bagged, or canned, must be kept free of poisons and contaminants, must be destroyed if infected or outdated, and must be stored in an area that is:

- raised at least 15 cm above the level of the deck, so as to facilitate cleaning
- accessible to inspection
- readily accessible for use
- kept clear of all cleansing or chemical agents
- locked when not in use
- used only for food items
- protected from rodent and insect contamination
- cool
- dry
- not liable to condensation
- not exposed to waste water.

Foods taken from the dry storage room to the day stores where they are unpacked must be protected from contamination.

After being loaded aboard ship, **boxed foods** should be:

- used quickly to minimize vermin infestation
- dated
- never left in storage.

Non-refrigerated **bulk items**, such as cereals, sugar, and vegetables, are extremely susceptible to contamination and to insect and rodent infestation. They must be protected by storage in easily cleaned, vermin-proof containers or bins.

Non-refrigerated **canned or bottled items** are usually stored in boxes or crates. They are best protected by:

- maintaining a rotating inventory
- keeping the units dry and cool
- eliminating damaged or distorted cans or tins.

Corrugated paper boxes should be emptied and removed from the ship as soon as possible, as they are apt to harbour insects.

REFRIGERATED ITEMS

The same basic requirements apply to the storage of refrigerated items. However, refrigerated storage is more confined and specific temperatures must be maintained.

Refrigerated foods fall into two general groups: frozen foods and cooled foods.

Frozen foods must be kept at between –18 °C and –23 °C from time of freezing until time of preparation. Under these conditions, food retains its normal taste and appearance and has a shelf-life of one to six months. Once thawed, such food must be used immediately and not re-frozen under any circumstances. Once food is thawed, it rapidly deteriorates and may become dangerous as a result of bacterial action. Frozen food is usually stored in packaged units. Once a package is opened, its contents must be wrapped, kept frozen in the day stores, and used at the earliest opportunity.

Cooled food items most often kept in storage include:

- fresh fruits
- vegetables
- processed and cooked meat products
- foods prepared for rapid use.

These foods, as well as leftovers, should be kept covered and stored at between 0 °C and 7 °C, depending on the product.

Freezer and cooler compartments should have accurate, adjustable thermostats for temperature control. Thermometers should be easily visible to persons working in passageways serving the refrigerated spaces and on the engineer's control panel.

In storage areas for cooled foods, humidity ranges from moderate to high. Cooled foods, properly handled, have a storage life of one day to four months, depending on the item. Leftover food is considered to have a shelf-life of not more than 48 hours because of the possibility of contamination.

Both frozen and cooled foods keep better when the refrigeration unit is:

- properly drained
- kept clean
- free of:
  - ice
  - frost
  - food spillage
  - residue
  - fungus
  - slime.

To maintain freezer efficiency, remove frost or ice before it reaches 5 mm in thickness.

When defrosting, wash the freezer with steam or heavily chlorinated, warm, soapy water to remove slime, dirt, grease, and fungus. Shelves, hooks, and grids should be removed and washed with a warm detergent solution, then steamed down, rinsed in hot water, and, if possible, sun-dried or heat-dried. The refrigerator decks should be cleaned and scrubbed with a hot detergent solution and then rinsed.

After cleaning, the refrigerator should be loaded so that stores are placed neatly, with no overloading, and separated to allow free circulation of air. Foods to be refrigerated should be stored in shallow metal pans or plastic containers covered with wax paper, plastic, or aluminium foil.

The chief steward must ensure the cleanliness of the storage areas and food storage equipment and the chief engineer must ensure the effective functioning of these units.

The galley (ship's kitchen)

The galley should be equipped, illuminated, and maintained in such a way as to ensure good sanitation. The equipment should be made of corrosion-resistant, non-toxic materials that are easy to clean. All galley areas, especially the cooking areas, should be protected against fire, easy to clean, and capable of being rapidly emptied of smoke, steam, odours, and gases.

Waste, particularly food scraps, should be kept in sturdy, tightly covered garbage cans.

Where possible, all galley equipment and utensils should be fixed in place. Non-fixed utensils should be hung or stored to avoid loss, damage, or injury when the ship rolls.

Foodstuffs, supplies, cookware, crockery, and utensils should be thoroughly cleaned after each use and stored in containers that can be secured when the contents are not in use.

Most raw meat is contaminated with microbes, which are destroyed by cooking and therefore do not cause disease. Undercooking can leave microbes alive. Meat should be cooked to a final temperature of at least 65 °C in the centre of the meat.

Cooked food can be recontaminated if it is placed on surfaces that have been used for preparing raw food. For this reason, utensils and chopping boards used to prepare raw food should be washed in hot soapy water after use.

Contaminated food, whether cooked or uncooked, is likely to cause disease if allowed to stand at room temperature for some time before being eaten. Some microbes produce toxins that are not destroyed by heat, so that even vigorous reheating of cooked food does not render the food safe. Cooked food that is not be eaten immediately, and leftovers, should, therefore be, refrigerated promptly and uncooked food should be prepared immediately before consumption.

Toilet and washing facilities

Adequate toilet facilities should be available for food-handlers (or for all crew in small vessels) near areas where food is prepared.

If possible, toilets should not open directly into areas where food is prepared, stored, or served. Where they do, the doors should be tight-fitting and self-closing. Wherever possible, there should be a ventilated space between the toilets and areas where there is food.

Adequate hand-washing facilities should be provided within or adjacent to toilets and should include:

- a single outlet for dispensing mixed (hot and cold) water;
- a single-service dispenser of paper or cloth towels;
- a drying device;
- soap, detergent, or alcohol-based gels;
- a sign over the basin reading:

WASH HANDS AFTER USING TOILET

WASH THE BASIN BEFORE AND AFTER USE

Signs urging personnel to wash their hands after using the toilet should also be conspicuously posted on the bulkhead adjacent to the toilet door.

Where a common washbasin serves both a food-handling space and a toilet for food-handlers, a sign should be posted above it reading

WASH HANDS OFTEN—WASH THE BASIN BEFORE AND AFTER USE

On ships where hand-washing facilities exist in a stateroom for food service employees and are easily accessible from the food-handling areas, additional facilities are not required in the food-handling areas. In such cases, individual cloth towels for food-handlers are acceptable.

Scullery sinks, slop sinks, laundry tubs, dish-washing sinks, and similar facilities should not be used for hand-washing.

Non-potable wash-water (see section below, *Liquid transport and potable water*) may be used for the hot water supply to washbasins, provided that it is heated to a temperature of 77 °C. Only potable water should be used for the cold water supply to washbasins.

LIQUID TRANSPORT AND POTABLE WATER

LIQUID TRANSPORT SYSTEMS

Special piping systems for ships include:

- the bilge system, which collects drainage that must be pumped overboard;
- the clean ballast system, which maintains the proper trim, stability, and immersion of the vessel;

- the fuel oil and oily ballast system, which stores and transfers clean oil to the ship's fuel system and also replaces used oil with sea water as part of the ballast system;
- the fire system, which supplies water under pressure to the ship's fire stations and to the deck and anchor wash areas;
- the sanitary system, which supplies water to the heads and other sanitary fixtures;
- the wash-water system, which supplies fresh water from skin and/or peak tanks:
  - the wash-water system must be independent of all other piping systems and its outlets should be labelled NOT FIT TO DRINK;
- the drinking-water system, which supplies potable water to drinking-fountains and to washing and culinary units:
  - the drinking-water system must be protected, and isolated from all other systems.

Potable water sources

The term **potable water** covers water used:

- for drinking
- for cooking
- for washing utensils used for cooking and eating
- in the ship's hospital.

To be potable, water should be free from pathogenic organisms and harmful chemicals. Its quality should comply with WHO guidelines, especially those relating to microbes (*Guidelines for drinking-water quality, Vol. I. Recommendations,* 3rd ed. Geneva, World Health Organization, 2004).

The handling of water must be rigidly controlled from source to consumer to avoid contamination.

Potable water on board ship is derived either from distillation or from natural sources. Distilled water is either fresh or comes from salt water that has been converted to steam and back to water. It is relatively free from impurities but has a flat taste. Natural water, or "shore water", is usually obtained from wells, springs, or freshwater sources ashore. It usually has to be treated, either ashore or afloat, to protect the health of the crew.

Potable water transport system

The water system of a port city is the usual source of potable water for ships. It is made available to a ship either through watering-points at dockside or from water-boats.

Each vessel should carry a sufficient length of special hose to load its potable water. This hose should be kept in a storage cabinet labelled POTABLE WATER HOSE ONLY and not used for any other purpose.

A deck officer should be responsible for the cleanliness and safety of a ship's filling hose and its extremities, as well as the connections of dockside, water-boat, or shipside filling lines. These connections – outlet and inlet – must be at least 40 cm above the dock, water-boat deck, and ship's deck, and housed with a proper fitting. Each watering-point connection must be labelled POTABLE WATER FILLING.

Potable water should be transported from storage areas to dispensing units through colour-coded, non-cross-connected pipes made of safe metals or plastic. All potable water outlets must be protected from back-siphonage by an air-gap or approved vacuum-breaker.

Potable water storage

To avoid contamination, a potable water tank should share no partitions with tanks containing non-potable liquids, including skin tanks. The potable water tank should be labelled POTABLE WATER and be accessible through a watertight, preferably side-mounted, manhole. The potable water tank must:

- have an overflow and relief valve or vent;
- be completely drainable from a bottom drain;
- be able to withstand pressure;
- have water-level gauges or petcocks;
- be emptied periodically for inspection and maintenance and then thoroughly scrubbed and flushed out; and the whole potable water system be disinfected with chlorine (see section below, *Disinfection of potable water*);
- be entered only by personnel wearing clean clothing and footwear and not suffering from a skin infection, diarrhoea, or a communicable disease.

Taking water on board

✔ ***What to do***

- Remember that however bright, clear, and sparkling water may be, it could easily contain disease organisms or harmful minerals.
- If you plan to take water for drinking from a new and/or doubtful source, consult the company agents about whether the water is likely to contain germs or harmful minerals.
- If you decide that the source is acceptable, check that the potable water storage tanks on board are in order.
- Check that the delivery cocks on shore and the receiving point on board have been properly cleaned.
- Examine the hose to ensure that it is clean, in good working order, and free from leaks (germs can enter through leaks in the hose).
- Ensure that the ends of the hose do not drag across the quay, fall into the sea, or trail across your deck.
- If you suspect that the water you have taken on board might be contaminated with disease organisms, disinfect it as described below under, *Disinfection of potable water*.

Disinfection of potable water

To disinfect water with chlorine effectively:

- use a chlorination unit in tandem with a distillation unit to ensure that drinking water is of acceptable hygienic quality;
- chlorinate the whole system after the tanks have been opened up and cleaned or after possible contamination of the water;
- filter the water carefully before chlorination to ensure that it is free from pathogenic protozoa (including *Cryptosporidium*) and helminths (worms), which are more resistant to chlorine disinfection than bacteria or viruses;

- ensure that water turbidity is less than 1 nephelometric turbidity unit;
- ensure that contact time is greater than 30 minutes and pH less than 8.0, resulting in a free chlorine residual of 0.2–0.5 mg/litre.

DISPOSAL OF LIQUID AND SOLID WASTES

Liquid wastes are organic materials that can be mixed with water, flushed from the sanitary water system, and carried out of the vessel by its waste pipes. Liquid wastes include:

- body excretions, such as faeces, urine, sputum, and vomit;
- sink, laundry, and washroom wastes;
- food, tank, bilge, and engine-room wastes;
- other degradable materials.

Solid wastes are discarded materials not readily degradable without heat or pressure. Solid wastes include such items as:

- surgical dressings;
- disposable containers;
- refuse.

Both liquid and solid wastes are health hazards. Contamination by these wastes can cause outbreaks of typhoid fever, paratyphoid fever, cholera, or dysentery. Rats, flies, and other vectors of disease thrive on solid wastes. These wastes must, therefore, be disposed of carefully so as not to endanger the health of persons aboard the vessel or in off-ship areas.

COMBATING DISEASE VECTORS

Disease vectors include:

- mosquitoes, which carry malaria, dengue, and yellow fever;
- fleas, which carry plague and typhus fever;
- lice, which carry epidemic typhus fever;
- ticks, which carry spotted fever and Lyme disease;
- animals (rats, mice, dogs, etc.);
- birds (parrots, for example, can transmit psittacosis to humans).

Rodents

Rats on a ship are a menace to health and a nuisance. They cause extensive damage to cargo and food, and can carry leptospirosis, a bacterial disease, and other dangerous diseases. Because rats usually forage in the galley and food storage areas, they can introduce disease organisms into food and water supplies. Rats also carry fleas, which can transmit plague and typhus fever. Ships heavily infested with rats must be fumigated. Fumigation is laborious, expensive, and dangerous: it can be avoided through adequate anti-rat measures, including frequent inspection of the ship for signs of rat life, such as trails or runs marked by dirt or droppings.

Despite precautions by the ship's personnel and port authorities, some rats may still be on board. However, their numbers can be kept down by ensuring that they do not have access to food and that there are no suitable nesting-places for them, and also by trapping or otherwise destroying them before they breed and develop colonies.

To keep a ship relatively free of rats:

- **prevent them from getting aboard by**:
  - placing and maintaining rat guards on all mooring lines and keeping the gangplank well lit;
- **rat-proof the ship** (at the same time curbing the proliferation of flies and cockroaches) by:
  - eliminating hidden and dead spaces where rats can hide;
  - keeping the ship in good repair;
  - preventing lockers, boxes, dunnage, or other movable equipment from providing temporary shelters for rodents;
- **starve rats by**:
  - keeping all food and garbage stored in metal containers with tightly fitting metal covers;
  - avoiding the accumulation of food scraps and cleaning up spilled food or edible waste;
- **kill rats by** trapping, poisoning, or fumigation:
  - for trapping:
    - set snap traps (more effective and easier to set than cage-type traps) along ledges, bulkheads, and other places used as rat runs;
    - for bait, use meat, bacon rind, or cheese, if rats cannot get at these foods in any other place, or apples, pears, dates, potatoes, and turnips;
    - point the bait trigger towards the bulkhead or rat run;
    - allow the rats to nibble at the bait for a few days before setting the trap;
    - do not flame or scald the trap after the rat is caught: the odour of the rat will help in catching others;
    - avoid touching a dead rat because of the danger of infected fleas;
  - for poisoning:
    - use anticoagulant rodenticides (rat poisons), such as warfarin and brodifacoum;
    - note that **these chemicals are poisonous to man**: keep them in their original container, properly labelled, and stored away from food;
    - bait trays or stations are recommended because they reduce the risk of poison being scattered and they allow remaining poison to be removed once rodents are controlled;
    - unpoisoned water placed next to the bait may increase consumption of the rodenticides by the rats;
    - surplus baits should be laid and then removed when rodents are controlled;
    - crew handling rat poisons should wear gloves and wash their hands carefully after laying baits;
  - for fumigation, which is the method of choice if the ship is badly infested:
    - have the operation carried out by experts from authorized agencies;
    - the gases most commonly used for fumigation are hydrogen cyanide and carbon monoxide;
    - note that **these gases are extremely poisonous to human beings**;

- before fumigation, have the ship tied up at a distance from other vessels;
- **make sure there is no one on board** other than the fumigation team;
- after fumigation, air the holds and superstructures;
- test for gas after about an hour of airing;
- thoroughly air beds and clothing on deck for at least two hours;
- destroy any food that has been exposed to the fumigant gas;
- note that **individuals have died because they returned too soon to compartments not completely aired and free of gas**;
- **a fumigated ship should not be boarded until authorization is given by the officer in charge of the fumigation**.

Insects

With so many varieties of insects, so many ways in which they gain access to the ship, and so powerful a capacity to evade or resist efforts to destroy them, keeping a ship completely free of insects is impossible. Note:

- flies and mosquitoes may board the vessel at wharves or in harbours;
- bedbugs, fleas, lice, and ticks may be brought aboard on the bodies, clothing, or personal gear of crew or passengers;
- fleas may also be carried aboard by rats:
- cockroaches may be present in provisions or in cargo brought aboard ship.

Insects occasionally transmit bacterial infections when germs on their bodies come in contact with food or other articles. More often, insects spread infection by biting: *Anopheles* mosquitoes transmit malaria and *Aedes* mosquitoes transmit yellow fever in this way. Disease-causing organisms are sometimes present in insect faeces, so that scratching an insect bite can allow these organisms to enter the body: typhus is acquired in this way.

The suppression of insect infestation on board ship calls for coordination between ship and shore personnel. Unless control efforts are continued at sea, the most thorough campaign to destroy insects and rodents on a ship in port will fail. It is easier and less costly to maintain constant controls than to apply sporadic intensive measures only in port. Continuing control efforts at sea will also improve living and working conditions on board.

Combating insects calls for a knowledge of the habits of each type. Note:

- body lice live on the human body and clothing:
  - personal cleanliness will reduce the risk of louse infestation;
- bedbugs seek shelter in cracks in walls and floors around beds:
  - cleanliness and frequent inspection are essential;
- cockroaches breed wherever food is available:
  - strict cleanliness is essential wherever food is stored, prepared, or eaten;
- flies are attracted to unprotected food and refuse:
  - avoid unnecessary exposure of food;
  - place refuse in clean, tightly covered cans for prompt disposal.

Personal cleanliness and cleanliness of the living and working environment are vital to keeping insect populations to a minimum. Insecticides provide short-term relief but are of little long-term value if unsanitary conditions persist. Insecticides can also contaminate drink, food, or surfaces used for food preparation. Some are dangerously flammable. Only properly trained personnel should be allowed to use insecticides, which must be stored in such a way as to prevent the insecticides from being stolen or picked up by accident. Regular maintenance and careful use of insecticide spraying equipment are imperative.

Note that failure to curb insect populations may be due to growing resistance of insects to insecticides. Using a different type of insecticide may be necessary.

Further information can be obtained from *Pesticides and their application for the control of vectors and pests of public health importance*, 6th ed. Geneva, World Health Organization, 2006, and also at www.who.int/whopes/.

Flies

Houseflies are a nuisance and may transmit diarrhoeal disease if they have access to faeces and food. Horseflies and deerflies cause painful bites, and sandflies can transmit a number of infections.

✔ *What to do*

- Store all refuse in durable cans with tight lids.
- Screen windows and doors.
- Use chemical sprays sparingly – widespread resistance limits their effectiveness and they may contaminate food:
  - do not use residual sprays: they promote the development of resistance;
  - cotton cords soaked in pyrethroids (0.5–10 g/l) and suspended from ceilings provide long-lasting fly control with less risk of resistance than residual spraying;
  - use one metre of cord for each square metre of floor area;
  - avoid placing cords over food containers or food preparation areas;
  - wear gloves when positioning cords.
- Space sprays are released as a fog or fine mist and kill on contact:
  - for space spraying use permethrin 0.025–0.05 g ai/m^2, natural pyrethrins 1–4 g/litre (0.1–0.4%), or chlorpyriphos-methyl;
  - where there is a risk of fire, use only space spraying dispensers that contain no propellant or a non-flammable propellant;
  - do not expose food or cooking utensils to insecticide sprays.

Mosquitoes

Several species of mosquito bite humans and may transmit malaria, dengue, yellow fever, encephalitis, filariasis, and other diseases.

✔ *What to do*

- Remove **all** potential receptacles or containers of standing water.
- Keep insect screens on windows and doors.
- When working outside, such as in ports where mosquito-borne diseases occur, use insect repellent lotions on exposed skin:

- DEET (N,N-diethyl-3-methylbenzamide) in 20–35% formulations is the best choice. DEET repels mosquitoes, flies, fleas, and ticks – higher concentrations last longer but are not more effective;
- picaridin and p-menthane-3,8-diol (PMD) are also effective insect repellents – they do not last as long as DEET and, therefore, have to be re-applied frequently;
- spray the hands with repellent lotion and use them to apply the lotion to the face;
- wash the hands after applying repellent so as to prevent contact with the eyes;
- spray permethrin and natural pyrethrins (which are not insect repellents but are toxic to insects) on the inside and outside of clothes and on socks, and allow to dry before wearing: protection against mosquito bites lasts up to one week, even after washing the clothes;
- at night, have the crew sleep under pyrethroid-treated bed nets;
- **DO NOT** use space spraying to control mosquitoes;
- **DO NOT** allow crew to rely on insect repellents other than those listed above.

Cockroaches

Cockroaches are often a mark of sub-standard cleaning and food storage but do not normally transmit disease.

✔ *What to do*

- Eliminate cracks, crevices, and dead spaces.
- Eliminate sources of moisture by repairing leaking taps and covering plug holes.
- Store food and garbage properly.
- Keep the entire ship scrupulously clean.
- Watch for, and destroy, all cockroaches and their egg cases, particularly those introduced with luggage, food stores, and furniture.
- Remove corrugated cardboard boxes and cartons from provision storerooms as soon as feasible.
- Use enclosed bait stations or gels containing chlorpyrifos 5 g/l in food storage and preparation areas.
- In other areas, spray with chlorpyrifos-methyl, 7–10 g/l.

Bedbugs

Bedbugs are common throughout the world, especially in tropical and sub-tropical zones and in poorer countries. They do not live in beds but in cracks and crevices around walls and roofs. They bite while the victim sleeps, most often just before dawn, and are rarely seen by the victim, who on waking notes the bites, usually on the hands, arms, and face. The bites cause itching, swelling, and redness of the skin, and can become infected. Typically, there are three bites closely spaced in a line.

✔ *What to do*

- To relieve itching, have the patient apply a 1% hydrocortisone cream.
- Hot-wash or dry-clean bedclothes, or place them in a plastic bag and then in a freezer (at –18 °C or less) for 24 hours.

- Early in the day (to allow the cabin or living space to dry before it is used again for sleeping) use a residual insecticide to spray on cracks and crevices in bulkheads and floors, bed bases, mattresses, slats and springs, and furniture, choosing from the following insecticides:
  - pirimiphos-methyl, 10 g/litre (1%)
  - d-phenothrin, 1–2 g/l.
- Dry insecticide-treated mattresses completely before covering them with sheets for reuse.
- Note that bedbugs do not transmit disease.
- Pyrethrin-impregnated mosquito nets also prevent bed-bug bites.

SANITARY INSPECTION

Regular inspections are necessary to maintain a vessel in good sanitary condition. Those making the inspections should be on the alert for signs of vermin and rodent infestation and should check general order and cleanliness. Frequent monitoring by the ship's master and senior officers will also help to keep the crew aware of the need to maintain scrupulous cleanliness.

Areas to be inspected thoroughly include:

- the forepeak
- the provision storeroom
- the galley
- the pantry
- the issue room
- the sickbay
- the scullery
- the garbage disposal area
- the brig spaces
- sewage disposal areas
- the washroom and head
- cold storage spaces
- the refrigeration space
- the mess space
- living spaces
- the shelter deck
- holds.

Preventing disease and promoting health in seafarers

Preventing disease is an important part of medicine and nowhere is it more important than on board ship. Conditions at sea are not as conducive to maintaining good health as those on shore: opportunities for exercise are necessarily restricted on board, living quarters may be cramped, and fresh food is less available. Boredom and stress may result, which may contribute to some of the illnesses that affect seafarers.

PREVENTING COMMUNICABLE DISEASES (see also Chapter 23, *Infectious diseases*)

Isolation (see Chapter 26, *Nursing care and medical procedures*)

Immunization

DIPHTHERIA AND TETANUS

Every seagoing person should be immunized against diphtheria and tetanus. A check should be made that full primary courses were given in childhood, or they should be repeated, and booster doses of adult diphtheria and tetanus vaccine should be given every 10 years.

Hepatitis A and hepatitis B

Immunization against hepatitis A and hepatitis B infections is a wise precaution for all crew, but is essential for any crew member assigned to medical care duties.

Other infections

The need for seafarers to be immunized against the following infections will depend on the route and destination of the vessel and also on the cargo it is carrying:

- cholera
- influenza
- Japanese encephalitis
- meningococcal disease
- poliomyelitis
- rabies
- typhoid fever
- yellow fever (vaccination required every 10 years in many tropical countries).

PREVENTING OTHER DISEASES (See also Chapter 26, *Nursing care and medical procedures;* Chapter 29, *Environmental control and hygiene,* under *Ventilation* and *Mosquitoes;* and Chapter 28, *Medical care for survivors at sea,* under *Cold exposure injuries*)

Stopping smoking

No other preventive measure offers anywhere near as much benefit to health as stopping smoking. Some facts:

- most smokers die prematurely;
- at 25 years of age, a healthy smoker is likely to have a remaining life expectancy 25% less than that of a non-smoker;
- stopping smoking before 50 years of age reduces by half the risk of dying over the next 15 years compared with continuing to smoke;
- one year without smoking halves the excess risk a smoker runs of dying from coronary heart disease, the commonest cause of death in smokers;
- the risk of lung cancer starts to decline as soon as a smoker stops: after 10 years the risk is one third to one half that of a smoker who continues to smoke;
- second-hand cigarette smoke ("passive smoking") has been proved to cause lung cancer and to increase the risk of coronary heart disease: smoking should not be permitted in any recreation area, common work area, or where food is prepared or eaten.

✔ *What to do*

- Nicotine is highly addictive: all regular smokers are nicotine addicts.
- Nicotine withdrawal causes:
  - a craving for nicotine
  - irritability
  - poor concentration
  - hunger.
- Nicotine replacement, with patches or chewing gum, relieves the withdrawal symptoms and doubles a smoker's chances of successfully quitting.
- The average smoker stops smoking and starts again four times before finally quitting: attempts to give up the habit should not be abandoned because of one failure.
- About three-quarters of smokers who stop and start again do so either when under stress or in social occasions, especially those that involve alcohol.
- Banning smoking in work areas and recreation rooms can help smokers who are trying to quit avoid relapse.

A balanced diet

A balanced diet is vital to maintaining good health. It should provide appropriate proportions of:

- protein, which is found in foods such as meat, poultry, fish, eggs, lentils, and nuts;
- carbohydrates, which are found in cereals, bread, and other starchy foods;
- fats, which are found in meat, milk, and other dairy foods;
- vitamins, such as vitamins A, B, C, D, E, B_{12}, and folate;
- minerals, such as iron, calcium, zinc, magnesium, and iodine, which are found mainly in protein-rich foods.

Nowadays, there is practically no risk of deficiency diseases occurring among ships' crews. However, overeating may present a health risk for some seafarers, particularly those whose work duties do not involve much physical exertion. Mild overweight is not a health hazard but severe obesity increases the risk of several diseases.

A healthy diet is one that provides:

- at least five servings a day of fruit and vegetables, especially lentils, citrus fruit, and dark-green, leafy vegetables (broccoli, Brussels sprouts, etc.);
- unprocessed cereals and fruit as sources of carbohydrates rather than sugar and starch;
- limited fat, preferably in the form of monounsaturated fat, such as olive oil:
  - polyunsaturated fat, as in margarine, is less desirable;
  - **avoid** "trans" fats, found in polyunsaturated fat packaged for deep frying and in commercially baked bread and biscuits;
- at least two fish meals a week, especially fast-swimming, ocean-dwelling fish;
- a moderate amount of alcohol (i.e. not more than five drinks per day for five days per week), which can reduce the risk of heart disease.

Personal hygiene

The health of a seafarer depends to a great extent on personal cleanliness, which includes:

- good care of:
  - skin
  - hair
  - nails
  - mouth
  - teeth, including dentures;
- proper maintenance of:
  - clothing
  - towels
  - other personal gear;
- a daily bath or shower, particularly in hot weather or after working in hot compartments;
- frequent washing of the hands, especially:
  - before eating
  - immediately after urinating or defecating.

Cleanliness aboard ship can be encouraged by ensuring that sufficient hot water is available in convenient wash places. A clothes laundry and drying room can contribute to maintaining a high standard of cleanliness. Each member of the crew should use only personal towels and be responsible for their cleanliness. Wet towels should not be folded and stowed away; dirty towels should be laundered as soon as possible and not allowed to accumulate.

Sleep

Adequate sleep is essential for health and efficiency. Sleep requirements and habits may vary considerably but everyone requires unbroken periods of rest.

Preventing illness from exposure to extremes of temperature (see also Chapter 28, *Medical care for survivors at sea*; Chapter 10, *Heat stroke and other heat disorders;* Chapter 26, *Nursing care and medical procedures*)

In hot conditions, a minimum of clothing should be worn indoors to allow the largest possible skin surface for free evaporation of sweat. In strong sun crew should wear light, loose, white, cotton clothing and a hat which shades the face and neck.

Sunburn and skin cancer

Sunburn is a skin burn caused by exposure to ultraviolet light from the sun. Like a heat burn, sunburn can be first, second or third degree. Severe sunburn should be assessed and treated in the same way as a heat burn (see Chapter 9, *Burns, chemical splashes, smoke inhalation, and electrocution*).

Prolonged exposure to ultraviolet light from the sun causes skin cancer: the risk is directly related to the duration and intensity of exposure and is greater for fair-skinned people. There is no safe level of exposure to ultraviolet light: discourage crew from sun tanning.

Crew working outdoors should work in the shade as much as possible. Try to arrange work so that crew do not spend long periods in the sun between 11:00 and 15:00. When exposed to the sun for long periods, crew should wear long-sleeved shirts and hats that shade the face and neck.

Sunscreens can reduce the effect of ultraviolet light on areas of skin that are difficult to cover, such as the face and hands. Sunscreens are **not** an alternative to shirts and hats, and **must not** be used to increase the amount of time crew spend unprotected in the sun. Zinc cream is cheaper, more effective and less prone to sweat off than lotions containing chemical sunscreens. If an invisible sunscreen is preferred choose one containing a physical agent such as titanium as well as chemical sunscreens.

Lifting heavy weights (see also Chapter 21, *Bone, joint, and muscle disorders*)

Backache, sciatica, lumbago, and slipped disc are often caused by attempts to lift heavy weights or by lifting weights incorrectly. The leg and thigh muscles should be used when lifting, with the torso and head held straight to avoid bending stresses.

Foot injuries

Injuries caused by dropping heavy weights on the feet are a common cause of lost work time on board ship, and can cause serious long-term problems.

All crew should wear safety boots when at risk of foot injuries.

Lack of exercise and boredom

Few seafarers exercise enough. Unused muscles become flabby and tend to atrophy. Regular, vigorous exercise reduces the risk of heart disease and stroke. Crew should be encouraged to spend 40 minutes every day exercising hard enough to raise their heart rate to three-quarters of their maximum heart rate (calculated by deducting the individual's age from 220): running, cycling, and stair climbing are excellent activities for this purpose.

On long, tedious voyages, boredom and lack of interest can lead to drug abuse. The ship's master should encourage exercise and recreational activities to keep the crew fit and occupied during off-duty hours at sea.

PREVENTING ILL-HEALTH FROM SEAFARING WORK

Seafaring is a high-risk occupation: although accidents at sea occur at about the same frequency as on shore, they tend to be more severe and are certainly more lethal – 10 to 20 times more lethal according to recent data. One reason why accidents are more severe among seafarers than among onshore workers is that seafaring tends to involve work with heavier equipment. Another reason is that seafarers, unlike land-based workers, are never entirely free of the risk of a shipwreck and the severe injuries and fatality with which it is associated. Moreover, research has shown that a seafarer who has been working from 10 to 40 years at sea runs a significantly increased risk of lifestyle-related disease – certain types of cancer, heart disease, alcoholic liver disease, hearing loss, and problems with the joints of the knees and back. The International Maritime Health Association provides information to seafarers on the risk of their occupation through the Seafarers Health Information Programme (www.seafarershealth.org).

GENERAL PRINCIPLES OF PROMOTING SAFETY ON BOARD SHIP

To reduce the frequency and severity of accidents and other adverse consequences to health from seafaring work:

- the shipping company must be dedicated to promoting a safety culture at all levels – from the chief executive officer in the board room to the captain and ratings on ship;

- the company's policy on health and safety must be clearly communicated to all personnel;
- the information and equipment needed to put the company health policies into practice should be made available on all company vessels;
- work procedures must be planned to ensure that they expose seafarers to the lowest possible risk of short-term and long-term damage to health.

The Health and Safety Committee

Safety on board must be the responsibility of a Health and Safety Committee. This entity should comprise one or more crew members, including one or more "safety representatives", as well as the captain or his deputies among senior officers. At least one safety representative should be available at all times during operation of a ship. All members should attend special courses on work safety that cover:

- prevention of "lost time accidents" (LTAs), i.e. injuries preventing the performance of duties for at least 24 hours;
- lessons learned from LTAs;
- reporting of "near-misses", i.e. accidents that nearly occurred in connection with the operation of a ship (also known as "hazardous incidents");
- exposure to potentially hazardous chemical, physical, or biological factors or circumstances, such as organic solvents, lifting heavy objects, noise, vibrations, and infectious microorganisms;
- general principles for the reduction of hazardous exposures;
- psychosocial factors, such as isolation, fatigue, ethnic heterogeneity of crews, and shift work.

Briefing for new tasks

Every ship must have a policy on providing crew members with proper instruction in performing new tasks. This policy should cover:

- a manual providing clear, detailed instructions on how to carry out seafaring tasks in the safest possible way;
- a written 'work permit' for every specific task to be done that:
  - ensures that the officer assigning the task has provided the seafarer chosen to perform the task with full instructions on how to carry out the task and how to do so as safely as possible;
  - ensures that the necessary tools are available to fulfil the task;
  - details all the risks entailed in carrying out the task and the precautions that have been taken to reduce those risks (such as providing a fire extinguisher or safety harness);
  - ensures that the seafarer is given only one task at a time, thereby reducing the risk of an accident that could occur when a seafarer is given more than one task to perform simultaneously;
- the right of other crew members, of whatever rank, to prevent a shipmate from continuing work they believe is hazardous or is being carried out in unsafe conditions.

Work place assessment

Work place assessment (WPA) is a useful tool for improving health and safety on board and an appropriate starting point in the briefing of crew members about new tasks. The WPA provides:

- a description of every job on board and of the measures required to ensure the maximum safety and protection of seafarers doing the job;
- a tool for identifying areas where occupational health and safety, as well as crew wellbeing and job satisfaction, could be improved.

Provision of good medical care

Medical care on board ship is usually the responsibility of a crew member – a senior officer in most cases – who has attended a training course for paramedical workers. The courses should be of a high standard and enable the responsible medical officer to treat the most common conditions and to judge when professional advice is needed from a medical service. The shipping company should ensure that refresher courses are provided for medical officers and that the ship's medical equipment, including the medical chest, is maintained and renewed at appropriate intervals.

Seafarers' lifestyles

Seafarers have been shown in many studies to be more likely to engage in unhealthy behaviour than people on shore. Such behaviour includes:

- **smoking and excessive alcohol consumption**:
  - greater awareness of the danger to health of these habits has certainly diminished their appeal among seafarers but many have not followed this trend;
- **an unhealthy diet and lack of exercise**:
  - together these factors can lead to excessive body weight, which is still a more common problem among seafarers than among onshore workers;
  - shipping companies in some countries have made efforts to deal with the problem of an unbalanced diet and lack of exercise, by providing, for example, less fatty food on board and well-equipped fitness rooms;
- **unsafe sex** (see Chapter 19, *Sexually transmitted infections*).

Anatomy and physiology

CELLS

- Cells are the building blocks of the human body: all the body's tissues and organs are composed of cells.
- Cells are thousandths of a millimetre in diameter – far too small to be seen without a microscope.
- All the cells of an adult's body come from the single cell that is formed when a sperm (spermatozoon) penetrates and fertilizes an egg (ovum): the single cell divides to produce two "daughter" cells, each of which divides to produce two more daughter cells, and so on until, over the nine months of a normal pregnancy, an entire fetus is created.
- After the birth of the baby, most cells lose their ability to divide, but some, even in an adult, retain their ability to divide and are capable of producing cells that replace dead or destroyed cells.
- Nearly all cells have:
    - a nucleus, which contains the cell's genetic material:
        - the red cells of the blood are the only cells that do not have a nucleus;
    - a cytoplasm, a jelly-like substance that fills the cell and in which the cell's activities (mainly chemical reactions) take place.

TISSUES

- Cells combine to form tissues, which in turn make up all the structures of the body, including organs and bones.
- A tissue is a group of similar cells, such as muscle cells, nerve cells, and so on, that work together to carry out a particular function, such as producing a muscle contraction or transmitting a nerve signal.

ORGANS

- An organ is a body structure that is made up of at least two types of tissue functioning together for a common purpose.
- The many different organs in the body include the liver, kidneys, and heart.
- The skin, which is composed of three tissue layers – the epidermis, dermis and subcutaneous layer – is the largest organ in the human body.

NOTE ON ANATOMICAL TERMS AND DESCRIPTIONS

- In anatomical descriptions, the body is always shown standing upright facing the observer, with the arms down and the palms of the hands facing forwards.
- In an anatomical description:
    - **up** means towards the head;
    - **down** means towards the feet;

- **in front of** and **forwards** mean towards the face side of the body;
- **behind** and **backwards** mean towards the back;
- **left** and **right** refer to the body's left and right, not the observer's;
- **median** means "exactly in the vertical midline of the body";
- **medial** means "closer to the vertical midline";
- **lateral** means "further away from the vertical midline"; for example:
  - "the lateral side of the arm" means the thumb side (with the arms down and the palms facing the observer).

THE SKELETAL SYSTEM

- **The skull** forms a casing that contains and protects the brain (Figure 31.1). It consists of many bones, firmly joined to each other, except for the lower jaw, which moves thanks to joints located in front of the ears. The skull rests on the upper end of the back bone.

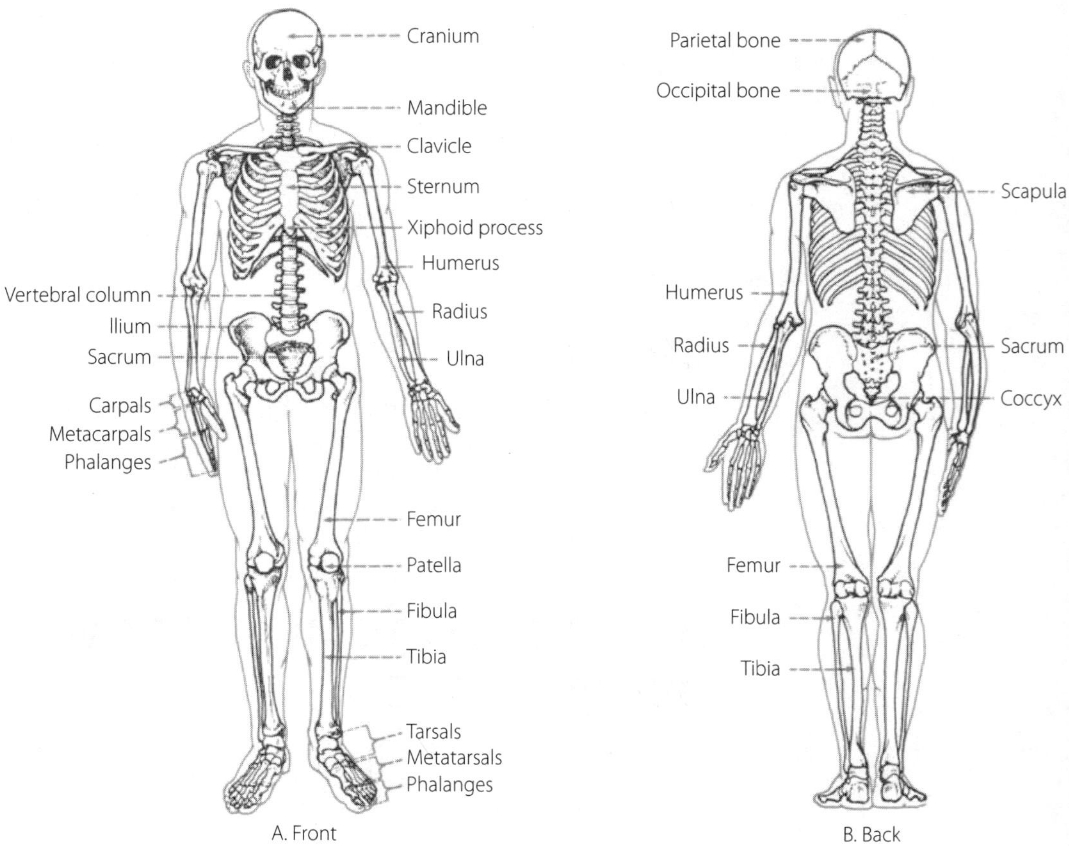

Figure 31.1 Skeleton.

- **The back bone** is made up of a series of small bones placed one on top of the other. These bones are called vertebrae and together form the spinal column. Within the spinal column is housed the spinal cord, from which nerves emerge at the level of each vertebra.
- **The ribs**, all 12 of them, are attached to the back bone on either side. Each rib, with the exception of the two lowermost ribs on either side, curves round the chest from the back bone to the sternum (breast bone) in front. The ribs protect the lungs, heart, and other internal organs. With every breath, the ribs move slightly upwards and outwards so as to expand the chest.
- **The sternum**, a flat, dagger-shaped bone, lies just under the skin at the front of the chest. Attached to the upper end of the sternum is a little square bone called the manubrium. An important landmark on the body is the junction between the manubrium and the sternum, which is marked by a ridge just below the inner ends of the collar bones.
- **The clavicle (collar bone)** joins the top edge of the manubrium and extends more or less horizontally to the point of the shoulder on either side.
- **The scapula (shoulder blade)**, to which the outer end of the collar bone is attached, is a triangular bone lying at the upper and outer sections of the back on either side. Each scapula has a shallow socket into which fits the rounded upper end of the humerus (arm bone).
- **The humerus** forms a hinge-like joint with the radius and ulna (the forearm bones) at the elbow, and these bones join with the hand at the wrist.
- **The wrist and hand**, like the foot, are made up of many small bones. There are two bones in the thumb and three in each finger.
- **The pelvis** is located at the lower end of the back bone. It is formed by the hip bones, one on either side. The pelvis looks like a basin, but it is angled so that the "top" of the basin points straight forward.
- **The hips** have, on their outer side, a cup-shaped socket into which the rounded head of the femur (or thigh bone) fits, forming a ball-and-socket joint.
- **The femur** ends at the knee, where it forms a hinge-like joint with the strong tibia (shin bone).
- **The tibia,** on its outer side, is attached to the slender fibula.
- **The patella (knee cap)** is located just above and in front of the knee joint.
- **The foot** is joined by a hinged joint at the ankle to the lower ends of both the tibia and the fibula. The foot is made up of many small bones of different shapes. There are two bones in the great toe and three in each of the other toes.

THE MUSCULAR SYSTEM

- Muscles are bundles of cells and fibres that can only contract (shorten) and relax (lengthen).
- There are 630 active muscles in the body and they work in groups (Figure 31.2).
- There are three types of muscle:
  - **skeletal, or voluntary, muscle**:
    - is attached to bones by fibrous tissue called a tendon;

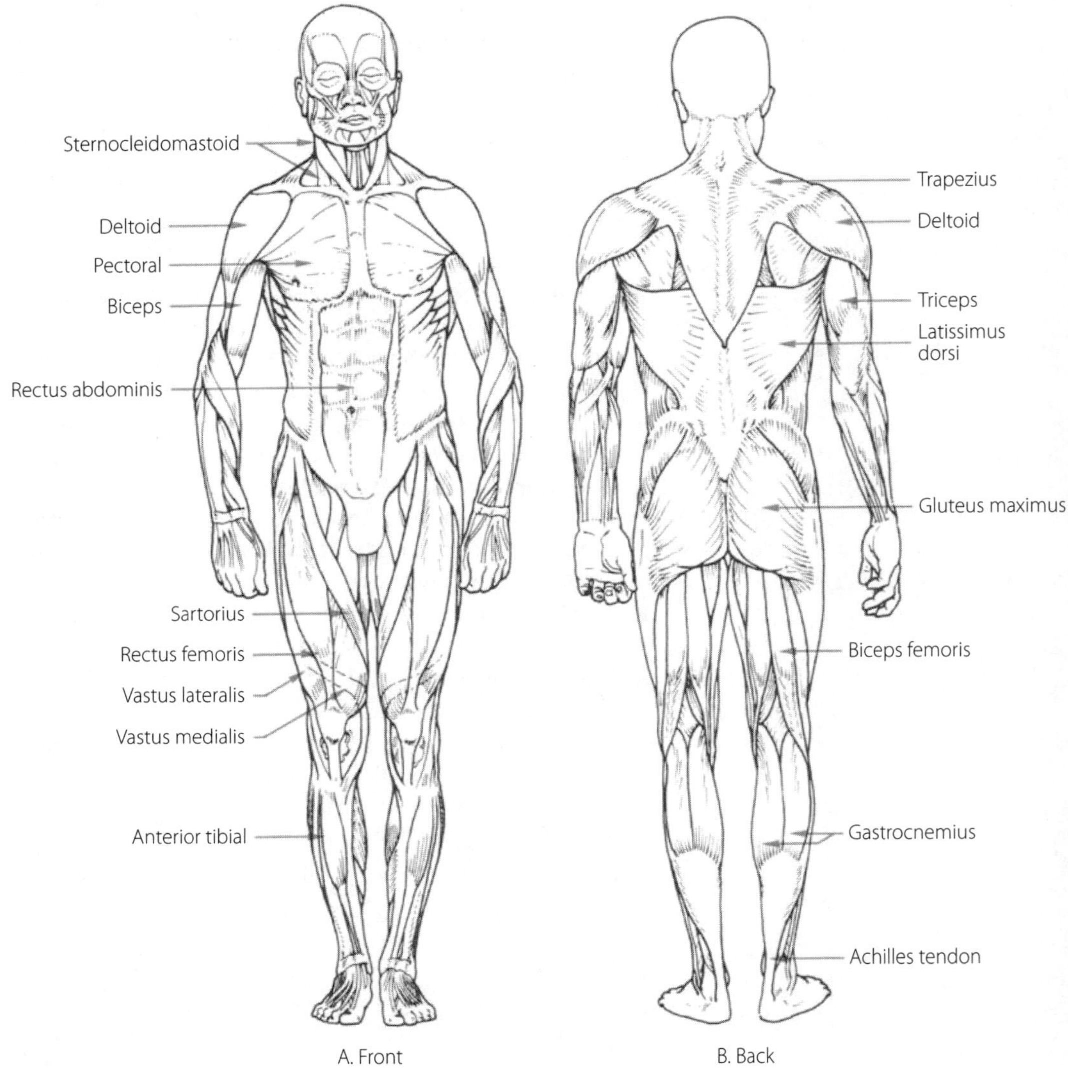

Figure 31.2 Major muscles of the body.

- contracts in response to an impulse sent from the brain through a nerve, thus becoming shorter and drawing the bones to which it is attached nearer to one another;
- is also called striated (or striped) muscle, because under a microscope the minute filaments within each muscle cell are aligned, giving the cells a striped appearance;

- **smooth, or involuntary, muscle**:
  - is located in the walls of internal organs, such as the stomach and intestines, blood vessels, urinary bladder, uterus, and airways;

    - is controlled by the autonomic (or involuntary) nervous system and is only to a limited extent influenced by the will;
- **cardiac muscle**:
    - is found only in the heart.

THE CIRCULATORY SYSTEM

- **Blood**, of which there are about five litres in the body, circulates to all the tissues of the body. Some of the blood passes to the stomach and intestines and, having taken up food products from these organs, flows into the liver, which regulates the many chemicals in the blood. Blood is also taken by arteries to the kidneys, which filter out waste products from the blood and pass them into the urine.
- **The heart**, a muscular pump about the size of a clenched fist, keeps the blood moving round the body. The heart is situated in the chest behind the breast bone: it lies between the lungs, slightly more to the left than to the right (Figure 31.3). The heart has two sides: the right side receives the venous blood coming back to it from the body and pumps it through the lungs, where it passes through minute tubes, gives up carbon dioxide, and takes up a supply of oxygen. The oxygenated blood now passes to the left side of the heart, which pumps it through the arteries to all parts of the body. This blood, which is bright red in colour, carries oxygen, food, water, and salts to the tissues.
- **Arteries** are like thick-walled tubes, whose diameter decreases the further away from the heart they are. As the blood passes along the arteries, they pulsate at the same rate as the heart is pumping. The average normal pulse rate is about 70 beats per minute, but it increases with exercise, nervousness, fear, fever, and various illnesses. The pulse is usually counted by feeling the artery at the front of the wrist just above the ball of the thumb.
- **Capillaries** are the smallest blood vessels in the body and are found in the tissues. Once the blood has supplied the tissues with oxygen and other substances and has taken up the carbon dioxide that had accumulated in the tissues, it becomes darker in colour. The capillaries take it into the veins.
- **Veins** are thin-walled tubes that carry the blood back to the right side of the heart.

THE RESPIRATORY SYSTEM

- **Breathing in** pulls air (containing oxygen) into the body: the air passes through the nose or mouth, then past the larynx (voice box) into the windpipe.
- **The windpipe** (trachea) divides into two tubes called the main bronchi.
- **The main bronchi** divide up into many smaller bronchi and then even smaller bronchioles that pass into the lung tissue. The air breathed in passes through the bronchioles into minute air cells called alveoli, each of which is surrounded by capillaries. The blood in the capillaries gives up carbon dioxide and takes up oxygen.
- **Breathing out** pushes air back along the same respiratory passages and out of the body through the nose or mouth.

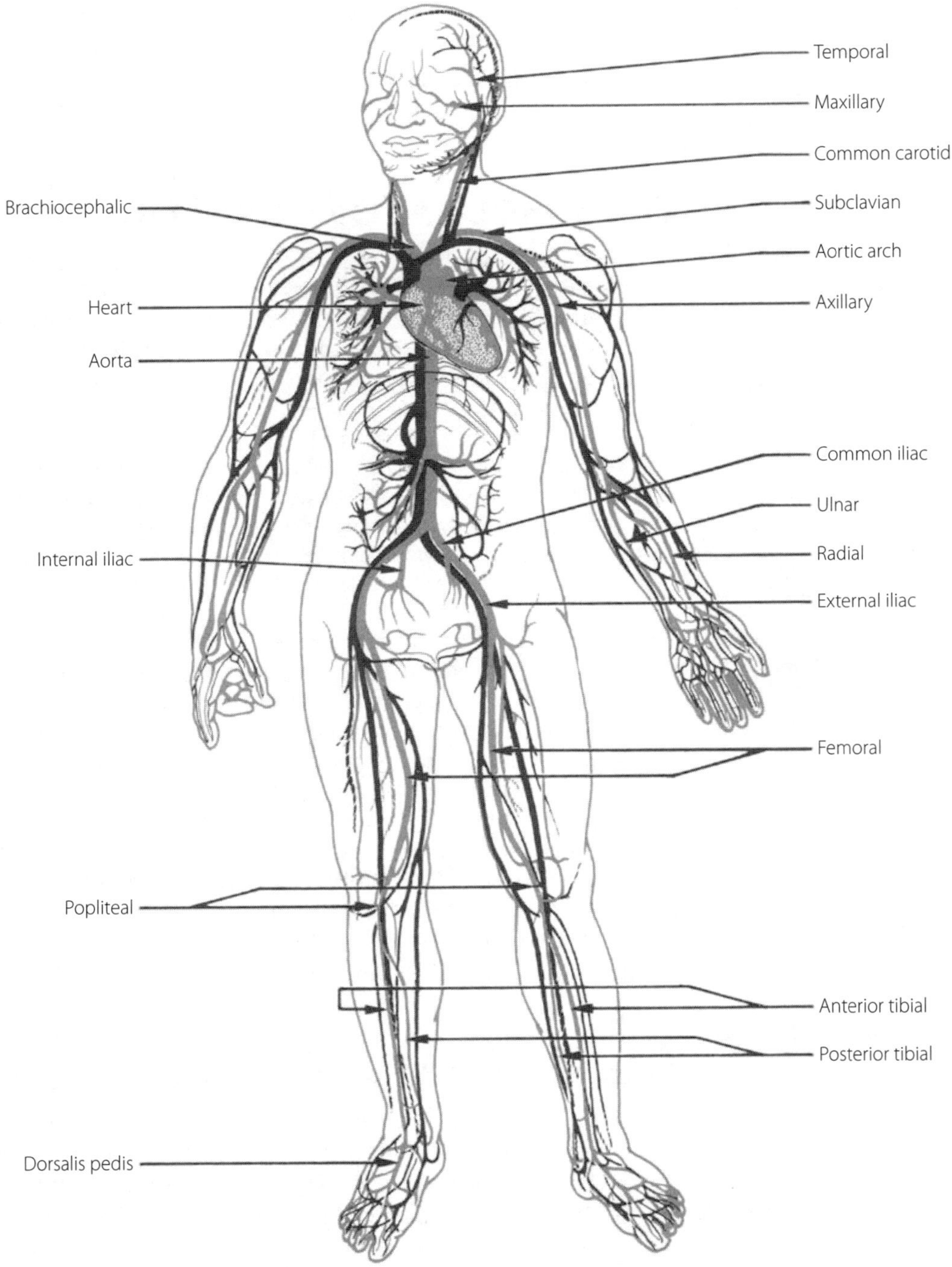

Figure 31.3 Circulatory system.

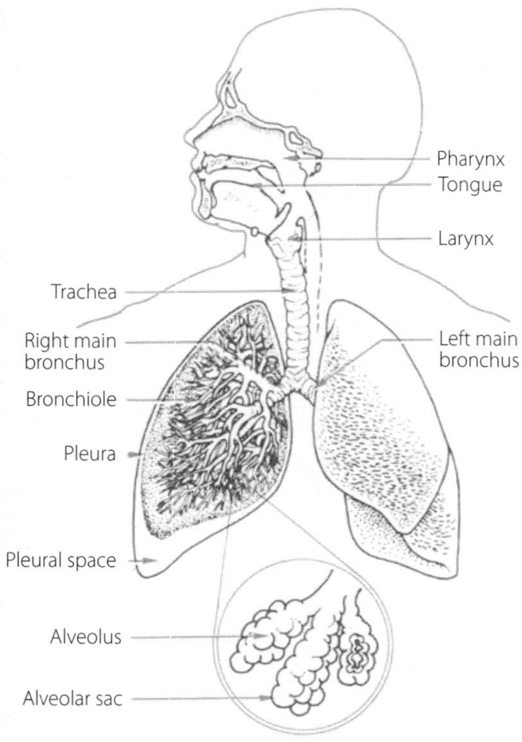

Figure 31.4 Respiratory system.

- **The pleurae** are two lubricated membranes, of which one lines the outer surface of the lungs and the other, the inner surface of the chest wall. These two pleural layers are in contact and slide smoothly over each other during breathing.
- **The lungs** are like elastic sponges, and the many air cells in them expand with breathing in and are compressed with breathing out (Figure 31.4). The rib movement that makes the chest bigger is powered by the diaphragm.
- **The diaphragm** is a large dome-shaped muscle that separates the chest from the abdominal cavity. The diaphragm is attached to the front and sides of the lower border of the rib cage. When it contracts it pulls the ribs up and forward so that the chest becomes larger and air is drawn in.
- **The breathing rate** at rest is 16 to 18 breaths a minute but increases considerably with exertion and also with some diseases, especially those affecting the heart and lungs.

THE DIGESTIVE SYSTEM

- **Food** in the mouth is broken up by chewing and tongue movements and mixed with saliva (spittle), which lubricates it and starts the digestive processes. When it is in a suitable state it passes to the back of the throat.
- **The throat**, through its muscular action, forces food down the oesophagus, or gullet.
- **The oesophagus** is a muscular tube in the neck behind the windpipe. It runs down the back of the chest between the lungs, then passes through the diaphragm into the stomach.
- **The stomach** lies mainly in the left upper part of the abdominal cavity, partly behind the lower left rib and just under the left part of the liver (Figures 31.5, 31.6). When food enters the stomach, various digestive juices act upon it, and the stomach muscles contract and relax, thoroughly mixing the food and juices. The food then passes into the duodenum.
- **The duodenum** produces more digestive juices that mix with the food. The most important of these digestive juices are bile and pancreatic juice.
- **Bile**, a yellowish fluid, is produced by the liver and passes to the bowel along the bile duct, which enters the duodenum alongside the pancreatic duct. Bile is especially important for digestion of fat. Blockage of the passage of bile from the liver to the bowel causes jaundice.
- **The pancreas** lies behind the stomach on the left of the upper abdomen (Figures 31.7, 31.8). Its juice breaks down proteins and fats. The pancreas also produces insulin and other hormones.
- **The liver**, the second-largest organ in the body, is a large triangular, reddish-brown organ in the upper abdomen. Most of its bulk is on the right and to the front, but it extends well backwards and to the left. It is situated immediately below the

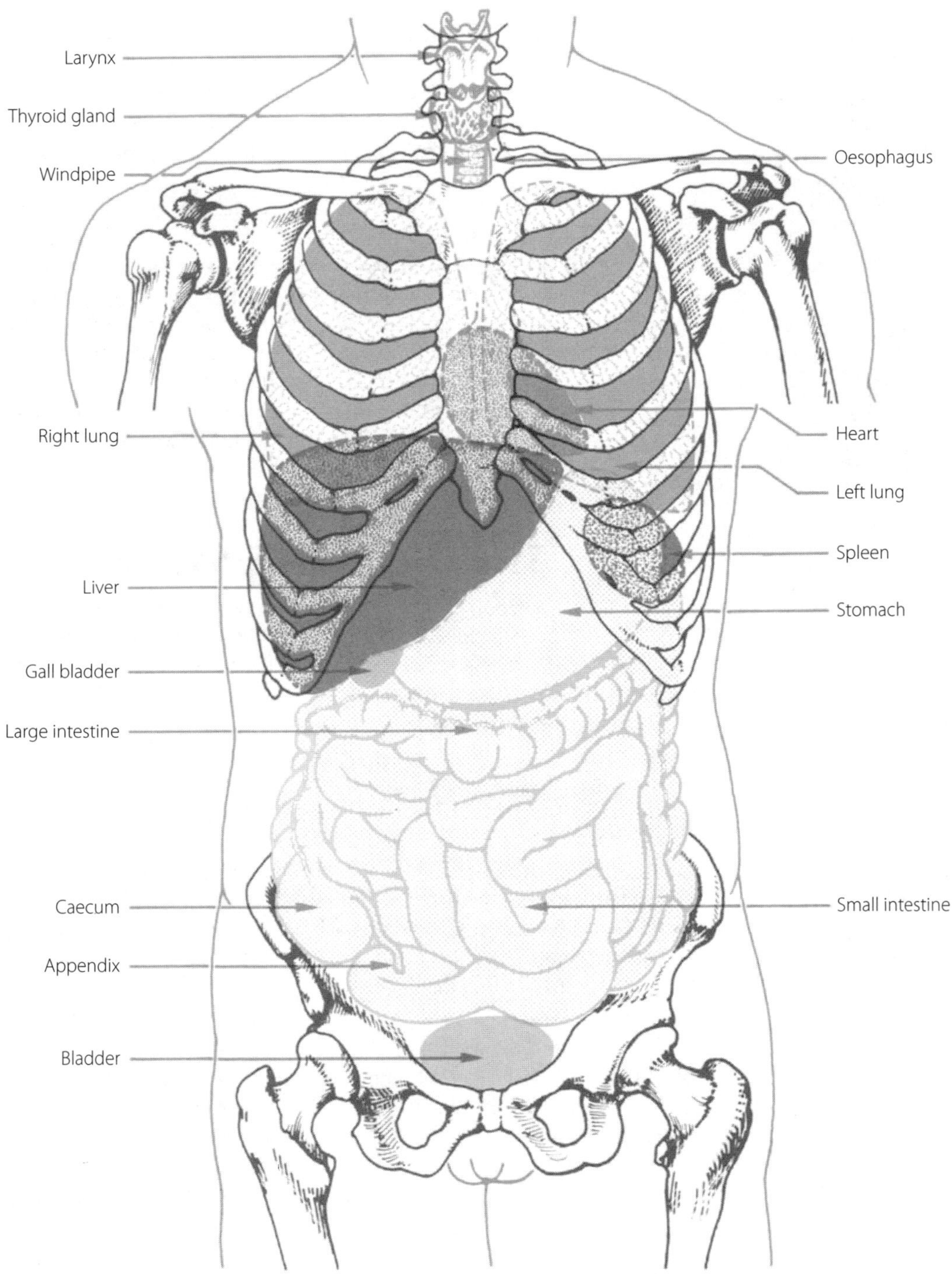

Figure 31.5 Organs of the chest and abdomen (seen from the front).

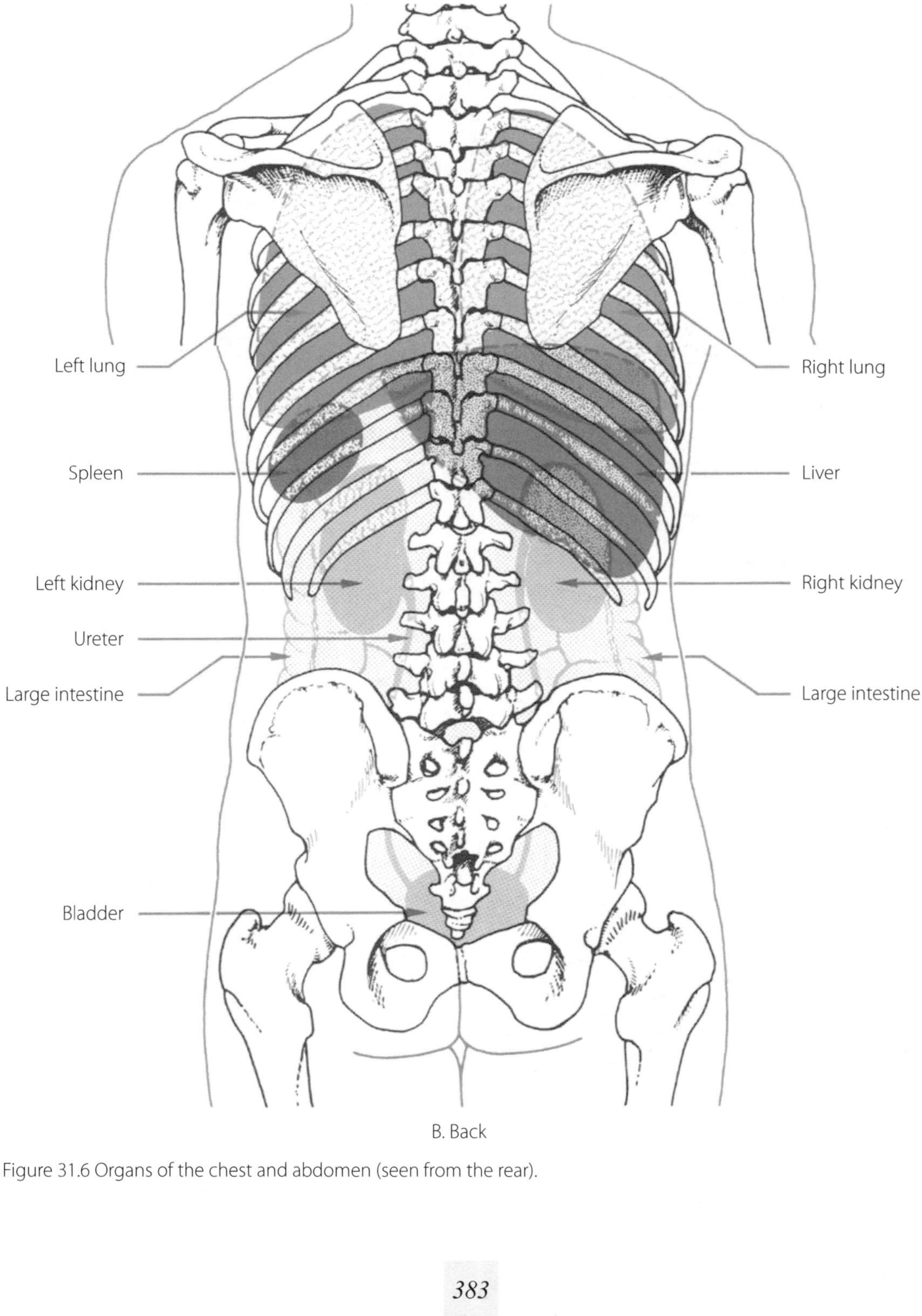

B. Back

Figure 31.6 Organs of the chest and abdomen (seen from the rear).

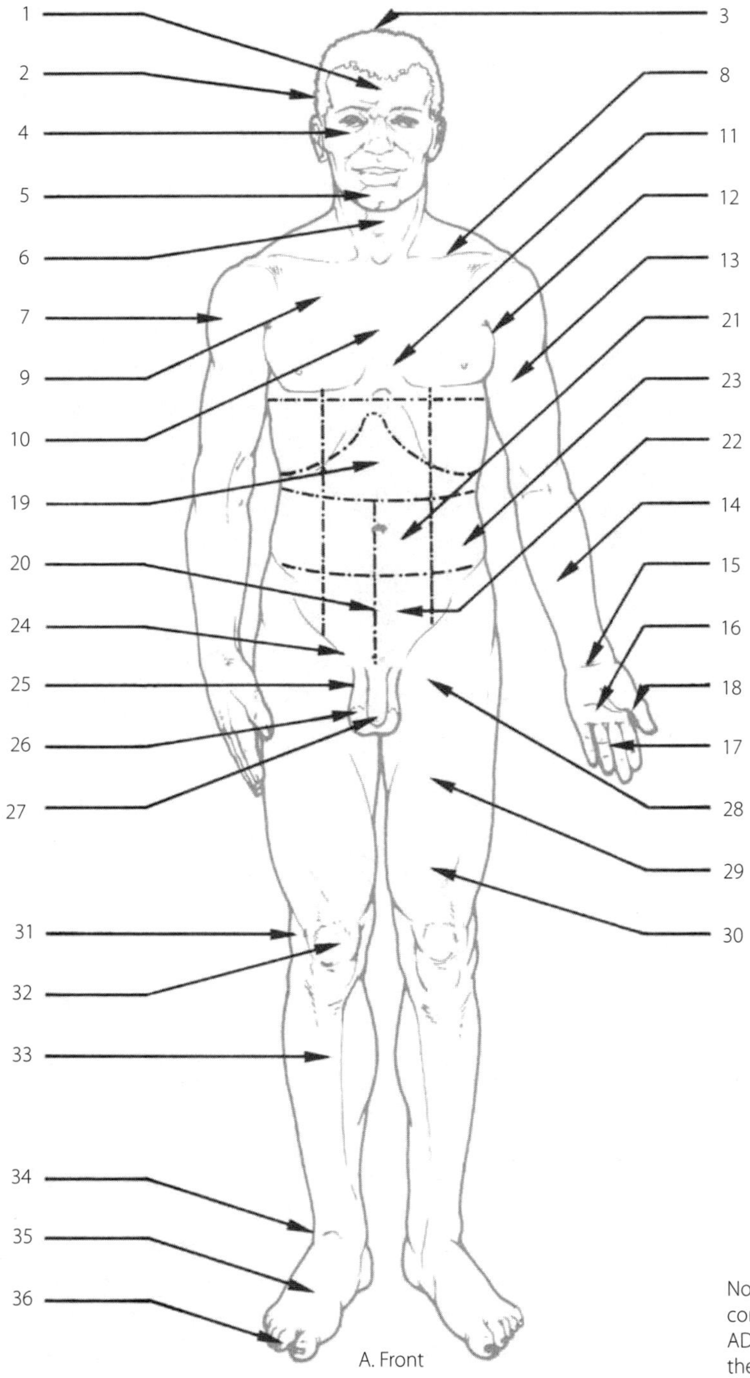

1. Frontal region of head
2. Side of head
3. Top of head
4. Face
5. Jaw
6. Neck (front)
7. Shoulder
8. Clavicle
9. Chest
10. Mid-chest
11. Heart
12. Armpit
13. Upper arm
14. Forearm
15. Wrist
16. Palm of hand
17. Fingers
18. Thumb
19. Central upper abdomen
20. Central lower abdomen
21. Upper abdomen
22. Lower abdomen
23. Lateral abdomen
24. Groin
25. Scrotum
26. Testicles
27. Penis
28. Upper thigh
29. Middle thigh
30. Lower thigh
31. Knee
32. Patella
33. Front of leg
34. Ankle
35. Foot
36. Toes

Note. When describing the patient's condition and getting RADIO MEDICAL ADVICE, the side (left or right) of the body, or the limb affected, should be clearly indicated.

Figure 31.7 Regions of the body (seen from the front).

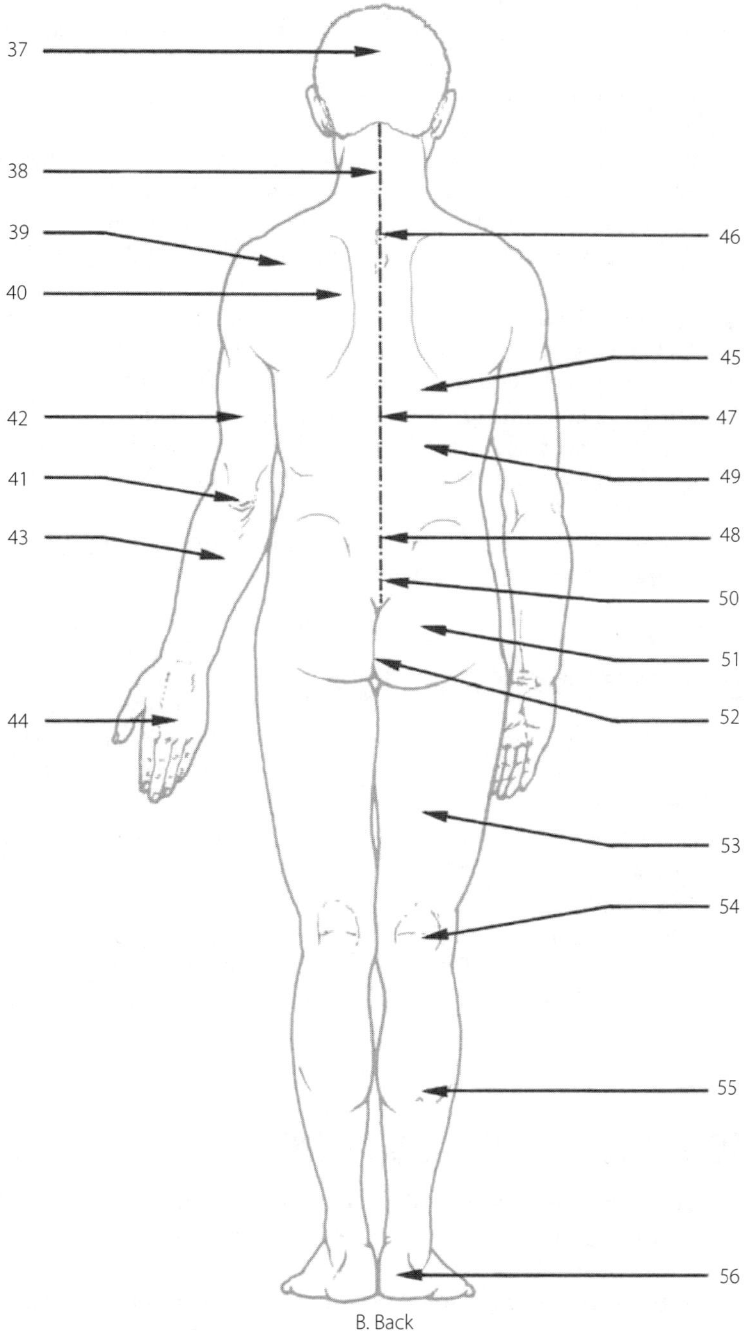

37. Back of head
38. Back of neck
39. Back of shoulder
40. Scapula regin
41. Elbow
42. Back upper arm
43. Back of lower arm
44. Back of hand
45. Lower chest region
46. Spinal column, upper
47. Spinal column, middle
48. Spinal column, lower
49. Lumbar (kidney) region
50. Sacral region
51. Buttock
52. Anus
53. Back of thigh
54. Back of knee
55. Calf
56. Heel

Figure 31.8 Regions of the body (seen from the rear).

diaphragm on the right and the heart on the left. The liver helps to break down protein, fat and carbohydrate, as well as many poisons and medicines, and stores digested food materials.

- **The gallbladder** is a small reservoir on the liver, where bile from the liver is stored and kept available.
- **The spleen**, although in the abdomen, is not part of the digestive system. It is a solid, oval-shaped organ in the upper part of the left side of the abdominal cavity at the back of the stomach, just above the kidney. Its functions are mainly to filter the blood and remove any foreign microbes that might be infecting the blood. The spleen may be enlarged in certain diseases.
- **The small bowel**, a coiled tube about six metres long, is where most nutrients and fluids are absorbed into the body. The first section of the small bowel, as it leaves the duodenum, is the **jejunum**. The next section is the **ileum**.
- **The large intestine (colon)** receives the residue of food at the point in the lower part of the right side of the abdomen where the **appendix** is situated. In the large intestine, moisture is extracted from the food residue. At its far end, the large intestine joins the rectum.
- **The rectum** is where the unwanted food residue collects and is then passed out of the body by the back passage, or anus.

THE URINARY SYSTEM

- **The kidneys** are located high up at the back of the abdominal cavity, one on either side of the spine. They remove water and certain waste products from the blood and produce urine.
- **Urine** leaves each kidney by a tube called a **ureter**, which passes along the back of the abdominal wall then turns sharply forward to reach the back of the bladder.
- **The bladder** is a muscular bag situated in the front part of the cavity of the pelvis. Urine collects in the bladder and is expelled from it through a tube, called the **urethra**. In the male, the last section of the urethra is contained in the penis.
- **The prostate gland** sits immediately below the bladder. Its function is to produce the liquid part of semen.

THE NERVOUS SYSTEM

- **The two main divisions of the nervous system** are:
  - **the voluntary nervous system**, which controls the muscles and carries sensation to the brain;
  - **the autonomic (or involuntary) nervous system**, which plays a central role in controlling the functions of the internal organs.
- **The autonomic nervous system** is divided into two parts: **the sympathetic and the parasympathetic nervous systems**. Many commonly used drugs have important effects, some beneficial, others unwanted, on the autonomic nervous system:

- **the sympathetic nervous system** controls what is sometimes called the "fight-or-flight response". Activation of the sympathetic system readies the body for action: the heart rate increases and the pulse becomes forceful; the face becomes flushed; the pupils dilate; blood vessels in organs such as the bowel become constricted so that blood is diverted to the muscles; and glucose is released from the liver;
- **the parasympathetic nervous system** slows the heart, increases the flow of saliva, constricts the pupils, and promotes bowel activity.

- **The brain** is a network of nerves and supporting tissue. It consists of:
  - **the cerebral cortex**, which is concerned with judgement and planning, with speech, and with movements that require planning; complex mental activities such as numbering and handling three-dimensional objects are also carried out in the cortex.
  - **the thalamus**, which coordinates the autonomic nervous system and executes automatic movements, such as walking;
  - **the brain stem**, which controls heart beating and breathing;
  - **the cerebellum**, which is responsible for balance and coordination of the body.
- **The spinal cord** is a bundle of long nerve tracts connecting the brain to each part of the body. The spinal cord leaves the under-surface of the brain through an opening in the base of the skull and passes down a canal in the vertebral column.
- **Nerve trunks** leave the spinal cord from each vertebra: each nerve trunk contains both motor and sensory fibres for that segment of the cord. The nerves make contact with muscles, which they cause to contract, and also with the skin and other organs:
  - **nerves of the sympathetic nervous system** (see above) leave their respective segments of the spinal cord in the chest and abdomen and travel to "**plexuses**", or way-stations, where they join the arteries that supply each organ. There are a number of plexuses, including the so-called "**solar plexus**" near the stomach;
  - **nerves of the parasympathetic nervous system** (see above) leave the spinal cord at its neck and sacral (tail bone) segments and also via the **vagus nerve**, which leaves the brain stem above the spinal cord, passes through the neck and chest, and supplies the heart and abdominal organs.

THE ENDOCRINE SYSTEM

- **The endocrine system** is a system of glands which produce chemicals, or hormones, that affect other "target" organs in the body – not immediately, as nerves do, but after they have been carried to the target organ by the blood.
- **The hypothalamus and the pituitary gland** together make up the "master gland" of the body in what is commonly referred to as "the hypothalamic–pituitary axis".
- **The hypothalamus** is at the base of the brain. It coordinates the control of body temperature, the balance of salt and water in the body, and the reproductive cycle. It also regulates the production of hormones by the pituitary gland.

- **The pituitary gland** lies in a niche within the base of the skull. It produces hormones which regulate the function of the testicles or ovaries, the thyroid gland, and the outer part (cortex) of the adrenal glands.
- **The testicles**, under the influence of the pituitary hormones, produce testosterone, which is responsible for male patterns of hair growth and body development.
- **The ovaries** produce oestrogen and progesterone, which control the menstrual cycle and produce female patterns of hair growth and body development.
- **The thyroid gland** produces hormones that control the rate of metabolism in the body.
- **The adrenal glands** produce hormones that control the kidney mechanisms for regulating salt and water balance. Adrenaline (epinephrine) comes from the inner part (medulla) of the adrenal gland. It is produced as part of the sympathetic nervous system (see above), and increases the force of contraction of the heart, dilates blood vessels so as to increase blood flow, and mobilizes fat and glucose to fuel the muscles.
- **The pancreas** produces insulin and several other hormones, which together regulate the use and storage of food.

THE BLOOD

- **Blood consists of**:
  - water, in which salts – mainly sodium chloride – are dissolved;
  - a large number of proteins;
  - cells.
- **Cells in the blood** are of three main types:
  - red cells, which carry oxygen;
  - white cells, which defend against infection;
  - platelets, which are the body's "first aid" response to a breach in a blood vessel.
- **Plasma** is blood from which the cells have been removed but which has been prevented from clotting: plasma accounts for about one half of the blood volume.
- **Red cells** account for the remaining half of the blood volume.
- **Serum** is the fluid that is left after blood has been allowed to clot.
- **Blood** proteins play a number of important roles:
  - **albumin**, the protein with the highest concentration in blood, helps to keep a balance between the amount of water leaving the blood to bathe the tissues of the body and the amount of water remaining in the blood;
  - **immunoglobulins** attack foreign cells, including disease-causing microbes;
  - **other blood proteins** play roles in blood clotting or as signals between cells and organs.

Blood and anaemia

Anaemia is a reduction in the number of red blood cells circulating in the body**.** The production of red blood cells, which takes place in the bone marrow, is regulated by erythropoietin, a hormone produced by the kidney. Red blood cells remain in the blood circulation for about 100 days before being removed from the blood by the spleen. This lag time means that a fall in red cell production does not cause anaemia immediately.

The main causes of anaemia are:

- reduced production of red blood cells, due to:
  - lack of the nutrients iron, folate, and vitamin B12;
  - damage to the bone marrow caused by cancer, drugs, or radiation;
  - low levels of erythropoietin, most often seen in long-standing kidney disease;
- increased destruction of red cells, due to:
  - inherited disorders (e.g. thalassaemia) of red cells or of haemoglobin;
  - immune reactions to red cells, as in a mismatched blood transfusion;
  - infections of red cells, such as by malaria;
- bleeding, which can be:
  - obvious and rapid, such as from a major wound;
  - obvious but slow, such as in menstruation;
  - not obvious (insidious), such as from bowel damage caused by hookworm.

The commonest cause of anaemia is iron deficiency due to slow loss of blood. Iron is needed to form haemoglobin, the pigment that carries oxygen to all the tissues of the body. If there is no bleeding, very little iron is lost from the body and there is enough iron in the diet to replace what is lost. When bleeding is copious or prolonged, there is often not enough iron in the diet to make up the losses, so that deficiency results. All other causes of anaemia do not cause iron deficiency because the body retains the iron.

Iron deficiency is common in women because of menstrual blood loss. Another important cause of iron deficiency in women in poor countries is having frequent pregnancies. In men, iron deficiency usually indicates blood loss from the bowel, which may be due to bowel cancer or peptic ulcer.

Because measuring a reduction in the number of red blood cells is difficult, anaemia is usually diagnosed by measuring the concentration in the blood of haemoglobin. WHO has defined anaemia as a blood haemoglobin concentration of less than 130 g/l in men and less than 120 g/l in women. However, some people with even lower concentrations may be healthy and some with higher concentrations may be seriously ill.

Anaemia typically causes few or no symptoms until it is quite severe. Moderate anaemia (i.e. haemoglobin 70–100 g/l) may cause tiredness and lack of energy, and shortness of breath on exercise. Once anaemia has become severe (haemoglobin below 70 g/l) symptoms of tiredness and shortness of breath are usual.

It is difficult to detect anaemia without testing the blood. Patients with severe anaemia may look pale, but most pale people are not anaemic. Pallor due to anaemia is best looked for on the inside of the lower eyelid and in the creases of the palms of the hand. If these areas are obviously paler than normal, anaemia is very likely to be the cause.

THE IMMUNE SYSTEM

The immune system consists of two components (or "arms"): humoral immunity and cellular immunity.

- Humoral immunity:
  - humoral immunity is the body's main defence against many common infections, including pneumonia, meningitis, diphtheria, and tetanus;
  - humoral immunity is provided by proteins called immunoglobulins (also known as gamma-globulins or antibodies), which circulate in the blood;
  - immunoglobulins are secreted into the blood by special cells in the bone marrow, called B lymphocytes;
  - each immunoglobulin reacts with only one kind of foreign material: for example, a special immunoglobulin exists for tetanus toxin, another for measles virus, and so on;
  - because immunoglobulins are present in the blood at all times they react very quickly.
- Cellular immunity:
  - cellular immunity is provided by T cells (or T lymphocytes), special cells which are processed in a gland (the thymus gland) located in the chest under the breastbone;
  - T lymphocytes take longer to react than immunoglobulins;
  - T lymphocytes play an important role in the body's defence against many viruses, certain bacteria (such as the bacterium that causes tuberculosis), and some forms of cancer;
  - T lymphocytes also play an important role in the rejection of transplants;
  - the HIV virus, which causes AIDS, reduces the body's defence against infection by destroying T-lymphocytes.

Allergy

Allergy is an immune response that some people develop to a substance (allergen) in the environment. The substance, in this type of immune response, is usually not one to which most people develop an immune response. Unlike humoral immunity, which involves mainly immunoglobulins of the G class (immunoglobulin G or IgG), in allergy, the immune response involves antibodies of the E class (immunoglobulin E or IgE). The interaction between allergen and immunoglobulin E triggers the special form of immune response that causes the symptoms of allergy.

Why some, but not other, individuals develop allergic responses to a given substance is not known, although heredity plays a role. People who develop allergies to many different things are called "atopic". The main diseases associated with atopic allergy are asthma and hay fever (see Chapter 15, *Respiratory diseases*), and also eczema (see Chapter 20, *Skin diseases*). However, many cases of asthma, hay fever, and dermatitis are not due to allergy.

Some drug reactions are forms of allergy (see Chapter 33. *The ship's medicine chest*). This is especially true of reactions to penicillin and related antibiotics. Most reactions to drugs, including penicillin, are not due to allergy: this is also true of skin rashes. A small percentage of reactions to food are allergic, especially those to peanuts and shellfish, but most food reactions are not allergic.

Anaphylaxis (anaphylactic shock) is an uncommon but very severe form of allergic reaction. It usually occurs when the allergen is injected directly into the body (penicillin injections and bee stings are two examples). On board ship injection of penicillin or a related antibiotic will be by far the commonest cause of anaphylaxis. Occasionally anaphylaxis follows the ingestion of the allergen (most often peanuts) but is very rare when the allergen is airborne (such as pollen). An anaphylactic-like reaction (anaphylactoid reaction) sometimes occurs in the absence of allergy. For treatment of anaphylaxis see Chapter 33, *The ship's medicine chest*.

International Health Regulations

The purpose of the International Health Regulations (2005) is to ensure maximum security against the international spread of disease, with minimum interference in world trade and travel. Administered by the World Health Organization (WHO), it is the only legally binding, global agreement which focuses on measures for preventing the transboundary spread of infectious disease.

The IHR (2005) provide a single code of procedures and practices for all participating countries, which include routine measures at airports and seaports for preventing the importation and exportation of disease and disease-transmitting agents (e.g. mosquitoes, rats, cockroaches, etc.). This chapter includes extracts from the IHR (2005) of articles which specifically pertain to ships – the full text of the Regulations is available from WHO.

INTERNATIONAL HEALTH REGULATIONS (2005)

PART I – DEFINITIONS, PURPOSE AND SCOPE, PRINCIPLES AND RESPONSIBLE AUTHORITIES

ARTICLE 1 DEFINITIONS

1. For the purposes of the International Health Regulations (hereinafter the "IHR" or "Regulations"):

"affected" means persons, baggage, cargo, containers, conveyances, goods, postal parcels or human remains that are infected or contaminated, or carry sources of infection or contamination, so as to constitute a public health risk;

"affected area" means a geographical location specifically for which health measures have been recommended by WHO under these Regulations;

"aircraft" means an aircraft making an international voyage;

"airport" means any airport where international flights arrive or depart;

"arrival" of a conveyance means:

(a) in the case of a seagoing vessel, arrival or anchoring in the defined area of a port;

(b) in the case of an aircraft, arrival at an airport;

(c) in the case of an inland navigation vessel on an international voyage, arrival at a point of entry;

(d) in the case of a train or road vehicle, arrival at a point of entry;

"baggage" means the personal effects of a traveller;

"cargo" means goods carried on a conveyance or in a container;

"competent authority" means an authority responsible for the implementation and application of health measures under these Regulations;

"container" means an article of transport equipment:

(a) of a permanent character and accordingly strong enough to be suitable for repeated use;

(b) specially designed to facilitate the carriage of goods by one or more modes of transport, without intermediate reloading;

(c) fitted with devices permitting its ready handling, particularly its transfer from one mode of transport to another; and

(d) specially designed so as to be easy to fill and empty;

"container loading area" means a place or facility set aside for containers used in international traffic;

"contamination" means the presence of an infectious or toxic agent or matter on a human or animal body surface, in or on a product prepared for consumption or on other inanimate objects, including conveyances, that may constitute a public health risk;

"conveyance" means an aircraft, ship, train, road vehicle or other means of transport on an international voyage;

"conveyance operator" means a natural or legal person in charge of a conveyance or their agent;

"crew" means persons on board a conveyance who are not passengers;

"decontamination" means a procedure whereby health measures are taken to eliminate an infectious or toxic agent or matter on a human or animal body surface, in or on a product prepared for consumption or on other inanimate objects, including conveyances, that may constitute a public health risk;

"departure" means, for persons, baggage, cargo, conveyances or goods, the act of leaving a territory;

"deratting" means the procedure whereby health measures are taken to control or kill rodent vectors of human disease present in baggage, cargo, containers, conveyances, facilities, goods and postal parcels at the point of entry;

"Director-General" means the Director-General of the World Health Organization;

"disease" means an illness or medical condition, irrespective of origin or source, that presents or could present significant harm to humans;

"disinfection" means the procedure whereby health measures are taken to control or kill infectious agents on a human or animal body surface or in or on baggage, cargo, containers, conveyances, goods and postal parcels by direct exposure to chemical or physical agents;

"disinsection" means the procedure whereby health measures are taken to control or kill the insect vectors of human diseases present in baggage, cargo, containers, conveyances, goods and postal parcels;

"event" means a manifestation of disease or an occurrence that creates a potential for disease;

"*free pratique*" means permission for a ship to enter a port, embark or disembark, discharge or load cargo or stores; permission for an aircraft, after landing, to embark or disembark, discharge or load cargo or stores; and permission for a ground transport vehicle, upon arrival, to embark or disembark, discharge or load cargo or stores;

"goods" mean tangible products, including animals and plants, transported on an international voyage, including for utilization on board a conveyance;

"ground crossing" means a point of land entry in a State Party, including one utilized by road vehicles and trains;

"ground transport vehicle" means a motorized conveyance for overland transport on an international voyage, including trains, coaches, lorries and automobiles;

"health measure" means procedures applied to prevent the spread of disease or contamination; a health measure does not include law enforcement or security measures;

"ill person" means an individual suffering from or affected with a physical ailment that may pose a public health risk;

"infection" means the entry and development or multiplication of an infectious agent in the body of humans and animals that may constitute a public health risk;

"inspection" means the examination, by the competent authority or under its supervision, of areas, baggage, containers, conveyances, facilities, goods or postal parcels, including relevant data and documentation, to determine if a public health risk exists;

"international traffic" means the movement of persons, baggage, cargo, containers, conveyances, goods or postal parcels across an international border, including international trade;

"international voyage" means:

(a) in the case of a conveyance, a voyage between points of entry in the territories of more than one State, or a voyage between points of entry in the territory or territories of the same State if the conveyance has contacts with the territory of any other State on its voyage but only as regards those contacts;

(b) in the case of a traveller, a voyage involving entry into the territory of a State other than the territory of the State in which that traveller commences the voyage;

"intrusive" means possibly provoking discomfort through close or intimate contact or questioning;

"invasive" means the puncture or incision of the skin or insertion of an instrument or foreign material into the body or the examination of a body cavity. For the purposes of these Regulations, medical examination of the ear, nose and mouth, temperature assessment using an ear, oral or cutaneous thermometer, or thermal imaging; medical inspection; auscultation; external palpation; retinoscopy; external collection of urine, faeces or saliva samples; external measurement of blood pressure; and electrocardiography shall be considered to be non-invasive;

"isolation" means separation of ill or contaminated persons or affected baggage, containers, conveyances, goods or postal parcels from others in such a manner as to prevent the spread of infection or contamination;

"medical examination" means the preliminary assessment of a person by an authorized health worker or by a person under the direct supervision of the competent authority, to determine the person's health status and potential public health risk to others, and may include the scrutiny of health documents, and a physical examination when justified by the circumstances of the individual case;

"National IHR Focal Point" means the national centre, designated by each State Party, which shall be accessible at all times for communications with WHO IHR Contact Points under these Regulations;

"Organization" or "WHO" means the World Health Organization;

"permanent residence" has the meaning as determined in the national law of the State Party concerned;

"personal data" means any information relating to an identified or identifiable natural person;

"point of entry" means a passage for international entry or exit of travellers, baggage, cargo, containers, conveyances, goods and postal parcels as well as agencies and areas providing services to them on entry or exit;

"port" means a seaport or a port on an inland body of water where ships on an international voyage arrive or depart;

"postal parcel" means an addressed article or package carried internationally by postal or courier services;

"public health emergency of international concern" means an extraordinary event which is determined, as provided in these Regulations:

(i) to constitute a public health risk to other States through the international spread of disease and

(ii) to potentially require a coordinated international response;

"public health observation" means the monitoring of the health status of a traveller over time for the purpose of determining the risk of disease transmission;

"public health risk" means a likelihood of an event that may affect adversely the health of human populations, with an emphasis on one which may spread internationally or may present a serious and direct danger;

"quarantine" means the restriction of activities and/or separation from others of suspect persons who are not ill or of suspect baggage, containers, conveyances or goods in such a manner as to prevent the possible spread of infection or contamination;

"recommendation" and "recommended" refer to temporary or standing recommendations issued under these Regulations;

"reservoir" means an animal, plant or substance in which an infectious agent normally lives and whose presence may constitute a public health risk;

"road vehicle" means a ground transport vehicle other than a train;

"scientific evidence" means information furnishing a level of proof based on the established and accepted methods of science;

"scientific principles" means the accepted fundamental laws and facts of nature known through the methods of science;

"ship" means a seagoing or inland navigation vessel on an international voyage;

"standing recommendation" means non-binding advice issued by WHO for specific ongoing public health risks pursuant to Article 16 regarding appropriate health measures for routine or periodic application needed to prevent or reduce the international spread of disease and minimize interference with international traffic;

"surveillance" means the systematic ongoing collection, collation and analysis of data for public health purposes and the timely dissemination of public health information for assessment and public health response as necessary;

"suspect" means those persons, baggage, cargo, containers, conveyances, goods or postal parcels considered by a State Party as having been exposed, or possibly exposed, to a public health risk and that could be a possible source of spread of disease;

"temporary recommendation" means non-binding advice issued by WHO pursuant to Article 15 for application on a time-limited, risk-specific basis, in response to a public health emergency of international concern, so as to prevent or reduce the international spread of disease and minimize interference with international traffic;

"temporary residence" has the meaning as determined in the national law of the State Party concerned;

"traveller" means a natural person undertaking an international voyage;

"vector" means an insect or other animal which normally transports an infectious agent that constitutes a public health risk;

"verification" means the provision of information by a State Party to WHO confirming the status of an event within the territory or territories of that State Party;

"WHO IHR Contact Point" means the unit within WHO which shall be accessible at all times for communications with the National IHR Focal Point.

2. Unless otherwise specified or determined by the context, reference to these Regulations includes the annexes thereto.

ARTICLE 2 PURPOSE AND SCOPE

The purpose and scope of these Regulations are to prevent, protect against, control and provide a public health response to the international spread of disease in ways that are commensurate with and restricted to public health risks, and which avoid unnecessary interference with international traffic and trade.

Article 18 Recommendations with respect to persons, baggage, cargo, containers, conveyances, goods and postal parcels

1. Recommendations issued by WHO to States Parties with respect to persons may include the following advice:
   - no specific health measures are advised;
   - review travel history in affected areas;
   - review proof of medical examination and any laboratory analysis;
   - require medical examinations;
   - review proof of vaccination or other prophylaxis;
   - require vaccination or other prophylaxis;
   - place suspect persons under public health observation;
   - implement quarantine or other health measures for suspect persons;
   - implement isolation and treatment where necessary of affected persons;
   - implement tracing of contacts of suspect or affected persons;
   - refuse entry of suspect and affected persons;
   - refuse entry of unaffected persons to affected areas; and
   - implement exit screening and/or restrictions on persons from affected areas.
2. Recommendations issued by WHO to States Parties with respect to baggage, cargo, containers, conveyances, goods and postal parcels may include the following advice:
   - no specific health measures are advised;
   - review manifest and routing;
   - implement inspections;
   - review proof of measures taken on departure or in transit to eliminate infection or contamination;

- implement treatment of the baggage, cargo, containers, conveyances, goods, postal parcels or human remains to remove infection or contamination, including vectors and reservoirs;
- the use of specific health measures to ensure the safe handling and transport of human remains;
- implement isolation or quarantine;
- seizure and destruction of infected or contaminated or suspect baggage, cargo, containers, conveyances, goods or postal parcels under controlled conditions if no available treatment or process will otherwise be successful; and
- refuse departure or entry.

PART IV – POINTS OF ENTRY

ARTICLE 19 GENERAL OBLIGATIONS

Each State Party shall, in addition to the other obligations provided for under these Regulations:

(a) ensure that the capacities set forth in Annex 1 for designated points of entry are developed within the time frame provided in paragraph 1 of Article 5 and paragraph 1 of Article 13;

(b) identify the competent authorities at each designated point of entry in its territory; and

(c) furnish to WHO, as far as practicable, when requested in response to a specific potential public health risk, relevant data concerning sources of infection or contamination, including vectors and reservoirs, at its points of entry, which could result in international disease spread.

ARTICLE 20 AIRPORTS AND PORTS

1. States Parties shall designate the airports and ports that shall develop the capacities provided in Annex 1.
2. States Parties shall ensure that Ship Sanitation Control Exemption Certificates and Ship Sanitation Control Certificates are issued in accordance with the requirements in Article 39 and the model provided in Annex 3.
3. Each State Party shall send to WHO a list of ports authorized to offer:

   (a) the issuance of Ship Sanitation Control Certificates and the provision of the services referred to in Annexes 1 and 3; or

   (b) the issuance of Ship Sanitation Control Exemption Certificates only; and

   (c) extension of the Ship Sanitation Control Exemption Certificate for a period of one month until the arrival of the ship in the port at which the Certificate may be received.

   Each State Party shall inform WHO of any changes which may occur to the status of the listed ports. WHO shall publish the information received under this paragraph.
4. WHO may, at the request of the State Party concerned, arrange to certify, after an appropriate investigation, that an airport or port in its territory meets the requirements referred to in paragraphs 1 and 3 of this Article. These certifications may be subject to periodic review by WHO, in consultation with the State Party.

5. WHO, in collaboration with competent intergovernmental organizations and international bodies, shall develop and publish the certification guidelines for airports and ports under this Article. WHO shall also publish a list of certified airports and ports.

ARTICLE 21 GROUND CROSSINGS

1. Where justified for public health reasons, a State Party may designate ground crossings that shall develop the capacities provided in Annex 1, taking into consideration:
   (a) the volume and frequency of the various types of international traffic, as compared to other points of entry, at a State Party's ground crossings which might be designated; and
   (b) the public health risks existing in areas in which the international traffic originates, or through which it passes, prior to arrival at a particular ground crossing.
2. States Parties sharing common borders should consider:
   (a) entering into bilateral or multilateral agreements or arrangements concerning prevention or control of international transmission of disease at ground crossings in accordance with Article 57; and
   (b) joint designation of adjacent ground crossings for the capacities in Annex 1 in accordance with paragraph 1 of this Article.

ARTICLE 22 ROLE OF COMPETENT AUTHORITIES

1. The competent authorities shall:
   (a) be responsible for monitoring baggage, cargo, containers, conveyances, goods, postal parcels and human remains departing and arriving from affected areas, so that they are maintained in such a condition that they are free of sources of infection or contamination, including vectors and reservoirs;
   (b) ensure, as far as practicable, that facilities used by travellers at points of entry are maintained in a sanitary condition and are kept free of sources of infection or contamination, including vectors and reservoirs;
   (c) be responsible for the supervision of any deratting, disinfection, disinsection or decontamination of baggage, cargo, containers, conveyances, goods, postal parcels and human remains or sanitary measures for persons, as appropriate under these Regulations;
   (d) advise conveyance operators, as far in advance as possible, of their intent to apply control measures to a conveyance, and shall provide, where available, written information concerning the methods to be employed;
   (e) be responsible for the supervision of the removal and safe disposal of any contaminated water or food, human or animal dejecta, wastewater and any other contaminated matter from a conveyance;
   (f) take all practicable measures consistent with these Regulations to monitor and control the discharge by ships of sewage, refuse, ballast water and other potentially disease-causing matter which might contaminate the waters of a port, river, canal, strait, lake or other international waterway;

(g) be responsible for supervision of service providers for services concerning travellers, baggage, cargo, containers, conveyances, goods, postal parcels and human remains at points of entry, including the conduct of inspections and medical examinations as necessary;

(h) have effective contingency arrangements to deal with an unexpected public health event; and

(i) communicate with the National IHR Focal Point on the relevant public health measures taken pursuant to these Regulations.

2. Health measures recommended by WHO for travellers, baggage, cargo, containers, conveyances, goods, postal parcels and human remains arriving from an affected area may be reapplied on arrival, if there are verifiable indications and/or evidence that the measures applied on departure from the affected area were unsuccessful.

3. Disinsection, deratting, disinfection, decontamination and other sanitary procedures shall be carried out so as to avoid injury and as far as possible discomfort to persons, or damage to the environment in a way which impacts on public health, or damage to baggage, cargo, containers, conveyances, goods and postal parcels.

PART V – PUBLIC HEALTH MEASURES

Chapter I – General provisions

ARTICLE 23 HEALTH MEASURES ON ARRIVAL AND DEPARTURE

1. Subject to applicable international agreements and relevant articles of these Regulations, a State Party may require for public health purposes, on arrival or departure:

(a) with regard to travellers:

(i) information concerning the traveller's destination so that the traveller may be contacted;

(ii) information concerning the traveller's itinerary to ascertain if there was any travel in or near an affected area or other possible contacts with infection or contamination prior to arrival, as well as review of the traveller's health documents if they are required under these Regulations; and/or

(iii) a non-invasive medical examination which is the least intrusive examination that would achieve the public health objective;

(b) inspection of baggage, cargo, containers, conveyances, goods, postal parcels and human remains.

2. On the basis of evidence of a public health risk obtained through the measures provided in paragraph 1 of this Article, or through other means, States Parties may apply additional health measures, in accordance with these Regulations, in particular, with regard to a suspect or affected traveller, on a case-by-case basis, the least intrusive and invasive medical examination that would achieve the public health objective of preventing the international spread of disease.

3. No medical examination, vaccination, prophylaxis or health measure under these Regulations shall be carried out on travellers without their prior express informed consent

or that of their parents or guardians, except as provided in paragraph 2 of Article 31, and in accordance with the law and international obligations of the State Party.

4. Travellers to be vaccinated or offered prophylaxis pursuant to these Regulations, or their parents or guardians, shall be informed of any risk associated with vaccination or with non-vaccination and with the use or non-use of prophylaxis in accordance with the law and international obligations of the State Party. States Parties shall inform medical practitioners of these requirements in accordance with the law of the State Party.

5. Any medical examination, medical procedure, vaccination or other prophylaxis which involves a risk of disease transmission shall only be performed on, or administered to, a traveller in accordance with established national or international safety guidelines and standards so as to minimize such a risk.

Chapter II – Special provisions for conveyances and conveyance operators

ARTICLE 24 CONVEYANCE OPERATORS

1. States Parties shall take all practicable measures consistent with these Regulations to ensure that conveyance operators:
   (a) comply with the health measures recommended by WHO and adopted by the State Party;
   (b) inform travellers of the health measures recommended by WHO and adopted by the State Party for application on board; and
   (c) permanently keep conveyances for which they are responsible free of sources of infection or contamination, including vectors and reservoirs. The application of measures to control sources of infection or contamination may be required if evidence is found.

2. Specific provisions pertaining to conveyances and conveyance operators under this Article are provided in Annex 4. Specific measures applicable to conveyances and conveyance operators with regard to vector-borne diseases are provided in Annex 5.

ARTICLE 25 SHIPS AND AIRCRAFT IN TRANSIT

Subject to Articles 27 and 43 or unless authorized by applicable international agreements, no health measure shall be applied by a State Party to:

(a) a ship not coming from an affected area which passes through a maritime canal or waterway in the territory of that State Party on its way to a port in the territory of another State. Any such ship shall be permitted to take on, under the supervision of the competent authority, fuel, water, food and supplies;

(b) a ship which passes through waters within its jurisdiction without calling at a port or on the coast; and

(c) an aircraft in transit at an airport within its jurisdiction, except that the aircraft may be restricted to a particular area of the airport with no embarking and disembarking or loading and discharging. However, any such aircraft shall be permitted to take on, under the supervision of the competent authority, fuel, water, food and supplies.

ARTICLE 27 AFFECTED CONVEYANCES

1. If clinical signs or symptoms and information based on fact or evidence of a public health risk, including sources of infection and contamination, are found on board a conveyance, the competent authority shall consider the conveyance as affected and may:

   (a) disinfect, decontaminate, disinsect or derat the conveyance, as appropriate, or cause these measures to be carried out under its supervision; and

   (b) decide in each case the technique employed to secure an adequate level of control of the public health risk as provided in these Regulations. Where there are methods or materials advised by WHO for these procedures, these should be employed, unless the competent authority determines that other methods are as safe and reliable.

   The competent authority may implement additional health measures, including isolation of the conveyances, as necessary, to prevent the spread of disease. Such additional measures should be reported to the National IHR Focal Point.

2. If the competent authority for the point of entry is not able to carry out the control measures required under this Article, the affected conveyance may nevertheless be allowed to depart, subject to the following conditions:

   (a) the competent authority shall, at the time of departure, inform the competent authority for the next known point of entry of the type of information referred to under subparagraph (b); and

   (b) in the case of a ship, the evidence found and the control measures required shall be noted in the Ship Sanitation Control Certificate.

   Any such conveyance shall be permitted to take on, under the supervision of the competent authority, fuel, water, food and supplies.

3. A conveyance that has been considered as affected shall cease to be regarded as such when the competent authority is satisfied that:

   (a) the measures provided in paragraph 1 of this Article have been effectively carried out; and

   (b) there are no conditions on board that could constitute a public health risk.

ARTICLE 28 SHIPS AND AIRCRAFT AT POINTS OF ENTRY

1. Subject to Article 43 or as provided in applicable international agreements, a ship or an aircraft shall not be prevented for public health reasons from calling at any point of entry. However, if the point of entry is not equipped for applying health measures under these Regulations, the ship or aircraft may be ordered to proceed at its own risk to the nearest suitable point of entry available to it, unless the ship or aircraft has an operational problem which would make this diversion unsafe.

2. Subject to Article 43 or as provided in applicable international agreements, ships or aircraft shall not be refused *free pratique* by States Parties for public health reasons; in particular they shall not be prevented from embarking or disembarking, discharging or loading cargo or stores, or taking on fuel, water, food and supplies. States Parties may subject the granting of *free pratique* to inspection and, if a source of infection

or contamination is found on board, the carrying out of necessary disinfection, decontamination, disinsection or deratting, or other measures necessary to prevent the spread of the infection or contamination.

3. Whenever practicable and subject to the previous paragraph, a State Party shall authorize the granting of *free pratique* by radio or other communication means to a ship or an aircraft when, on the basis of information received from it prior to its arrival, the State Party is of the opinion that the arrival of the ship or aircraft will not result in the introduction or spread of disease.

4. Officers in command of ships or pilots in command of aircraft, or their agents, shall make known to the port or airport control as early as possible before arrival at the port or airport of destination any cases of illness indicative of a disease of an infectious nature or evidence of a public health risk on board as soon as such illnesses or public health risks are made known to the officer or pilot. This information must be immediately relayed to the competent authority for the port or airport. In urgent circumstances, such information should be communicated directly by the officers or pilots to the relevant port or airport authority.

5. The following shall apply if a suspect or affected aircraft or ship, for reasons beyond the control of the pilot in command of the aircraft or the officer in command of the ship, lands elsewhere than at the airport at which the aircraft was due to land or berths elsewhere than at the port at which the ship was due to berth:
   (a) the pilot in command of the aircraft or the officer in command of the ship or other person in charge shall make every effort to communicate without delay with the nearest competent authority;
   (b) as soon as the competent authority has been informed of the landing it may apply health measures recommended by WHO or other health measures provided in these Regulations;
   (c) unless required for emergency purposes or for communication with the competent authority, no traveller on board the aircraft or ship shall leave its vicinity and no cargo shall be removed from that vicinity, unless authorized by the competent authority; and
   (d) when all health measures required by the competent authority have been completed, the aircraft or ship may, so far as such health measures are concerned, proceed either to the airport or port at which it was due to land or berth, or, if for technical reasons it cannot do so, to a conveniently situated airport or port.

6. Notwithstanding the provisions contained in this Article, the officer in command of a ship or pilot in command of an aircraft may take such emergency measures as may be necessary for the health and safety of travellers on board. He or she shall inform the competent authority as early as possible concerning any measures taken pursuant to this paragraph.

ARTICLE 29 CIVILIAN LORRIES, TRAINS AND COACHES AT POINTS OF ENTRY

WHO, in consultation with States Parties, shall develop guiding principles for applying health measures to civilian lorries, trains and coaches at points of entry and passing through ground crossings.

Chapter III – Special provisions for travellers

ARTICLE 30 TRAVELLERS UNDER PUBLIC HEALTH OBSERVATION

Subject to Article 43 or as authorized in applicable international agreements, a suspect traveller who on arrival is placed under public health observation may continue an international voyage, if the traveller does not pose an imminent public health risk and the State Party informs the competent authority of the point of entry at destination, if known, of the traveller's expected arrival. On arrival, the traveller shall report to that authority.

ARTICLE 31 HEALTH MEASURES RELATING TO ENTRY OF TRAVELLERS

1. Invasive medical examination, vaccination or other prophylaxis shall not be required as a condition of entry of any traveller to the territory of a State Party, except that, subject to Articles 32, 42 and 45, these Regulations do not preclude States Parties from requiring medical examination, vaccination or other prophylaxis or proof of vaccination or other prophylaxis:
   - (a) when necessary to determine whether a public health risk exists;
   - (b) as a condition of entry for any travellers seeking temporary or permanent residence;
   - (c) as a condition of entry for any travellers pursuant to Article 43 or Annexes 6 and 7; or
   - (d) which may be carried out pursuant to Article 23.
2. If a traveller for whom a State Party may require a medical examination, vaccination or other prophylaxis under paragraph 1 of this Article fails to consent to any such measure, or refuses to provide the information or the documents referred to in paragraph 1(a) of Article 23, the State Party concerned may, subject to Articles 32, 42 and 45, deny entry to that traveller. If there is evidence of an imminent public health risk, the State Party may, in accordance with its national law and to the extent necessary to control such a risk, compel the traveller to undergo or advise the traveller, pursuant to paragraph 3 of Article 23, to undergo:
   - (a) the least invasive and intrusive medical examination that would achieve the public health objective;
   - (b) vaccination or other prophylaxis; or
   - (c) additional established health measures that prevent or control the spread of disease, including isolation, quarantine or placing the traveller under public health observation.

ARTICLE 32 TREATMENT OF TRAVELLERS

In implementing health measures under these Regulations, States Parties shall treat travellers with respect for their dignity, human rights and fundamental freedoms and minimize any discomfort or distress associated with such measures, including by:

(a) treating all travellers with courtesy and respect;

(b) taking into consideration the gender, sociocultural, ethnic or religious concerns of travellers; and

(c) providing or arranging for adequate food and water, appropriate accommodation and clothing, protection for baggage and other possessions, appropriate medical treatment, means of necessary communication if possible in a language that they can understand and other appropriate assistance for travellers who are quarantined, isolated or subject to medical examinations or other procedures for public health purposes.

Chapter IV – Special provisions for goods, containers and container loading areas

ARTICLE 33 GOODS IN TRANSIT

Subject to Article 43 or unless authorized by applicable international agreements, goods, other than live animals, in transit without transhipment shall not be subject to health measures under these Regulations or detained for public health purposes.

ARTICLE 34 CONTAINER AND CONTAINER LOADING AREAS

1. States Parties shall ensure, as far as practicable, that container shippers use international traffic containers that are kept free from sources of infection or contamination, including vectors and reservoirs, particularly during the course of packing.
2. States Parties shall ensure, as far as practicable, that container loading areas are kept free from sources of infection or contamination, including vectors and reservoirs.
3. Whenever, in the opinion of a State Party, the volume of international container traffic is sufficiently large, the competent authorities shall take all practicable measures consistent with these Regulations, including carrying out inspections, to assess the sanitary condition of container loading areas and containers in order to ensure that the obligations contained in these Regulations are implemented.
4. Facilities for the inspection and isolation of containers shall, as far as practicable, be available at container loading areas.
5. Container consignees and consignors shall make every effort to avoid cross-contamination when multiple-use loading of containers is employed.

PART VI – HEALTH DOCUMENTS

ARTICLE 35 GENERAL RULE

No health documents, other than those provided for under these Regulations or in recommendations issued by WHO, shall be required in international traffic, provided however that this Article shall not apply to travellers seeking temporary or permanent residence, nor shall it apply to document requirements concerning the public health status of goods or cargo in international trade pursuant to applicable international agreements. The competent authority may request travellers to complete contact information forms and questionnaires on the health of travellers, provided that they meet the requirements set out in Article 23.

ARTICLE 36 CERTIFICATES OF VACCINATION OR OTHER PROPHYLAXIS

1. Vaccines and prophylaxis for travellers administered pursuant to these Regulations, or to recommendations and certificates relating thereto, shall conform to the provisions of Annex 6 and, when applicable, Annex 7 with regard to specific diseases.
2. A traveller in possession of a certificate of vaccination or other prophylaxis issued in conformity with Annex 6 and, when applicable, Annex 7, shall not be denied entry as a consequence of the disease to which the certificate refers, even if coming from an affected area, unless the competent authority has verifiable indications and/or evidence that the vaccination or other prophylaxis was not effective.

ARTICLE 37 MARITIME DECLARATION OF HEALTH

1. The master of a ship, before arrival at its first port of call in the territory of a State Party, shall ascertain the state of health on board, and, except when that State Party does not require it, the master shall, on arrival, or in advance of the vessel's arrival if the vessel is so equipped and the State Party requires such advance delivery, complete and deliver to the competent authority for that port a Maritime Declaration of Health which shall be countersigned by the ship's surgeon, if one is carried.
2. The master of a ship, or the ship's surgeon if one is carried, shall supply any information required by the competent authority as to health conditions on board during an international voyage.
3. A Maritime Declaration of Health shall conform to the model provided in Annex 8.
4. A State Party may decide:
   (a) to dispense with the submission of the Maritime Declaration of Health by all arriving ships; or
   (b) to require the submission of the Maritime Declaration of Health under a recommendation concerning ships arriving from affected areas or to require it from ships which might otherwise carry infection or contamination.

   The State Party shall inform shipping operators or their agents of these requirements.

ARTICLE 39 SHIP SANITATION CERTIFICATES

1. Ship Sanitation Control Exemption Certificates and Ship Sanitation Control Certificates shall be valid for a maximum period of six months. This period may be extended by one month if the inspection or control measures required cannot be accomplished at the port.
2. If a valid Ship Sanitation Control Exemption Certificate or Ship Sanitation Control Certificate is not produced or evidence of a public health risk is found on board a ship, the State Party may proceed as provided in paragraph 1 of Article 27.
3. The certificates referred to in this Article shall conform to the model in Annex 3.
4. Whenever possible, control measures shall be carried out when the ship and holds are empty. In the case of a ship in ballast, they shall be carried out before loading.
5. When control measures are required and have been satisfactorily completed, the competent authority shall issue a Ship Sanitation Control Certificate, noting the evidence found and the control measures taken.

6. The competent authority may issue a Ship Sanitation Control Exemption Certificate at any port specified under Article 20 if it is satisfied that the ship is free of infection and contamination, including vectors and reservoirs. Such a certificate shall normally be issued only if the inspection of the ship has been carried out when the ship and holds are empty or when they contain only ballast or other material, of such a nature or so disposed as to make a thorough inspection of the holds possible.
7. If the conditions under which control measures are carried out are such that, in the opinion of the competent authority for the port where the operation was performed, a satisfactory result cannot be obtained, the competent authority shall make a note to that effect on the Ship Sanitation Control Certificate.

PART VII – CHARGES

ARTICLE 40 CHARGES FOR HEALTH MEASURES REGARDING TRAVELLERS

1. Except for travellers seeking temporary or permanent residence, and subject to paragraph 2 of this Article, no charge shall be made by a State Party pursuant to these Regulations for the following measures for the protection of public health:
   (a) any medical examination provided for in these Regulations, or any supplementary examination which may be required by that State Party to ascertain the health status of the traveller examined;
   (b) any vaccination or other prophylaxis provided to a traveller on arrival that is not a published requirement or is a requirement published less than 10 days prior to provision of the vaccination or other prophylaxis;
   (c) appropriate isolation or quarantine requirements of travellers;
   (d) any certificate issued to the traveller specifying the measures applied and the date of application; or
   (e) any health measures applied to baggage accompanying the traveller.
2. State Parties may charge for health measures other than those referred to in paragraph 1 of this Article, including those primarily for the benefit of the traveller.
3. Where charges are made for applying such health measures to travellers under these Regulations, there shall be in each State Party only one tariff for such charges and every charge shall:
   (a) conform to this tariff;
   (b) not exceed the actual cost of the service rendered; and
   (c) be levied without distinction as to the nationality, domicile or residence of the traveller concerned.
4. The tariff, and any amendment thereto, shall be published at least 10 days in advance of any levy thereunder.
5. Nothing in these Regulations shall preclude States Parties from seeking reimbursement for expenses incurred in providing the health measures in paragraph 1 of this Article:
   (a) from conveyance operators or owners with regard to their employees; or
   (b) from applicable insurance sources.

6. Under no circumstances shall travellers or conveyance operators be denied the ability to depart from the territory of a State Party pending payment of the charges referred to in paragraphs 1 or 2 of this Article.

ARTICLE 41 CHARGES FOR BAGGAGE, CARGO, CONTAINERS, CONVEYANCES, GOODS OR POSTAL PARCELS

1. Where charges are made for applying health measures to baggage, cargo, containers, conveyances, goods or postal parcels under these Regulations, there shall be in each State Party only one tariff for such charges and every charge shall:
   (a) conform to this tariff;
   (b) not exceed the actual cost of the service rendered; and
   (c) be levied without distinction as to the nationality, flag, registry or ownership of the baggage, cargo, containers, conveyances, goods or postal parcels concerned. In particular, there shall be no distinction made between national and foreign baggage, cargo, containers, conveyances, goods or postal parcels.
2. The tariff, and any amendment thereto, shall be published at least 10 days in advance of any levy thereunder.

ANNEX 1

B. CORE CAPACITY REQUIREMENTS FOR DESIGNATED AIRPORTS, PORTS AND GROUND CROSSINGS

1. At all times

   The capacities:

   (a) to provide access to (i) an appropriate medical service including diagnostic facilities located so as to allow the prompt assessment and care of ill travellers, and (ii) adequate staff, equipment and premises;

   (b) to provide access to equipment and personnel for the transport of ill travellers to an appropriate medical facility;

   (c) to provide trained personnel for the inspection of conveyances;

   (d) to ensure a safe environment for travellers using point of entry facilities, including potable water supplies, eating establishments, flight catering facilities, public washrooms, appropriate solid and liquid waste disposal services and other potential risk areas, by conducting inspection programmes, as appropriate; and

   (e) to provide as far as practicable a programme and trained personnel for the control of vectors and reservoirs in and near points of entry.

2. For responding to events that may constitute a public health emergency of international concern

   The capacities:

   (a) to provide appropriate public health emergency response by establishing and maintaining a public health emergency contingency plan, including the nomination of a coordinator and contact points for relevant point of entry, public health and other agencies and services;

   (b) to provide assessment of and care for affected travellers or animals by establishing arrangements with local medical and veterinary facilities for their isolation, treatment and other support services that may be required;

   (c) to provide appropriate space, separate from other travellers, to interview suspect or affected persons;

   (d) to provide for the assessment and, if required, quarantine of suspect travellers, preferably in facilities away from the point of entry;

   (e) to apply recommended measures to disinsect, derat, disinfect, decontaminate or otherwise treat baggage, cargo, containers, conveyances, goods or postal parcels including, when appropriate, at locations specially designated and equipped for this purpose;

   (f) to apply entry or exit controls for arriving and departing travellers; and

   (g) to provide access to specially designated equipment, and to trained personnel with appropriate personal protection, for the transfer of travellers who may carry infection or contamination.

ANNEX 2

DECISION INSTRUMENT FOR THE ASSESSMENT AND NOTIFICATION OF EVENTS THAT MAY CONSTITUTE A PUBLIC HEALTH EMERGENCY OF INTERNATIONAL CONCERN

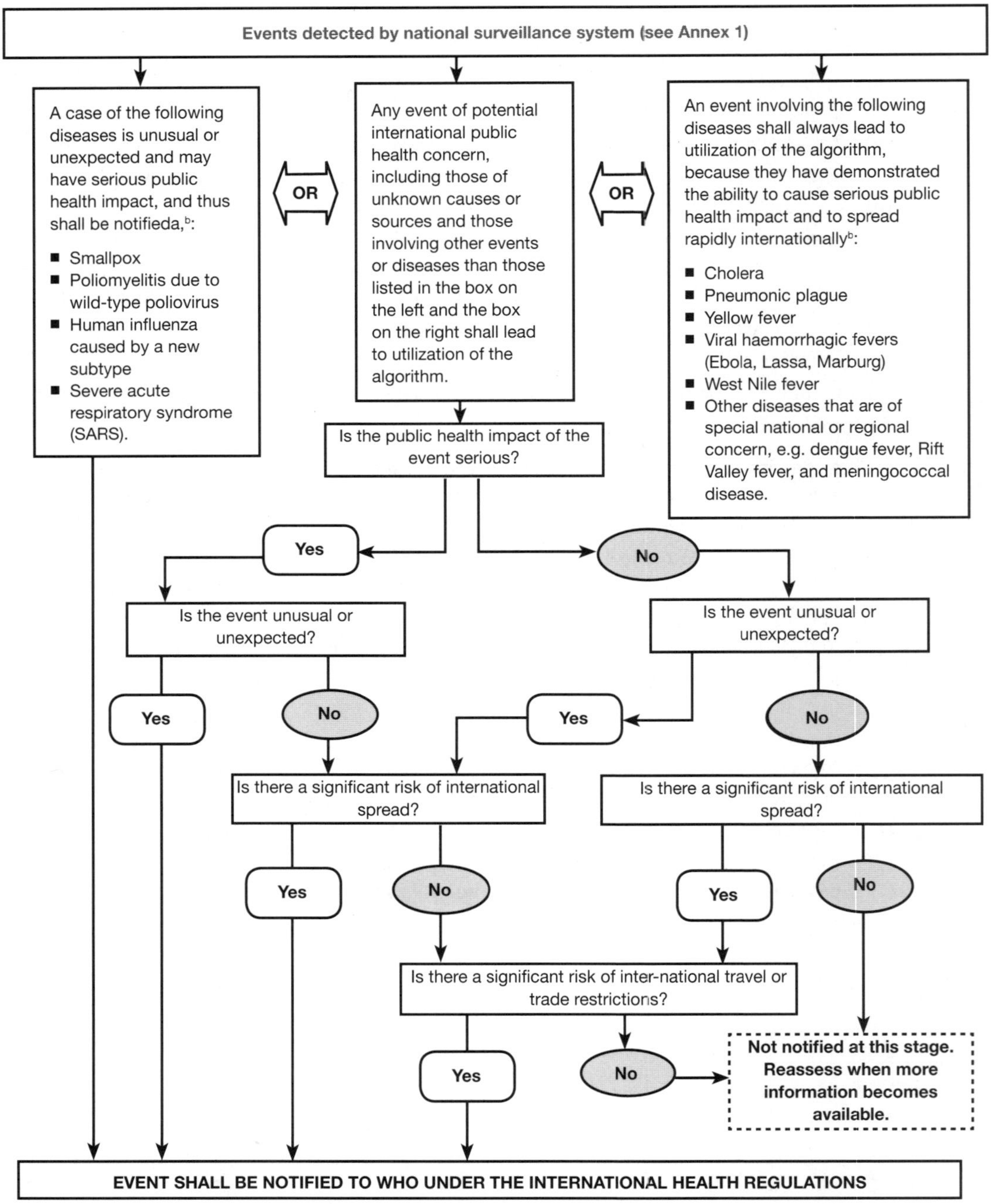

Examples for the application of the decision instrument for the assessment and notification of events that may constitute a public health emergency of international concern

The examples appearing in this Annex are not binding and are for indicative guidance purposes to assist in the interpretation of the decision instrument criteria.

DOES THE EVENT MEET AT LEAST TWO OF THE FOLLOWING CRITERIA?

<table>
<tr><td rowspan="4">Is the public health impact of the event serious?</td><td>I. Is the public health impact of the event serious?</td></tr>
<tr><td>1. Is the number of cases and/or number of deaths for this type of event large for the given place, time or population?</td></tr>
<tr><td>2. Has the event the potential to have a high public health impact?

THE FOLLOWING ARE EXAMPLES OF CIRCUMSTANCES THAT CONTRIBUTE TO HIGH PUBLIC HEALTH IMPACT:
✓ Event caused by a pathogen with high potential to cause epidemic (infectiousness of the agent, high case fatality, multiple transmission routes or healthy carrier).
✓ Indication of treatment failure (new or emerging antibiotic resistance, vaccine failure, antidote resistance or failure).
✓ Event represents a significant public health risk even if no or very few human cases have yet been identified.
✓ Cases reported among health staff.
✓ The population at risk is especially vulnerable (refugees, low level of immunization, children, elderly, low immunity, undernourished, etc.).
✓ Concomitant factors that may hinder or delay the public health response (natural catastrophes, armed conflicts, unfavourable weather conditions, multiple foci in the State Party).
✓ Event in an area with high population density.
✓ Spread of toxic, infectious or otherwise hazardous materials that may be occurring naturally or otherwise that has contaminated or has the potential to contaminate a population and/or a large geographical area.</td></tr>
<tr><td>3. Is external assistance needed to detect, investigate, respond and control the current event, or prevent new cases?
The following are examples of when assistance may be required:

✓ Inadequate human, financial, material or technical resources – in particular:
■ Insufficient laboratory or epidemiological capacity to investigate the event (equipment, personnel, financial resources)
■ Insufficient antidotes, drugs and/or vaccine and/or protective equipment, decontamination equipment, or supportive equipment to cover estimated needs
■ Existing surveillance system is inadequate to detect new cases in a timely manner.</td></tr>
<tr><td></td><td>IS THE PUBLIC HEALTH IMPACT OF THE EVENT SERIOUS?
Answer "yes" if you have answered "yes" to questions 1, 2 or 3 above.</td></tr>
</table>

	II. Is the event unusual or unexpected?
	4. Is the event unusual? THE FOLLOWING ARE EXAMPLES OF UNUSUAL EVENTS: ✓ The event is caused by an unknown agent or the source, vehicle, route of transmission is unusual or unknown. ✓ Evolution of cases more severe than expected (including morbidity or case-fatality) or with unusual symptoms. ✓ Occurrence of the event itself unusual for the area, season or population.
	5. Is the event unexpected from a public health perspective? THE FOLLOWING ARE EXAMPLES OF UNEXPECTED EVENTS: ✓ Event caused by a disease/agent that had already been eliminated or eradicated from the State Party or not previously reported.
	IS THE EVENT UNUSUAL OR UNEXPECTED? **Answer "yes" if you have answered "yes" to questions 4 or 5 above.**

Is there a significant risk of international spread?	**III. Is there a significant risk of international spread?**
	6. Is there evidence of an epidemiological link to similar events in other States?
	7. Is there any factor that should alert us to the potential for cross border movement of the agent, vehicle or host? THE FOLLOWING ARE EXAMPLES OF CIRCUMSTANCES THAT MAY PREDISPOSE TO INTERNATIONAL SPREAD: ✓ Where there is evidence of local spread, an index case (or other linked cases) with a history within the previous month of: ■ international travel (or time equivalent to the incubation period if the pathogen is known) ■ participation in an international gathering (pilgrimage, sports event, conference, etc.) ■ close contact with an international traveller or a highly mobile population. ✓ Event caused by an environmental contamination that has the potential to spread across international borders. ✓ Event in an area of intense international traffic with limited capacity for sanitary control or environmental detection or decontamination.
	IS THERE A SIGNIFICANT RISK OF INTERNATIONAL SPREAD? **Answer "yes" if you have answered "yes" to questions 6 or 7 above.**

Risk of international restrictions ?	**IV. Is there a significant risk of international travel or trade restrictions?**
	8. Have similar events in the past resulted in international restriction on trade and/or travel?
	9. Is the source suspected or known to be a food product, water or any other goods that might be contaminated that has been exported/imported to/from other States?
	10. Has the event occurred in association with an international gathering or in an area of intense international tourism?
	11. Has the event caused requests for more information by foreign officials or international media?
	IS THERE A SIGNIFICANT RISK OF INTERNATIONAL TRADE OR TRAVEL RESTRICTIONS? **Answer "yes" if you have answered "yes" to questions 8, 9, 10 or 11 above.**

States Parties that answer "yes" to the question whether the event meets any two of the four criteria (I-IV) above, shall notify WHO under Article 6 of the International Health Regulations.

ANNEX 3

MODEL SHIP SANITATION CONTROL EXEMPTION CERTIFICATE/SHIP SANITATION CONTROL CERTIFICATE

Port of......... Date: ....

This Certificate records the inspection and 1) exemption from control or 2) control measures applied

Name of ship or inland navigation vessel........................Flag........................ Registration/IMO No. ....

At the time of inspection the holds were unladen/laden with ...... tonnes of .... cargo

Name and address of inspecting officer......................

Ship Sanitation Control Exemption Certifica

Areas , [systems, and services] inspected	Evidence found1	Sample results 2	Documents reviewed
Galley			Medical log
Pantry			Ship's log
Stores			Other
Hold(s)/cargo			
Quarters:			
- crew			
- officers			
- passengers			
- deck			
Potable water			
Sewage			
Ballast tanks			
Solid and medical waste			
Standing water			
Engine room			
Medical facilities			
Other areas specified - see attached			
Note areas not applicable, by marking N/A.			

No evidence found. Ship/vessel is exempted from control measures.

Ship Sanitation Control Certificate

Control measures applied	Re-inspection date	Comments regarding conditions found

Control measures indicated were applied on the date below.

Name and designation of issuing officer .... Signature and seal .... Date ....

[1] (a) Evidence of infection or contamination, including: vectors in all stages of growth; animal reservoirs for vectors; rodents or other species that could carry human disease, microbiological, chemical and other risks to human health; signs of inadequate sanitary measures. (b) Information concerning any human cases (to be included in the Maritime Declaration of Health).

[2] Results from samples taken on board. Analysis to be provided to ship's master by most expedient means and, if re-inspection is required, to the next appropriate port of call coinciding with the re-inspection date specified in this certificate.

Sanitation Control Exemption Certificates and Sanitation Control Certificates are valid for a maximum of six months, but the validity period may be extended by one month if inspection cannot be carried out at the port and there is no evidence of infection or contamination.

ATTACHMENT TO MODEL SHIP SANITATION CONTROL EXEMPTION CERTIFICATE/SHIP SANITATION CONTROL CERTIFICATE

Areas/facilities/systems inspected	Evidence found	Sample results	Documents reviewed	Control measures applied	Re-inspection date	Comments regarding conditions found
Food						
Source						
Storage						
Preparation						
Service						
Water						
Source						
Storage						
Distribution						
Waste						
Holding						
Treatment						
Disposal						
Swimming pools/spas						
Equipment						
Operation						
Medical facilities						
Equipment and medical devices						
Operation						
Medicines						
Other areas inspected						

Indicate when the areas listed are not applicable by marking N/A.

ANNEX 4

TECHNICAL REQUIREMENTS PERTAINING TO CONVEYANCES AND CONVEYANCE OPERATORS

Section A Conveyance operators

1. Conveyance operators shall facilitate:
   (a) inspections of the cargo, containers and conveyance;
   (b) medical examinations of persons on board;
   (c) application of other health measures under these Regulations; and
   (d) provision of relevant public health information requested by the State Party.
2. Conveyance operators shall provide to the competent authority a valid Ship Sanitation Control Exemption Certificate or a Ship Sanitation Control Certificate or a Maritime Declaration of Health, or the Health Part of an Aircraft General Declaration, as required under these Regulations.

Section B Conveyances

1. Control measures applied to baggage, cargo, containers, conveyances and goods under these Regulations shall be carried out so as to avoid as far as possible injury or discomfort to persons or damage to the baggage, cargo, containers, conveyances and goods. Whenever possible and appropriate, control measures shall be applied when the conveyance and holds are empty.
2. States Parties shall indicate in writing the measures applied to cargo, containers or conveyances, the parts treated, the methods employed, and the reasons for their application. This information shall be provided in writing to the person in charge of an aircraft and, in case of a ship, on the Ship Sanitation Control Certificate. For other cargo, containers or conveyances, States Parties shall issue such information in writing to consignors, consignees, carriers, the person in charge of the conveyance or their respective agents.

ANNEX 5

SPECIFIC MEASURES FOR VECTOR-BORNE DISEASES

1. WHO shall publish, on a regular basis, a list of areas where disinsection or other vector control measures are recommended for conveyances arriving from these areas. Determination of such areas shall be made pursuant to the procedures regarding temporary or standing recommendations, as appropriate.
2. Every conveyance leaving a point of entry situated in an area where vector control is recommended should be disinsected and kept free of vectors. When there are methods and materials advised by the Organization for these procedures, these should be employed. The presence of vectors on board conveyances and the control measures used to eradicate them shall be included:
   (a) in the case of aircraft, in the Health Part of the Aircraft General Declaration, unless this part of the Declaration is waived by the competent authority at the airport of arrival;
   (b) in the case of ships, on the Ship Sanitation Control Certificates; and
   (c) in the case of other conveyances, on a written proof of treatment issued to the consignor, consignee, carrier, the person in charge of the conveyance or their agent, respectively.
3. States Parties should accept disinsecting, deratting and other control measures for conveyances applied by other States if methods and materials advised by the Organization have been applied.
4. States Parties shall establish programmes to control vectors that may transport an infectious agent that constitutes a public health risk to a minimum distance of 400 metres from those areas of point of entry facilities that are used for operations involving travellers, conveyances, containers, cargo and postal parcels, with extension of the minimum distance if vectors with a greater range are present.
5. If a follow-up inspection is required to determine the success of the vector control measures applied, the competent authorities for the next known port or airport of call with a capacity to make such an inspection shall be informed of this requirement in advance by the competent authority advising such follow-up. In the case of ships, this shall be noted on the Ship Sanitation Control Certificate.
6. A conveyance may be regarded as suspect and should be inspected for vectors and reservoirs if:
   (a) it has a possible case of vector-borne disease on board;
   (b) a possible case of vector-borne disease has occurred on board during an international voyage; or
   (c) it has left an affected area within a period of time where on-board vectors could still carry disease.
7. A State Party should not prohibit the landing of an aircraft or berthing of a ship in its territory if the control measures provided for in paragraph 3 of this Annex or otherwise recommended by the Organization are applied. However, aircraft or ships coming from an affected area may be required to land at airports or divert to another port specified by the State Party for that purpose.
8. A State Party may apply vector control measures to a conveyance arriving from an area affected by a vector-borne disease if the vectors for the foregoing disease are present in its territory.

ANNEX 6

VACCINATION, PROPHYLAXIS AND RELATED CERTIFICATES

1. Vaccines or other prophylaxis specified in Annex 7 or recommended under these Regulations shall be of suitable quality; those vaccines and prophylaxis designated by WHO shall be subject to its approval. Upon request, the State Party shall provide to WHO appropriate evidence of the suitability of vaccines and prophylaxis administered within its territory under these Regulations.
2. Persons undergoing vaccination or other prophylaxis under these Regulations shall be provided with an international certificate of vaccination or prophylaxis (hereinafter the "certificate") in the form specified in this Annex. No departure shall be made from the model of the certificate specified in this Annex.
3. Certificates under this Annex are valid only if the vaccine or prophylaxis used has been approved by WHO.
4. Certificates must be signed in the hand of the clinician, who shall be a medical practitioner or other authorized health worker, supervising the administration of the vaccine or prophylaxis. The certificate must also bear the official stamp of the administering centre; however, this shall not be an accepted substitute for the signature.
5. Certificates shall be fully completed in English or in French. They may also be completed in another language, in addition to either English or French.
6. Any amendment of this certificate, or erasure, or failure to complete any part of it, may render it invalid.
7. Certificates are individual and shall in no circumstances be used collectively. Separate certificates shall be issued for children.
8. A parent or guardian shall sign the certificate when the child is unable to write. The signature of an illiterate shall be indicated in the usual manner by the person's mark and the indication by another that this is the mark of the person concerned.
9. If the supervising clinician is of the opinion that the vaccination or prophylaxis is contraindicated on medical grounds, the supervising clinician shall provide the person with reasons, written in English or French, and where appropriate in another language in addition to English or French, underlying that opinion, which the competent authorities on arrival should take into account. The supervising clinician and competent authorities shall inform such persons of any risk associated with non-vaccination and with the non-use of prophylaxis in accordance with paragraph 4 of Article 23.
10. An equivalent document issued by the Armed Forces to an active member of those Forces shall be accepted in lieu of an international certificate in the form shown in this Annex if:

    (a) it embodies medical information substantially the same as that required by such form; and

    (b) it contains a statement in English or in French and where appropriate in another language in addition to English or French recording the nature and date of the vaccination or prophylaxis and to the effect that it is issued in accordance with this paragraph.

MODEL INTERNATIONAL CERTIFICATE OF VACCINATION OR PROPHYLAXIS

This is to certify that [name] ...., date of birth ...., sex ....,

nationality ...., national identification document, if applicable ....

whose signature follows ....

has on the date indicated been vaccinated or received prophylaxis against:

(name of disease or condition) ....

in accordance with the International Health Regulations.

Vaccine or prophylaxis	Date	Signature and professional status of supervising clinician	Manufacturer and batch No. of vaccine or prophylaxis	Certificate valid from .... until	Official stamp of administering centre
1.					
2.					

This certificate is valid only if the vaccine or prophylaxis used has been approved by the World Health Organization.

This certificate must be signed in the hand of the clinician, who shall be a medical practitioner or other authorized health worker, supervising the administration of the vaccine or prophylaxis. The certificate must also bear the official stamp of the administering centre; however, this shall not be an accepted substitute for the signature.

Any amendment of this certificate, or erasure, or failure to complete any part of it, may render it invalid.

The validity of this certificate shall extend until the date indicated for the particular vaccination or prophylaxis. The certificate shall be fully completed in English or in French. The certificate may also be completed in another language on the same document, in addition to either English or French.

ANNEX 7

REQUIREMENTS CONCERNING VACCINATION OR PROPHYLAXIS FOR SPECIFIC DISEASES

1. In addition to any recommendation concerning vaccination or prophylaxis, the following diseases are those specifically designated under these Regulations for which proof of vaccination or prophylaxis may be required for travellers as a condition of entry to a State Party:

Vaccination against yellow fever.

2. Recommendations and requirements for vaccination against yellow fever:
   (a) For the purpose of this Annex:
      (i) the incubation period of yellow fever is six days;
      (ii) yellow fever vaccines approved by WHO provide protection against infection starting 10 days following the administration of the vaccine;
      (iii) this protection continues for 10 years; and
      (iv) the validity of a certificate of vaccination against yellow fever shall extend for a period of 10 years, beginning 10 days after the date of vaccination or, in the case of a revaccination within such period of 10 years, from the date of that revaccination.
   (b) Vaccination against yellow fever may be required of any traveller leaving an area where the Organization has determined that a risk of yellow fever transmission is present.
   (c) If a traveller is in possession of a certificate of vaccination against yellow fever which is not yet valid, the traveller may be permitted to depart, but the provisions of paragraph 2(h) of this Annex may be applied on arrival.
   (d) A traveller in possession of a valid certificate of vaccination against yellow fever shall not be treated as suspect, even if coming from an area where the Organization has determined that a risk of yellow fever transmission is present.
   (e) In accordance with paragraph 1 of Annex 6 the yellow fever vaccine used must be approved by the Organization.
   (f) States Parties shall designate specific yellow fever vaccination centres within their territories in order to ensure the quality and safety of the procedures and materials employed.
   (g) Every person employed at a point of entry in an area where the Organization has determined that a risk of yellow fever transmission is present, and every member of the crew of a conveyance using any such point of entry, shall be in possession of a valid certificate of vaccination against yellow fever.
   (h) A State Party, in whose territory vectors of yellow fever are present, may require a traveller from an area where the Organization has determined that a risk of yellow fever transmission is present, who is unable to produce a valid certificate of vaccination against yellow fever, to be quarantined until the certificate becomes valid, or until a period of not more than six days, reckoned from the date of last possible exposure to infection, has elapsed, whichever occurs first.
   (i) Travellers who possess an exemption from yellow fever vaccination, signed by an authorized medical officer or an authorized health worker, may nevertheless be allowed entry, subject to the provisions of the foregoing paragraph of this Annex and to being provided with information regarding protection from yellow fever vectors. Should the travellers not be quarantined, they may be required to report any feverish or other symptoms to the competent authority and be placed under surveillance.

Chapter 32

ANNEX 8

MODEL OF MARITIME DECLARATION OF HEALTH

To be completed and submitted to the competent authorities by the masters of ships arriving from foreign ports.

Submitted at the port of .... Date ....

Name of ship or inland navigation vessel .... Registration/IMO No .... arriving from ....sailing to ....

(Nationality) (Flag of vessel) .... Master's name ....

Gross tonnage (ship).................

Tonnage (inland navigation vessel).....................

Valid Sanitation Control Exemption/Control Certificate carried on board? yes........... no........... Issued at.................. date.....................

Re-inspection required? yes....... no.......

Has ship/vessel visited an affected area identified by the World Health Organization? yes..... no.....

Port and date of visit ....

List ports of call from commencement of voyage with dates of departure, or within past thirty days, whichever is shorter:

....

Upon request of the competent authority at the port of arrival, list crew members, passengers or other persons who have joined ship/vessel since international voyage began or within past thirty days, whichever is shorter, including all ports/countries visited in this period (add additional names to the attached schedule):

(1) Name .... joined from: (1)................(2)................(3)................

(2) Name .... joined from: (1)................(2)................(3)................

(3) Name .... joined from: (1)................(2)................(3)................

Number of crew members on board...........

Number of passengers on board...............

Health questions

(1) Has any person died on board during the voyage otherwise than as a result of accident?
yes.... no.....

If yes, state particulars in attached schedule. Total no. of deaths ....

(2) Is there on board or has there been during the international voyage any case of disease which you suspect to be of an infectious nature? yes........ no........ If yes, state particulars in attached schedule.

(3) Has the total number of ill passengers during the voyage been greater than normal/expected?
yes.... no.....

How many ill persons? ....

(4) Is there any ill person on board now? yes........ no........ If yes, state particulars in attached schedule.

(5) Was a medical practitioner consulted? yes....... no...... If yes, state particulars of medical treatment or advice provided in attached schedule.

(6) Are you aware of any condition on board which may lead to infection or spread of disease? yes........ no........

If yes, state particulars in attached schedule.

(7) Has any sanitary measure (e.g. quarantine, isolation, disinfection or decontamination) been applied on board? yes .... no......

If yes, specify type, place and date...

(8) Have any stowaways been found on board? yes .... no...... If yes, where did they join the ship (if known)? ....

(9) Is there a sick animal or pet on board? yes .... no........

Note: In the absence of a surgeon, the master should regard the following symptoms as grounds for suspecting the existence of a disease of an infectious nature:

(a) fever, persisting for several days or accompanied by (i) prostration; (ii) decreased consciousness; (iii) glandular swelling; (iv) jaundice; (v) cough or shortness of breath; (vi) unusual bleeding; or (vii) paralysis.

(b) with or without fever: (i) any acute skin rash or eruption; (ii) severe vomiting (other than sea sickness); (iii) severe diarrhoea; or (iv) recurrent convulsions.

I hereby declare that the particulars and answers to the questions given in this Declaration of Health (including the schedule) are true and correct to the best of my knowledge and belief.

Signed ....

Master

Countersigned ....

Ship's Surgeon (if carried)

Date ....

ATTACHMENT TO MODEL OF MARITIME DECLARATION OF HEALTH

Name	Class or rating	Age	Sex	Nationality	Port, date joined ship/vessel	Nature of illness	Date of onset of symptoms	Reported to a port medical officer?	Disposal of case*	Drugs medicines or other treatment given to patient	Comments

* State: (1) whether the person recovered, is still ill or died; and (2) whether the person is still on board, was evacuated (including the name of the port or airport), or was buried at sea.

The ship's medicine chest

INTRODUCTION

All ships subject to the regulations established by the International Maritime Organization (IMO) and International Labour Organization (ILO) must have adequate medical supplies, that are periodically inspected, kept in good condition, and are ready for use whenever required. The quantities needed on board will depend on the duration and destination of the voyage, the number of crew members, and the nature of the cargo.

The medicine chest is designed to hold a range of medicinal products needed for the most common medical emergencies likely to occur on board ship, however distant it is from shore.

Different communities have different methods of treatment. Items specific to national requirements and customs can be added to the list of recommended medicines and medical supplies provided at the end of this chapter. The added items, however, should not be used to replace any of the recommended medicines or medical supplies on the list, but should be integrated into the list together with detailed information about their actions and unwanted effects.

The list assumes that on-board medical treatment is dispensed by an officer working under the responsibility of the master. Ships with a doctor on board may carry an expanded range of medicines and other medical equipment and supplies.

Some of the listed medicines are available only on prescription. As regulations differ from country to country, no advice is given here about obtaining these medicines.

BASIC RULES FOR MANAGING THE MEDICINE CHEST

RESPONSIBILITY

The ship's master is responsible for managing medical supplies kept on board, although he may delegate responsibility for their use and maintenance to a properly trained crew member. Nevertheless, however well-trained, crew members are not medically qualified. A doctor should always be consulted about serious illness or injury or when any doubt exists about the proper action to take in treating a patient.

KEEPING RECORDS

A list of medicines and medical supplies should be carried on board and be regularly updated. The list should include, for each item, such details as expiry date, storage conditions, and quantities remaining after purchase or use. A record of treatment given to any person on board, including the type and quantity of any medicines administered, must be entered in the ship's log. In some countries, it is compulsory to keep such a record.

In addition, the master of the vessel is required to maintain a register of controlled drugs and this register must not be discarded before two years have elapsed after the date of the last entry.

IDENTIFICATION OF MEDICINES

All medicines listed in this guide are identified by their generic or approved name, since local brand (or proprietary) names may differ from country to country. The box or package for every medicine, therefore, should be labelled with its generic name. The dose per tablet, capsule, or vial/ampoule, and the expiry date of each item should be clearly indicated on the package or container. If the label is illegible or if the contents of an opened or unlabelled package or container cannot be identified, the medicine should be destroyed.

STORAGE

Drawers or medicine cabinets should be large enough to store medicines and equipment in an orderly manner so that they are easily identified and available for immediate use. This is particularly important for medicines and equipment used in emergencies: these should be kept separately in the most accessible place. Generally, items of the same type or category should be stored in a box, shelf or drawer, properly labelled. Controlled medicines must be kept apart in a locked compartment, preferably the master's safe, in a room that is locked when unoccupied (see below, under *Controlled drugs*).

All medicines must be kept in good condition and protected against humidity and temperature extremes. When not otherwise specified, they should be stored at room temperature (15–25 °C). A refrigerator should be available nearby for storage of items that must be kept at 2–8 °C. This refrigerator should not be used for any other purpose and should be equipped with a lock.

EXPIRY DATE

An expiry date for a medicine corresponds to the average maximum shelf life for that medicine, given appropriate storage conditions. Medicines must be inspected regularly to make sure they have not reached or exceeded their expiry dates: those that have, should be replaced and then taken to a pharmacy to be destroyed. Certain types of medical equipment also have expiry dates. Moreover, some countries impose fines on ships entering their territory with expired medicinal items on board.

PREGNANCY

Before any medicine is given to a female patient, the ship's doctor or officer designated as health provider should know if the patient is pregnant or breast-feeding and can safely take the medicine.

UNWANTED EFFECTS AND DRUG INTERACTIONS

All medicines have unwanted effects that must be evaluated case-by-case – by the patient, the responsible officer and the consulting doctor – in relation to their benefits. Severe unwanted effects can occur when certain medicines administered simultaneously to a patient interact with each other. A doctor should always be consulted if a patient is already taking medication or if several medicines from the list in this guide have to be used together.

DRUG ALLERGY

Before any drug is administered, the patient should be asked whether he or she knows about or has experienced in the past any allergy, intolerance, or sensitivity to medicines. The patient's answer should be noted in the patient's record. If the patient is unable to answer for whatever reason, that fact should also be recorded. A patient who believes he or she is, or is likely to be, allergic to a medicine should not be given the medicine without medical advice.

Anaphylaxis

Anaphylaxis is one of the most serious, and often life-threatening, forms of allergic reaction. It can occur within a few minutes of exposure to an allergy-causing substance (allergen), which may be a medicine. In some cases the reaction may be delayed for an hour or so. The most common symptoms are urticaria (see Chapter 20, *Skin diseases*) and swelling of the lips, face and throat. The patient may feel flushed and itchy all over. In about half the patients there is breathlessness, wheezing, and swelling of the larynx, which can cause choking. In about a third of cases, there is a marked fall in blood pressure (anaphylactic shock).

Wheezing, difficulty breathing, or low blood pressure calls for immediate treatment, which can be life-saving. The patient should be given:

- adrenaline (epinephrine), 0.3–0.5 ml of 1/1000 solution, intramuscularly on the lateral or anterior thigh, repeated every five minutes if necessary; **PLUS**
- oxygen, at the highest possible flow rate, using a reservoir mask if possible; **PLUS**
- salbutamol (albuterol) inhaler, four puffs via a plastic spacer, repeated every 10 minutes if wheezing and breathlessness persist; **PLUS**
- dexamethasone 4 mg, intravenously if possible, or intramuscularly, then prednisone, 50 mg orally at once and then daily for four days; **PLUS**
- cetirizine, 10 mg orally at once; **PLUS**
- 1–2 litres of normal saline over 30 minutes given by intravenous drip: if blood pressure stays low, this fluid administration may need to be repeated;
- seek medical advice as soon as possible, but **DO NOT** delay giving adrenaline.

If the patient responds and remains well for eight hours, further problems are unlikely without further exposure to the allergen. Patients should be seen by a doctor at the next port to identify the responsible allergen and to develop a plan to prevent recurrent anaphylaxis.

Drug rash and other drug-related skin problems

The commonest type of drug rash resembles the rash of measles: pale-red, irregular blotches. It is most marked on the lower parts of the body.

Any drug can cause this rash, and the drugs given most often – penicillin especially – are the commonest causes. The rash appears within three weeks of starting the drug, but not usually in the first few days. It is not clear whether drug rashes are due to an allergic process. They often clear up even if the drug is continued. Nevertheless, it is safer to stop the drug. If stopping the drug may be dangerous, such as during treatment of a severe infection, medical advice should be sought before stopping it.

Drugs are common causes of urticaria and exfoliative dermatitis (see Chapter 20, *Skin diseases*), in which the skin is red and peeling, like the late stages of a bad sunburn. Some drugs, especially ibuprofen and related drugs, and ciprofloxacin and doxycycline, can cause phototoxicity, in which the effect of ultraviolet light is exacerbated. Patients have a typical sunburn in areas exposed to the sun but it is much more severe than can be accounted for by the sun exposure.

A very severe form of drug reaction is called Stevens-Johnson Syndrome, or Toxic Epidermal Necrolysis: the patient rapidly develops a rash consisting of sharp-edged, dark-red spots, and also large blisters, painful ulcers in the mouth, and fever. This condition is often fatal: **any patient who develops a rash with blistering after taking a drug must be evacuated at once**.

Controlled drugs

Controlled (or "scheduled") drugs are those that, in most countries, are subject to prescription requirements limiting their distribution and use, because of their liability to be abused. Controlled drugs should be obtained only from a pharmacist or other person licensed to supply these medicines. The supplier will need a handwritten order, signed by the master, and formulated according to national requirements. The master has also to sign a receipt for the goods.

The 1961 United Nations Single Convention on Narcotic Drugs includes provisions stipulating that "the international carriage by ships or aircraft of such limited amounts of drugs as may be needed during their journey or voyage for first-aid purposes or emergency cases shall not be considered to be import, export or passage through a country". A second provision stipulates that "appropriate safeguards shall be taken by the country of registry to prevent the improper use of [these] drugs ... or their diversion for illicit purposes".

National regulations of the country visited, however, predominate and must be respected. National authorities of many countries require ships' masters to produce a general declaration of medicines on board and a separate declaration of controlled drugs and to keep a drug register for two years after the date of the last entry in it. The *Maritime Labour Convention (2006)* contains guidance on national authority responsibilities in this matter. Smaller vessels should carry medical supplies in accordance with the relevant national guidelines and in relation to their needs, as determined by length of voyage, and number of crew.

A ship must not carry quantities of controlled drugs larger than those specified by the appropriate national regulations, unless required by a doctor.

Regulations relating to records to be kept concerning the use of controlled drugs vary from country to country. Generally speaking, these records should be kept separate from patients' ordinary medical charts and should give the following information:

- doses given, including the name of the person ordering the dose, the name of the person giving it, and the name of the person receiving it;
- date and time when a dose is lost or spoiled (e.g. broken ampoule, drug prepared but not injected, and so on);

- a running count of remaining stocks, updated after each use;
- a count, made at least weekly, of remaining ampoules, tablets, etc., in store, to be checked against the records of use and the running count.

Ships carrying dangerous goods

Ships carrying dangerous goods have additional medicines, specific antidotes, and special equipment on board, as prescribed in the International Maritime Organization's *Medical First Aid Guide for Use in Accidents Involving Dangerous Goods (MFAG)*[1]. These special items, which are not listed in this guide, should be stored and registered together with the regular medicines and medical supplies carried on board.

SPECIFIC CATEGORIES OF MEDICINES

ANTIBIOTICS

Inflammations or infectious diseases of bacterial origin may be treated with antibiotics, which, however, are ineffective for colds, flu, or other viral infections. Unnecessary administration of antibiotics puts the patient at risk of allergic reactions, unwanted effects, and possible super-infection with resistant organisms. Unnecessary antibiotic use also contributes to the worldwide development of resistant strains of bacteria.

ANTIMALARIAL MEDICINES

Prevention (prophylaxis) of malaria is a continuing process whereby preventive measures and medication change frequently with developments in scientific, particularly pharmacological, capabilities and with growing knowledge of local malaria epidemiology, including risk of infection. It is, therefore, not efficient and certainly not cost-effective to have prophylactic antimalarials in the medical chest on all voyages.

As each tropical or sub-tropical region requires its specific malarial prophylaxis, the master and ship owner must decide, in planning a voyage to potentially malarious areas, what antimalarial medication should be carried on board. The WHO website (http://www.who.int/en/) can be consulted for recommended malarial prophylaxis in specific countries.

ANALGESICS

Pain is a mental phenomenon that may be influenced by psychological and environmental factors. Individual patients vary in their response to treatment. Careful judgement, therefore, should be used in deciding on the best dose and medicine or combination of medicines required to provide pain relief in a given situation. It is important to prescribe with confidence and to assure the patient that the medicine will bring relief. Patients should not be allowed to suffer because of reluctance on the part of a caregiver to administer analgesics.

The analgesics to be carried on board are:

- paracetamol
- acetylsalicylic acid (Aspirin®)
- ibuprofen

- tramadol
- morphine.

These analgesics should cover most pain situations encountered at sea. Once the analgesic drug and starting dose have been decided and the treatment has begun, the patient's pain should be reviewed after two doses. If the pain is not under control, administration of a stronger drug should be started or the dose of the first drug increased if it is less than the recommended maximum.

Fluids for intravenous infusion

PARENTERAL SOLUTIONS

Sodium chloride 0.9%, also called normal saline solution, serves to replace loss of fluid and electrolytes in the body. It may be used in cases of bleeding, dehydration due to severe vomiting or diarrhoea, or when an unconscious patient is unable to drink sufficient fluids. A possible unwanted effect is fluid overload resulting in pulmonary oedema – a risk particularly for patients with underlying heart disease if large quantities of the solution are administered at a high flow rate. The risk is minimal for a young, healthy person with no heart or kidney problems.

QUANTITIES

The amount of fluid to be administered is specified in this guide where appropriate or by the consulting doctor, when outside advice is sought.

FLOW RATE

Rate of flow (drops per minute) should be carefully regulated and monitored at frequent intervals to prevent fluctuations in flow. To prevent air from entering the vein, flow should be stopped before all the solution has been administered. The number of drops per millilitre (ml) varies with the administration set but is usually indicated on the packaging. A rule of thumb is 20 drops per millilitre. If a set delivers 20 drops per ml and the quantity to be administered is 500 ml, i.e. 10 000 (500 × 20) drops of solution, over a four-hour (240 minute) period, the rate of flow would be 42 (10 000 ÷ 240) drops per minute. The volume of solution in the infusion bag should be checked after 15 minutes and the drop rate adjusted if necessary. The solution in the infusion bag should be checked at frequent intervals in order to verify the actual flow rate.

OXYGEN

Oxygen is administered to a patient when the body is not receiving enough from the air or if poisoning from a toxic gas has occurred (see Chapter 11, *Poisoning*). Oxygen should be treated as a drug: the amount to be given, the type of mask to be used, and the duration of use should be prescribed on the medication record.

Oxygen should be given during resuscitation efforts (see Chapter 1, *First aid*). In all other circumstances it should only be administered when advised in this guide or prescribed by a doctor.

Oxygen is usually given by mask to a patient who is breathing without assistance, whether unconscious or conscious.

OXYGEN CYLINDERS

The oxygen cylinder should be carefully identified as such. The colour of the cylinder may vary from country to country, as it has not been stipulated in any international code. To reduce the risk of explosion or fire, the oxygen cylinder should be kept at a distance from sources of heat, sparks or smoking, and its screw thread should not be greased.

Oxygen can be dangerous to patients who have a long-standing history of chronic bronchitis or emphysema. Regular examination of seafarers should ensure that such patients are not on board. Administering oxygen to a passenger always requires prior consultation with a doctor, except in emergencies.

The gas in the cylinder is 100% oxygen. The oxygen concentration that the patient actually breathes will depend on the degree to which the oxygen is diluted with air. The oxygen leaving the cylinder is cold and dry.

NASAL CANNULA

A nasal cannula is more comfortable than a mask, especially in hot climates. It is still unpleasant for patients, especially with flow rates greater than 2 l per minute. High flows of dry oxygen cause drying and possible crusting of the nasal mucous membrane.

OXYGEN MASKS

Different types of oxygen masks may be on board, each with specific operating instructions. There are three main types of mask:

- **standard simple face mask**: with the oxygen tube connected directly to the mask: during respiration the patient draws air around the sides of the mask, thereby diluting the inspired oxygen concentration: a patient taking small, shallow breaths will get a relatively high concentration of oxygen and a patient taking deep breaths a lower concentration;
- **Venturi (or high flow) mask**: offers a choice of seven levels of oxygen concentration, from 24% to 50%, with corresponding flow rate settings for each level: the actual concentration delivered still varies depending on the patient's rate and depth of breathing;
- **mask with reservoir bag**: by adding a reservoir bag, inhalation of air from the room is reduced and the concentration of oxygen breathed in by the patient is increased.

QUANTITIES AND FLOW RATE

The amount of oxygen to be administered is specified in the appropriate sections of this guide or by the doctor consulted where outside advice is sought. Rate of flow (litres per minute) must be carefully regulated by checking the top of the flowmeter ball. The pressure gauge should be verified at frequent intervals and the bottle replaced before it is empty. A 2 litre/200 bar oxygen cylinder contains at most 400 litres of oxygen. At a flow rate of 4 l per minute, it takes 100 minutes to empty the bottle.

LIST OF RECOMMENDED MEDICINES AND EQUIPMENT

ORDER OF LISTING

Medicines are listed in alphabetical order of their generic names.

RECOMMENDED MEDICINE

The choice of medications given in the list below is based on effect, unwanted effects, route of administration, shelf life, worldwide availability, price, storage conditions, and the medical skills officers on board are presumed to possess.

STORAGE

If an item has to be kept "cool" this means that the item deteriorates in quality and efficacy if it is not kept refrigerated.

If an item has to be stored in a "safe", it should be kept in a locked compartment, separate from other medicines and preferably in the master's safe.

Where no indication is given whether a drug has to be taken with food or on an empty stomach, it may be taken with or without food.

ABBREVIATIONS

SC:	subcutaneously
IM:	intramuscularly
IV:	intravenously
IMGS3:	*International Medical Guide for Ships*, 3rd edition (this guide)
MFAG:	*Medical First Aid Guide for Use in Accidents Involving Dangerous Goods*, IMO/WHO/ILO, 2004
ND:	not determined
NSAID:	nonsteroidal anti-inflammatory drug

Generic name	Acetylsalicylic acid
Also known as	■ Aspirin®, Aspro®
Dosage form, strength	■ tablet 300 mg
Indications (on board ship)	■ high dose (600–900 mg): to reduce pain, fever, inflammation ■ low dose (100–150 mg) to inhibit formation of blood clots in angina pectoris, myocardial infarction, stroke
Contraindications	■ peptic ulcer, history of gastrointestinal bleeding, haemophilia, fever in patients under 18, trauma
Consult doctor before using	■ no
Adult dosage	■ for pain and inflammation: 2–3 tablets every 4–6 hours ■ for thrombosis: half a tablet daily
Unwanted effects	■ indigestion ■ gastric bleeding ■ increased bleeding during surgery
Remarks	■ to be used with caution in cardiac failure ■ not to be used if past use has exacerbated asthma ■ not to be used if surgery may be required within 7 days

Generic name	Aciclovir
Also known as	■ Zovirax®, acyclovir
Dosage form, strength	■ tablet 400 mg
Indications (on board ship)	■ treatment of primary or recurrent herpes simplex virus infection ■ may be useful for severe varicella and herpes zoster (doctor should be consulted)
Contraindications	ND
Consult doctor before using	■ not if used according to IMGS3 recommendations
Adult dosage	■ 400 mg 3 times daily for 5–10 days for primary infection or for 3–5 days for recurrence
Unwanted effects	ND
Remarks	■ patient should drink more than 2 l of fluid daily

Generic name	Adrenaline
Also known as	■ epinephrine, adrenaline 1:1000
Dosage form, strength	■ ampoule 1 ml = 1 mg
Indications (on board ship)	■ to raise blood pressure in anaphylaxis ■ to dilate airways in severe asthma or anaphylaxis
Contraindications	■ none in emergencies
Consult doctor before using	■ yes, if possible, but do not delay use in emergency
Adult dosage	■ for anaphylaxis: 0.5 ml, IM, repeated every 5 minutes if needed ■ for severe asthma: 0.5 ml, IM, repeated every 5 minutes if needed
Unwanted effects	■ palpitations ■ cardiac arrhythmia ■ hypertension (high blood pressure) ■ chest pain ■ headache ■ restlessness
Remarks	ND

Generic name	Amethocaine 0.5% eye drops
Also known as	■ tetracaine
Dosage form, strength	■ single-use vial 1 ml
Indications (on board ship)	■ for eye examination and procedures
Contraindications	ND
Consult doctor before using	■ no
Adult dosage	■ 2 drops inside lower eyelid
Unwanted effects	■ transitory burning sensation soon after application
Remarks	■ unused portion to be discarded immediately after use

Generic name	Amoxicillin + clavulanate
Also known as	■ Augmentin®, co-amoxyclav
Dosage form, strength	■ tablet 875 mg/125 mg
Indications (on board ship)	■ to treat infections responsive to this antibiotic
Contraindications	■ allergy to penicillin and beta-lactam antibiotics ■ glandular fever (infectious mononucleosis) ■ liver disease
Consult doctor before using	■ no, if used according to IMGS3 recommendations
Adult dosage	■ one tablet twice daily, taken with food.
Unwanted effects	■ diarrhoea ■ hepatitis due to clavulanate is rare but may be serious
Remarks	■ for ships carrying dangerous goods see MFAG (204) Table 9 ■ to be used with caution in liver disease

Generic name	Artemether
Also known as	■ Larither®
Dosage form, strength	■ ampoule 1 ml (= 80 mg)
Indications (on board ship)	■ treatment of severe malaria
Contraindications	ND
Consult doctor before using	■ as soon as possible but, in emergencies, treatment must be carried out without delay in accordance with IMGS3 recommendations
Adult dosage	■ see under *Malaria* in IMGS3, Chapter 23, *Infectious diseases*
Unwanted effects	■ pain at injection site ■ slow pulse rate ■ fits (convulsions)
Remarks	■ required only for voyages to areas where malaria transmission is a risk

Generic name	Artemether + Lumefantrine
Also known as	■ Riamet ®
Dosage form, strength	■ tablets 20 mg + 120 mg
Indications (on board ship)	■ treatment of malaria
Contraindications	■ not to be used in women in early pregnancy without medical advice
Consult doctor before using	■ not if used according to IMGS3 recommendation
Adult dosage	■ see under *Malaria* in Chapter 23, *Infectious diseases*
Unwanted effects	■ headache ■ dizziness ■ sleep disorder ■ palpitations ■ anorexia ■ nausea ■ vomiting ■ diarrhoea ■ itch ■ rash ■ arthralgia (joint pain) ■ myalgia (muscle pain) ■ weakness ■ fatigue
Remarks	■ not for prophylaxis ■ should not be used together with haloperidol or azithromycin ■ required only for voyages to areas where malaria transmission is a risk

The ship's medicine chest

Generic name	Atropine
Also known as	ND
Dosage form, strength	■ ampoule 1.2 mg/ml
Indications (on board ship)	■ to treat slow heart rate in myocardial infarction ■ to treat organophosphate insecticide poisoning
Contraindications	■ none in emergencies
Consult doctor before using	■ no, in emergencies; yes, in organophosphate insecticide poisoning
Adult dosage	■ for slow heart rate in myocardial infarction: 0.6 mg IM or IV
Unwanted effects	■ dry mouth ■ blurred vision ■ urinary retention ■ hallucinations and psychosis (with very large doses)
Remarks	■ in organophosphate poisoning huge doses may be needed

Generic name	Azithromycin
Also known as	■ Zithromax®
Dosage form, strength	■ tablet 500 mg
Indications (on board ship)	■ to treat infections responsive to this antibiotic
Contraindications	■ allergy to erythromycin or similar (macrolide) antibiotics
Consult doctor before using	■ no, if used according to instructions in IMGS3
Adult dosage	■ as recommended in IMGS3 for the specific infection
Unwanted effects	■ diarrhoea ■ vomiting ■ stomach pain
Remarks	■ for ships carrying dangerous goods, see MFAG (1998) Table 9 ■ not to be given with artemether/lumefantrine or haloperidol ■ to be used with caution in liver disease

Generic name	Ceftriaxone
Also known as	■ Rocephin®
Dosage form, strength	■ ampoule 1 g powder for injection (dissolve in water for injection)
Indications (on board ship)	■ to treat infections responsive to this antibiotic
Contraindications	■ allergy to cephalosporin or penicillin antibiotics
Consult doctor before using	■ no, if used according to IMGS3 instructions
Adult dosage	■ as recommended in IMGS3 for the specific infection
Unwanted effects	■ diarrhoea ■ pain at injection site ■ formation of biliary sludge and kidney stones
Remarks	■ for ships carrying dangerous goods see MFAG (1998), Table 10 ■ if administered IV, no other drug should be given via the same tubing

Generic name	Cetirizine
Also known as	■ Zyrtec®
Dosage form, strength	■ tablet 10 mg
Indications (on board ship)	■ to treat allergy symptoms in hay fever, hives, allergic dermatitis, etc.
Contraindications	■ allergy to cetirizine
Consult doctor before using	■ no
Adult dosage	■ 10 mg daily up to a maximum of 20 mg daily
Unwanted effects	■ drowsiness (in 10–15% of cases) ■ dry mouth ■ headache ■ nausea
Remarks	■ not effective for seasickness ■ relatively non-sedating but may still make crew unsafe to operate machinery or take watch ■ not to be combined with alcohol or sedatives

Generic name	Charcoal, activated
Also known as	ND
Dosage form, strength	■ 50 g in 300 ml purified water
Indications (on board ship)	■ to absorb ingested poisons
Contraindications	■ bowel obstruction
Consult doctor before using	■ yes
Adult dosage	■ 1 g/kg orally up to a maximum of 100 g for first dose ■ for repeat doses, 50 g every 4 hours, if advised by a doctor
Unwanted effects	■ abdominal pain ■ vomiting ■ constipation
Remarks	■ not effective in poisoning with ethanol, methanol, organic solvents, or iron

Generic name	Ciprofloxacin
Also known as	■ Ciproxin®, Cipro®
Dosage form, strength	■ tablet 250 mg
Indications (on board ship)	■ to treat infections responsive to this antibiotic
Contraindications	■ allergy to quinolones
Consult doctor before using	■ no, if used according to IMGS3 instructions
Adult dosage	■ as recommended in IMGS3 for the specific infection ■ to be taken 1 hour before or 2 hours after meals ■ milk and other dairy products to be avoided
Unwanted effects	■ vomiting ■ diarrhoea ■ depression ■ ankle pain ■ makes sunburn worse ■ may increase the effect of caffeine, with headache, palpitations, and nausea
Remarks	ND

Generic name	Cloves, oil of
Also known as	■ *Syzygium aromaticum*
Dosage form, strength	■ oil
Indications (on board ship)	■ toothache
Contraindications	ND
Consult doctor before using	■ no
Adult dosage	■ to be applied to affected tooth with cotton wool soaked in oil of cloves
Unwanted effects	■ irritation of the mucous membranes
Remarks	■ not to be used for more than 48 hours

Generic name	Dexamethasone
Also known as	■ Decadron®
Dosage form, strength	■ ampoule 4mg/ml
Indications (on board ship)	■ to treat life-threatening and severe asthma ■ to treat anaphylaxis ■ to treat severe allergic reactions
Contraindications	■ none in emergencies
Consult doctor before using	■ not in anaphylaxis or in life-threatening asthma; yes, otherwise
Adult dosage	■ for anaphylaxis and life-threatening asthma: 4 mg IM or IV ■ otherwise as advised by a doctor
Unwanted effects	■ with repeated doses exacerbates peptic ulcer ■ euphoria or depression ■ exacerbates diabetes mellitus
Remarks	ND

Generic name	Diazepam
Also known as	■ Valium®
Dosage form, strength	■ tablet 5 mg
Indications (on board ship)	■ to treat alcohol withdrawal
Contraindications	■ severe respiratory disease ■ opioid intoxication ■ severe liver disease ■ myasthenia gravis
Consult doctor before using	■ no
Adult dosage	■ see IMGS3, Chapter 22, *Tobacco, alcohol, and drug use*
Unwanted effects	■ drowsiness ■ confusion
Remarks	■ not to be used in combination with alcohol or opioids ■ operating machinery or taking watch to be avoided for 24 hours after use

Generic name	Docusate with Senna (or equivalent)
Also known as	■ Coloxyl®
Dosage form, strength	■ tablet 50 mg + 8 mg
Indications (on board ship)	■ to avoid straining in patients with anal fissure and haemorrhoids ■ to prevent constipation caused by opioid use
Contraindications	■ suspected bowel obstruction ■ inflammatory bowel disease ■ appendicitis
Consult doctor before using	■ no
Adult dosage	■ 1–2 tablets at bedtime, may be increased to up to 2 tablets twice daily if required
Unwanted effects	■ flatulence ■ abdominal cramps (rare) ■ diarrhoea
Remarks	■ not to be used for longer than 1 week ■ may cause yellow-brown discolouration of urine

Generic name	Doxycycline
Also known as	■ Neo-Dagracycline®, Unidox®, Vibra-S®, Vibramycine®, Doryx®
Dosage form, strength	■ tablet 100 mg
Indications (on board ship)	■ as recommended in IMGS3 for the specific infection
Contraindications	■ allergy to tetracyclines ■ severe liver disease ■ not to be used in children under eight years or pregnant women
Consult doctor before using	■ no, if used according to IMGS3 instructions
Adult dosage	■ as recommended in IMGS3 for the specific infection ■ 1 tablet with 300 ml water ■ to be taken with meals ■ patient to remain sitting or standing for 30 minutes after a dose
Unwanted effects	■ vomiting ■ diarrhoea ■ makes sunburn worse ■ ulceration of the oesophagus (rare)
Remarks	

Generic name	Ethanol 70%, hand cleanser gel
Also known as	ND
Dosage form, strength	■ gel
Indications (on board ship)	■ an alternative to hand-washing when hands are not obviously soiled
Contraindications	■ soiled hands
Consult doctor before using	■ no
Adult dosage	■ enough should be used to cover hands thoroughly and allowed to dry
Unwanted effects	■ dryness, but less than with soap and water
Remarks	■ 70% alcohol liquid hand-cleanser may be used instead

Generic name	Ethanol 70%, liquid
Also known as	ND
Dosage form, strength	■ liquid
Indications (on board ship)	■ to disinfect instruments and surfaces
Contraindications	ND
Consult doctor before using	ND
Adult dosage	■ topical use only
Unwanted effects	ND
Remarks	■ contact with eyes and mucous membranes to be avoided ■ inflammable

Generic name	Fluorescein 1%, strips
Also known as	ND
Dosage form, strength	ND
Indications (on board ship)	■ to detect damage to cornea: damaged area stains yellow/green
Contraindications	ND
Consult doctor before using	ND
Adult dosage	ND
Unwanted effects	ND
Remarks	■ fluorescent effect easier to see if illuminated by a penlight torch fitted with a blue cap ■ for ships carrying dangerous goods, see MFAG (1998) Table 7

Generic name	Frusemide
Also known as	■ Lasix®, furosemide
Dosage form, strength	■ ampoule 4 ml = 40 mg
Indications (on board ship)	■ to treat severe fluid retention in lungs (pulmonary oedema) due to cardiac failure
Contraindications	■ none in an emergency
Consult doctor before using	■ yes, after first dose
Adult dosage	■ 40 mg IV over 10 minutes or (less desirable) IM ■ repeat in 1 hour if necessary
Unwanted effects	■ dehydration ■ loss of potassium ■ hearing loss if given too quickly IV
Remarks	■ onset of action: a few minutes ■ duration of effectiveness: 2–3 hours. ■ for ships carrying dangerous goods see MFAG (2004), Tables 2 and 9

Generic name	Glucagon, ready to use
Also known as	■ Gulcagen®
Dosage form, strength	■ ampoule 1 mg
Indications (on board ship)	■ to treat low blood sugar (hypoglycaemia) due to insulin when oral intake is impossible and intravenous glucose cannot be given
Contraindications	ND
Consult doctor before using	■ not if used in accordance with IMGS3 recommendations
Adult dosage	■ 1 mg IM or SC: response should occur within 15 minutes
Unwanted effects	ND
Remarks	■ effect short-lived ■ glucose to be given orally when patient regains consciousness

Generic name	Haloperidol
Also known as	■ Haldol®
Dosage form, strength	■ ampoule 1 ml = 5 mg
Indications (on board ship)	■ to treat psychotic hallucinations and delusions ■ to treat severe agitation and aggressiveness
Contraindications	■ coma of whatever cause ■ severe alcohol intoxication
Consult doctor before using	■ yes, except in emergencies
Adult dosage	■ 2–10 mg IM, repeated every 2–6 hours if needed ■ maximum: 15 mg in 24 hours
Unwanted effects	■ drowsiness ■ low blood pressure ■ confusion ■ dry mouth ■ urine retention
Remarks	■ not to be used in combination with alcohol ■ not to be used in patients receiving artemether/lumefantrine or azithromycin

Generic name	Hydrocortisone 1% cream
Also known as	ND
Dosage form, strength	■ cream
Indications (on board ship)	■ to treat allergy and some other inflammatory skin conditions
Contraindications	■ open wounds or skin infections caused by bacteria, viruses or fungi
Consult doctor before using	■ no, unless use exceeds one week
Adult dosage	■ to be applied sparingly twice daily ■ after a few days, application to be reduced to once a day
Unwanted effects	■ minimal with short-term use ■ thinning of skin with long-term use
Remarks	■ not to be applied to the eyes

The ship's medicine chest

Generic name	Ibuprofen
Also known as	■ Advil®, Actifen®, Nerofen®, Genpril®, Haltran®, Medipren®, Brufen®
Dosage form, strength	■ coated tablet 400 mg
Indications (on board ship)	■ to treat inflammation ■ to reduce mild-to-moderate pain, especially if associated with inflammation
Contraindications	■ peptic ulcer ■ gastrointestinal bleeding ■ kidney failure ■ liver failure ■ history of exacerbation of asthma after taking aspirin
Consult doctor before using	■ no
Adult dosage	■ 400–800 mg every 6 hours ■ maximum 3200 mg (= 8 tablets) per 24 hours ■ take with food
Unwanted effects	■ stomach pain ■ vomiting ■ diarrhoea ■ headache ■ oedema ■ hypertension
Remarks	■ to be used with caution in asthma ■ not to be used if asthma has been worsened by aspirin

Generic name	Isosorbide dinitrate
Also known as	■ Cedocard®, Isordil®
Dosage form, strength	■ tablet 5 mg
Indications (on board ship)	■ to treat angina pectoris (chest pain) ■ to treat myocardial infarction
Contraindications	■ hypotension (low blood pressure) ■ known heart valve disease ■ head injury ■ treatment with sildenafil (Viagra) and similar drugs
Consult doctor before using	■ no
Adult dosage	■ 1 tablet, sublingual, repeated once after 10 minutes if pain persists ■ to be used preventively if possible before activity likely to cause angina ■ patient to sit or lie down when using ■ tablet to be placed under tongue, patient must not swallow tablet ■ if pain resolves, patient spits out remaining tablet so as to reduce risk of headache
Unwanted effects	■ headache ■ flushing ■ dizziness or fainting ■ palpitations.
Remarks	■ if 2 sublingual tablets over 15 minutes do not relieve pain, treat as for myocardial infarction (see IMGS3, Chapter 14, *Chest pain and other disorders of the heart and circulation*)

Generic name	Lignocaine 1% (without adrenaline)
Also known as	■ Xylocaine®, lidocaine
Dosage form, strength	■ ampoule 5 ml
Indications (on board ship)	■ for local anaesthesia when suturing wounds or performing minor surgery
Contraindications	■ allergy to local anaesthetics
Consult doctor before using	■ no
Adult dosage	■ maximum 200 mg (20 ml of 1% solution) ■ after maximum dose, give no more for 2 hours
Unwanted effects	■ stinging on injection
Remarks	■ intravenous injection must be avoided ■ an ampoule must not be used for more than one patient

Generic name	Loperamide
Also known as	■ Imodium®, Diacure®
Dosage form, strength	■ tablet 2 mg
Indications (on board ship)	■ to treat symptoms of diarrhoea
Contraindications	■ bowel obstruction ■ dysentery ■ acute ulcerative colitis
Consult doctor before using	■ no
Adult dosage	■ starting dose 4 mg ■ then 2 mg with each diarrhoeal motion up to 16 mg (= 8 capsules) per 24 hours
Unwanted effects	■ abdominal pain ■ bloating ■ constipation
Remarks	■ not to be used in children ■ use only when diarrhoea is severe or is hampering with the safe operation of the vessel

Generic name	Mebendazole
Also known as	■ Vermox®
Dosage form, strength	■ tablet 100 mg
Indications (on board ship)	■ to treat intestinal worm infections ■ not effective for tapeworm infection or hydatid disease
Contraindications	■ allergy to mebendazole
Consult doctor before using	■ no, if used according to IMGS3 instructions
Adult dosage	■ as recommended in IMGS3 for the specific infection ■ to be taken with food
Unwanted effects	■ diarrhoea ■ stomach pain
Remarks	ND

Generic name	Metoprolol
Also known as	■ Selokeen®, Lopresor®, Toprol XL®, Betaloc®
Dosage form, strength	■ tablet 100 mg
Indications (on board ship)	■ to treat hypertension (high blood pressure) ■ to treat atrial fibrillation (irregular or rapid heart rate) ■ to treat angina pectoris (chest pain) ■ to prevent migraine.
Contraindications	■ asthma ■ shock ■ heart rate less than 50 beats/min ■ cardiac failure
Consult doctor before using	■ yes
Adult dosage	■ oral, with food ■ for hypertension: 100 mg once daily ■ for angina pectoris: 50 mg twice daily: on medical advice, may be increased to 100 mg twice daily ■ for atrial fibrillation: 50 mg twice daily: on medical advice, may be gradually increased to 100 mg twice daily ■ for migraine: 50 mg twice daily
Unwanted effects	■ tiredness ■ light-headedness ■ cold hands and feet ■ slow heart rate ■ shortness of breath ■ wheezing ■ fainting due to low blood pressure
Remarks	■ to be used with caution in smokers and patients with diabetes mellitus

Generic name	Metronidazole
Also known as	■ Flagyl®
Dosage form, strength	■ tablet 500 mg
Indications (on board ship)	■ to treat infections responsive to this antibiotic
Contraindications	■ allergy to metronidazole
Consult doctor before using	■ no, if used according to IMGS3 instructions
Adult dosage	■ as recommended in IMGS3 for the specific infection ■ to be taken with food if possible to minimize unwanted effects
Unwanted effects	■ metallic taste in the mouth ■ nausea ■ vomiting ■ diarrhoea ■ nerve damage (rare)
Remarks	■ alcohol not to be consumed while taking metronidazole (to avoid flushing, vomiting and diarrhoea) ■ to be used with caution in patients with epilepsy or severe liver disease

Generic name	Miconazole 2% cream
Also known as	■ Daktarin®, Dermacure®, Monistat®
Dosage form, strength	■ cream
Indications (on board ship)	■ to treat fungal skin infections
Contraindications	■ allergy to miconazole
Consult doctor before using	■ no
Adult dosage	■ a thin film to be applied twice daily then for 2 weeks after symptoms have gone ■ hands should be washed promptly after use
Unwanted effects	ND
Remarks	ND

Generic name	Midazolam
Also known as	■ Hypnovel®
Dosage form, strength	■ ampoule 1 ml (= 5 mg)
Indications (on board ship)	■ to terminate epileptic fits
Contraindications	ND
Consult doctor before using	■ no, for emergencies, yes, for repeated use
Adult dosage	■ 0.1–0.2 mg/kg body weight IM or 10 mg intranasally ■ two ampoules should be opened and one drop allowed to drip into alternate nostrils until ampoules are empty
Unwanted effects	■ sedation
Remarks	■ can be used as alternative to haloperidol for sedation of violent patients, who should be given the same dose as used IM for epilepsy

Generic name	Misoprostol
Also known as	■ Cytotec®
Dosage form, strength	■ tablet 200 μg
Indications (on board ship)	■ to prevent post-partum haemorrhage
Contraindications	■ none if given according to IMGS3 recommendations
Consult doctor before using	■ no
Adult dosage	■ 600 μg orally immediately after delivery
Unwanted effects	■ diarrhoea
Remarks	ND

Generic name	Morphine (injectable)
Also known as	ND
Dosage form, strength	■ ampoule 1 ml = 10 mg
Indications (on board ship)	■ to reduce severe pain ■ to reduce pain not relieved by other analgesics
Contraindications	■ coma, unless the patient is dying of a clearly-documented illness, such as cancer ■ severe liver disease ■ asthma ■ severe respiratory disease except pneumonia or pleurisy associated with severe pain ■ to be used with caution in patients known to have epilepsy, head injury, acute alcohol intoxication, withdrawal, shock (of whatever cause)
Consult doctor before using	■ yes, if doses exceeding those recommended in IMGS3 are needed or if duration of treatment exceeds 48 hours
Adult dosage	■ see IMGS3, Chapter 3, *Pain management*
Unwanted effects	■ sedation ■ confusion ■ nausea ■ vomiting ■ low blood pressure ■ respiratory depression ■ small pupils ■ constipation
Remarks	■ onset of action: 15–30 minutes ■ duration of effectiveness: 2–3 hours ■ controlled drug: must comply with regulations ■ overdose reversed with naloxone 0.8 mg IM repeated as required ■ laxative to be given early if use for over 48 hours likely ■ for ships carrying dangerous goods see MFAG (2004) Tables 7, 8, 10 and 13

Generic name	Morphine (oral)
Also known as	ND
Dosage form, strength	■ liquid 1 mg/ml
Indications (on board ship)	■ to reduce severe pain likely to last several days in patients able to eat and drink
Contraindications	■ as for morphine given by injection
Consult doctor before using	■ not if used according to IMGS3 recommendations
Adult dosage	■ see IMGS3, Chapter 3, *Pain management*
Unwanted effects	■ as for morphine given by injection
Remarks	■ should be preferred to injected morphine for patients able to take medication orally

Generic name	Naloxone
Also known as	■ Narcan®
Dosage form, strength	■ ampoule 1 ml (= 0.4 mg)
Indications (on board ship)	■ to reverse effects of opioids, especially in cases of overdose
Contraindications	ND
Consult doctor before using	■ not in emergencies
Adult dosage	■ 0.4 mg IM, repeated as needed ■ response should be rapid: if no response to 5 doses, diagnosis is not opioid overdose
Unwanted effects	ND
Remarks	■ for use only in emergencies

Generic name	Omeprazole
Also known as	■ Losec®, Prilosec®
Dosage form, strength	■ tablet 20 mg
Indications (on board ship)	■ to treat gastro-oesophageal reflux ■ to treat peptic ulcer disease
Contraindications	ND
Consult doctor before using	■ no
Adult dosage	■ starting dose 20 mg once daily before a meal, preferably in the evening ■ dose increased to 40 mg daily if symptoms persist ■ in gastrointestinal haemorrhage: 40 mg twice daily
Unwanted effects	■ nausea ■ diarrhoea
Remarks	ND

Generic name	Ondansetron
Also known as	■ Zofran®
Dosage form, strength	■ tablet 4 mg
Indications (on board ship)	■ to prevent vomiting ■ to prevent seasickness
Contraindications	ND
Consult doctor before using	■ not for single doses
Adult dosage	■ one tablet, preferably taken before the stimulus to vomiting
Unwanted effects	■ headache ■ fatigue ■ constipation
Remarks	■ non-sedating

Generic name	Oral rehydration salts
Also known as	■ Repolyte®, Gastrolyte®, Dioralyte®
Dosage form, strength	■ sachets of powder for reconstitution
Indications (on board ship)	■ to prevent or treat dehydration, especially due to diarrhoea
Contraindications	ND
Consult doctor before using	■ no
Adult dosage	■ as recommended in IMGS3 ■ correct amount of boiled, cooled tap water (not less water than specified) to be added to the entire contents of one sachet, shaken or stirred until all the powder dissolved ■ solution keeps for 24 hours
Unwanted effects	■ vomiting
Remarks	■ the patient should drink plain water when thirsty between doses ■ for ships carrying dangerous goods, see MFAG (1998) Tables 8, 10 and 11

Generic name	Oxymetazoline 0.5% (or equivalent)
Also known as	■ Drixine®
Dosage form, strength	■ drops
Indications (on board ship)	■ to treat nasal obstruction due to allergies or viral infection ■ to improve sinus drainage in sinusitis
Contraindications	■ use of anti-depressants
Consult doctor before using	■ no
Adult dosage	■ 2–3 drops in each nostril twice daily or only at night if disturbed sleep is the main complaint
Unwanted effects	■ stinging or burning in nose or throat ■ dry nasal mucosa ■ rebound obstruction
Remarks	■ not to be used for more than 5 days ■ not for use in the eye

Generic name	Paracetamol
Also known as	■ acetaminophen, Tylenol®, Panadol®
Dosage form, strength	■ tablet 500 mg
Indications (on board ship)	■ to reduce pain and fever (but not inflammation)
Contraindications	■ liver disease
Consult doctor before using	■ no
Adult dosage	■ 1000 mg every 6 hours ■ maximum 4000 mg (= 8 tablets) per 24 hours
Unwanted effects	■ rare at normal doses
Remarks	■ doses greater than 150 mg/kg can cause severe liver damage ■ many over-the-counter products contain paracetamol: if patient is taking one of these products, care must be taken not to exceed maximum dose ■ for ships carrying dangerous goods, see MFAG Tables 7, 8 and 13

Generic name	Permethrin 1% lotion
Also known as	■ Loxazol®, Elimite®, Nix®
Dosage form, strength	■ lotion
Indications (on board ship)	■ to eliminate hair, pubic, and body lice
Contraindications	ND
Consult doctor before using	■ no
Adult dosage	■ to be applied to washed, damp hair or skin, rubbed in, left for 10 minutes, then rinsed off ■ a fine-tooth comb should be used to remove eggs ■ to be repeated after one week ■ hands to be washed to remove lotion
Unwanted effects	■ increased likelihood of skin irritation in cases of scabies
Remarks	■ for external use only ■ not to be applied to the eyes or mucous membranes ■ to treat clothes and bed linen see IMGS3, Chapter 20, *Skin diseases*

Generic name	Permethrin 5% lotion
Also known as	■ Lyclear®
Dosage form, strength	■ lotion
Indications (on board ship)	■ to treat scabies
Contraindications	ND
Consult doctor before using	■ no
Adult dosage	■ to be applied to clean, dry skin from chin down, left on for 12 hours, then washed with soapy water and rinsed ■ to be repeated after 7 days
Unwanted effects	■ increased likelihood of skin irritation
Remarks	■ for external use only ■ not to be applied to the eyes or mucous membranes ■ to treat clothes and bed linen see IMGS3, Chapter 20, *Skin diseases*

Generic name	Povidone iodine ointment 10% and solution 10%
Also known as	■ Betadine®, Povidine®
Dosage form, strength	■ ointment, liquid
Indications (on board ship)	■ to disinfect skin and wounds
Contraindications	■ allergy to iodine
Consult doctor before using	■ no
Adult dosage	■ ointment to be applied thinly with gauze 1–2 times a day
Unwanted effects	■ skin irritation
Remarks	■ contact with eyes and mucous membranes to be avoided ■ not to be used with serious burns or deep puncture wounds ■ not to be used for more than 1 week

The ship's medicine chest

Generic name	Prednisone
Also known as	■ prednisolone
Dosage form, strength	■ tablet 25 mg
Indications (on board ship)	■ to treat severe asthma ■ to treat other inflammatory conditions (on medical advice)
Contraindications	ND
Consult doctor before using	■ not if used in accordance with IMGS3 recommendations
Adult dosage	■ see under *Asthma* in IMGS3, Chapter 15, *Respiratory diseases* ■ to be taken with food
Unwanted effects	■ exacerbates diabetes mellitus, depression or euphoria
Remarks	ND

Generic name	Salbutamol aerosol
Also known as	■ albuterol, Ventolin®, Proventil®
Dosage form, strength	■ inhaler 0.1 mg/dose with volume spacer
Indications (on board ship)	■ to treat asthma ■ to treat chronic bronchitis ■ to treat emphysema ■ to treat other lung diseases
Contraindications	ND
Consult doctor before using	■ no
Adult dosage	■ for symptoms: 2 puffs every 4 hours up to 12 puffs maximum per day ■ in severe asthma, up to 10 puffs repeated every 15 minutes
Unwanted effects	■ dry mouth ■ throat irritation ■ tremor ■ nervousness ■ dizziness ■ excitement ■ rapid heartbeat ■ headache
Remarks	■ inhaler should be shaken well before use ■ plastic spacer (Volumatic ®) should always be used ■ for ships carrying dangerous goods, see MFAG (2004) Table 9

Generic name	Sodium chloride 0.9% infusion
Also known as	■ NaCl 0.9%, saline solution
Dosage form, strength	■ plastic bottle, 1 litre
Indications (on board ship)	■ for fluid replacement
Contraindications	ND
Consult doctor before using	■ as soon as possible but not in emergencies if used in accordance with IMGS3 recommendations
Adult dosage	■ see appropriate IMGS3 text or as advised by a doctor
Unwanted effects	■ cardiac overload and pulmonary oedema if large doses are administered at a high flow rate
Remarks	■ for ships carrying dangerous goods see MFAG (1998) Table 7 (eye bath to treat chemicals in the eye)

Generic name	Tetracycline 1% ointment
Also known as	ND
Dosage form, strength	■ ointment
Indications (on board ship)	■ to treat minor eye infections ■ to prevent infection following damage to the cornea
Contraindications	■ allergy to tetracyclines
Consult doctor before using	■ not if used according to IMGS3 recommendations
Adult dosage	■ 1 cm ointment to be applied twice daily to inner surface of lower eyelid
Unwanted effects	ND
Remarks	■ to be kept refrigerated once opened ■ applicator tip should not be touched ■ use of a tube to be limited to one patient ■ for ships carrying dangerous goods, see MFAG (1998) Annex 7

Generic name	Vitamin K
Also known as	■ Konakion®, phytomenadione
Dosage form, strength	■ ampoule 1 ml = 10 mg
Indications (on board ship)	■ to reverse excessive or unwanted effect of warfarin or related drugs
Contraindications	ND
Consult doctor before using	■ yes
Adult dosage	■ for life-threatening situations (trauma, major bleeding): 10 mg orally or IM ■ for minor bleeding: 1–2 mg orally
Unwanted effects	■ pain at the injection site if given IM ■ anaphylaxis, if given IV
Remarks	■ not effective for bleeding disorders in liver failure ■ for ships carrying dangerous goods, see MFAG Table 14

Generic name	Water for injection
Also known as	ND
Dosage form, strength	■ ampoule 5 ml
Indications (on board ship)	■ reconstitution of injectable drugs provided as powders
Contraindications	ND
Consult doctor before using	ND
Adult dosage	ND
Unwanted effects	ND
Remarks	■ ampoule to be discarded if not used immediately

Generic name	Zidovudine plus Lamivudine
Also known as	■ Combivir®
Dosage form, strength	■ tablet, 300 mg + 150 mg
Indications (on board ship)	■ prophylaxis against HIV infection after needle-stick injury
Contraindications	■ allergy to either component ■ pre-existing HIV infection
Consult doctor before using	■ yes
Adult dosage	■ one tablet twice daily for four weeks
Unwanted effects	■ Common: headache, fatigue and malaise, insomnia, nausea, vomiting, diarrhoea or constipation, cough, loss of appetite, muscle soreness or weakness ■ Uncommon but potentially serious: low white blood cell count, anaemia, hepatitis, severe muscle weakness, pancreatitis
Remarks	■ Seek medical advice if severe or sustained abdominal pain occurs during treatment

Generic name	Zinc oxide
Also known as	ND
Dosage form, strength	■ paste or ointment, 20%
Indications (on board ship)	■ protection of irritated skin
Contraindications	ND
Consult doctor before using	■ no
Adult dosage	■ apply liberally to affected skin twice daily and after washing
Unwanted effects	■ soiling of clothes
Remarks	■ a 500 g jar should be carried

The ship's medicine chest

		Category	Recommended item	Quantity per 10 crew
	1	RESUSCITATION EQUIPMENT		
		Appliance for the administration of oxygen	Portable oxygen set, complete, containing:	1
			1 oxygen cylinder, 2 l/200 bar	1
			1 spare oxygen cylinder, 2 l/200 bar	1
			Pressure regulating unit and flow meter with tubes such that ship's industrial oxygen can also be used	1
			3 disposable face masks of choice: including simple face mask and non-rebreathing mask	3
		Oropharyngeal airway	Guedel airway (Mayo-tube): sizes medium and large	2
		Mechanical aspirator	Manual aspirator to clear upper airways, including 2 catheters	1
		Bag and mask resuscitator	Ambubag (or equivalent); supplied with large, medium and small masks	1
		Cannula for mouth-to-mouth resuscitation	Brook Airway, Lifeway, pocket face mask or equivalent	1
	2	DRESSING MATERIAL AND SUTURING EQUIPMENT		
		Adhesive dressings	Assorted wound-plaster or plaster strips, water-resistant	200
		Sterile gauze compresses	Sterile gauze compresses, 5 x 5 cm, sterile	100
			Sterile gauze compresses, 10 x 10 cm, sterile	100
		Gauze roll	Gauze roll, 5cm and 90 cm or 60 cm x 100 m, non sterile	1
		Gauze dressing with non-adherent surface	Non-adherent gauze dressing, square, 10 cm	100
		Vaseline gauze	Paraffin gauze dressing, 10 x 10 cm, sterile	50
		Bandage	Elastic fixation bandage, 4 m x 6 cm	3
		Sterile compression bandages	First-aid absorbent gauze-covered cotton pad sewn onto a cotton bandage (ambulance dressing), small/medium/large	5
		Tubular gauze for finger bandage	Tubular gauze bandage for finger bandage with applicator, 5 m	1
		Adhesive elastic bandage	Adhesive elastic bandage, 4 m x 6 cm	10
		Triangular sling	Triangular sling	5
		Sterile sheet for burn victims	Sterile sheet for burn patients	1
		Honey for dressing burns	1 kg	1
		Adhesive sutures or zinc oxide bandages	Adhesive tape, waterproof, skin-friendly, 5 x 1.25 cm	10
		Q-tips	Q-tips (wooden)	100
		Safety pins	Safety pins (stainless steel) 12 pcs	50

The ship's medicine chest

		Butterfly sutures	Butterfly sutures, Steristrip® or Leukostrip®, sterile	20
		Skin adhesive	2-octyl cyanoacrylate liquid, 0.5 ml	2
		Suturing equipment	Sutures, absorbable with curved non-traumatic needles, 1-O, 3-O & 4-O or 5-O	10 each
				10
		Gloves	Disposable examination gloves	50
			Surgical gloves sizes 6.5, 7.5, 8.5, sterile, in pairs	3 of each size
	3	INSTRUMENTS		
		Disposable scalpels	Scalpel, sterile, disposable	20
		Stainless-steel instrument box	Instrument box (stainless steel)	1
		Scissors	Operating scissors, straight (stainless steel)	1
			Bandage scissors (stainless steel)	1
		Forceps	Splinter forceps, pointed (stainless steel)	3
			Teeth tissue forceps (stainless-steel)	1
		Needle holder	Needle holder, Mayo-Hegar, 180 mm, straight	1
		Haemostatic clamps	Haemostatic clamp, Halstead mosquito, 125 mm, stainless steel	3
		Disposable razors	Razor, disposable	50
	4	EXAMINATION AND MONITORING EQUIPMENT		
		Disposable tongue depressors	Tongue depressors, disposable	100
		Reactive strips for urine analysis	Reactive strips for urine analysis: blood/glucose/protein/ nitrite/leukocytes, 50 paper strips	100
		Microscope slides	Microscope slides	100
		Stethoscope	Stethoscope	1
		Aneroid sphygmomanometer	Sphygmomanometer (blood pressure set), preferably automatic	1
		Standard thermometer	Thermometer, digital if possible	1
		Rectal thermometer	Thermometer, digital if possible	1
		Hypothermic thermometer	Thermometer 32°–34°, digital if possible	1
		Penlight	Penlight + blue cover	1
	5	EQUIPMENT FOR INJECTION, INFUSION, AND CATHETERIZATION		
		Equipment for injection	Syringes, Luer connection, 2 ml, sterile, disposable	50
			Syringes, Luer connection, 5 ml, sterile, disposable	50
			Hypodermic subcutaneous needle, Luer connection, 16 x 0.5 mm, sterile, disposable	20
			Hypodermic intramuscular needle, Luer connection, 40 x 0.8 mm, sterile, disposable	20
			Needles, 19G, blunt, "drawing up" type	20
		Equipment for infusion	Intravenous infusion cannula 16G (1.2 mm) and 22G (0.8 mm), Luer-lock connection, sterile non-recap type	10 each
			Intravenous giving set, Luer-lock connection, sterile	3

			Tourniquet, blood-taking type, to be used with intravenous infusion cannula	1
		Bladder drainage equipment	Penile sheath set with condom catheter, tube, and bag	2
			Short-term urine catheter with soft-eye straight tip Thieman No.12 and No.16 or equivalent, sterile, individually packed, prelubricated or with additional lignocaine/chlorhexidine lubricant	2
			Urine collecting bag and tube	2
	6	GENERAL MEDICAL AND NURSING EQUIPMENT		
		Eye protection	Plastic goggles or full-face masks	2
		Plastic apron	Disposable	20
		Kidney dish	Kidney dish, stainless steel, 825 ml	2
		Plastic backed towels	Towels, plastic backed, absorbent, 600 x 500 mm	10
		Safety box	Safety box for sharps disposal, 5 l	1
		Mask	Mask, duckbill type, disposable	50
		Tape measure	Tape measure, vinyl coated, 1.5 m	1
		Draw sheets	Draw sheet, plastic 90 x 180 cm	2
		Bedpan	Bedpan, stainless steel	1
		Hot-water bottle	Hot-water bag	1
		Urine bottle	Urinal, male (plastic)	1
		Ice bag	ColdHotpack Maxi	1
		Aluminium foil blanket	Aluminium foil blanket	1
		Condoms	Male condoms	100
		Wash bottle	Plastic wash bottle, 250 ml	1
		Plastic bottle	Bottle, 1 litre, plastic with screw top	3
		Dressing tray	Stainless steel dressing tray, 300 x 200 x 30 mm	1
		Plastic apron	Apron, protection, plastic, disposable	20
		Bowl	Bowl, stainless steel, 180 ml	3
		Specimen jars	Jars, plastic, with lids and labels, 100 ml	10
		Plaster-of-Paris bandage	Bandages, POP, 5 cm and 10 cm x 2.7 m	12 each
		Stockinet	Sizes for arm and leg splints, 10 m roll	1 each
		Cotton wool	Cotton wool roll, 500 g	10
		Alcohol swabs	70% alcohol swabs for skin cleansing prior to injection	200
		Nail brush	Nail brush	1
	7	IMMOBILIZATION AND TRANSPORTATION EQUIPMENT		
		Malleable splints	Malleable finger splint	
			Malleable forearm/hand splint	

Endnote

1. *Medical first aid guide for use in accidents involving dangerous goods (MFAG)*, London, International Maritime Organization, 2004.

Forms for case reporting, referral, and evacuation

Information about a seafarer's injury or illness should be recorded on standardized forms to ensure that all important medical details are provided to medical care providers, whether on board or shore-based, or to officials, such as coroners and the police.

This information may also be of interest to others, including insurers, legal representatives, or ship owners. However interested these parties may be, they do not have a right to any medical information about the patient. These forms, therefore, should not be used to communicate with anyone not concerned with the medical care of the crew member.

Four sample forms are proposed here:

- **A ship master's report form**, to be completed by the ship's master assisted by the ship's doctor or crew member assigned to basic medical duties: this form, which should be filed in the ship's medical log, provides a brief but sufficiently comprehensive record of every medical case managed on board.
- **A ship's identity and navigational status form**, to be used when requesting evacuation of an injured or sick seafarer.
- **A patient health status form**, providing the most important aspects of the medical history, medical treatment, and other pertinent medical information that should accompany a patient being evacuated to an on-shore medical facility.
- **A primary physician's report form**, which an on-shore physician assigned to the care of a sick or injured seafarer should use to note all pertinent details of the case.

Ship master's report form

Date of report ______________________________

****

Ship's identity and navigation status

Name ______________________________

Owner ______________________________

Name and address of on-shore agent ______________________________
____

Position (latitude, longitude) at onset of illness ______________________________

Destination and ETA (expected time of arrival) ______________________________
____

****

The patient and the medical problem

Surname and first name ______________________________

Sex ______________ Male ☐ Female ☐

Date of birth (dd-mm-yyyy) ______________________________

Nationality ____________________

Seafarer registration number ______________________

Shipboard job title ______________________

Hour and date when taken off work ______________________

Hour and date when returned to work ______________________

****

Injury or illness

Hour and date of injury or onset of illness ____________________

Hour and date of first examination or treatment ____________________

Location on ship where injury occurred ____________________

Circumstances of injury ____________________

____

Symptoms ____________________

Findings of physical examination ____________________

____

Findings of X-ray or laboratory tests ____________________

Overall clinical impression before treatment ____________________

____

Treatment given on board ____________________

____

Overall clinical impression after treatment ____________________

____

****

Telemedical consultation

Hour and date of initial contact ____________________

Mode of communication (radio, telephone, fax, other) ____________________

Surname and first name of telemedical consultant ____________________

Details of telemedical advice given ____________________

____

****

N.B. Attach all relevant medical reports to this report form.

Ship's identity and navigational status form

(To be used when calling for medical evacuation)

Vessel name ______________________________

Call sign ______________________________

Date and time (GMT) ______________________________

Communications resources ______________________________

Flag of registry ______________________________

Home port ______________________________

Vessel classification ______________________________

Helicopter deck ______________Yes ☐ No ☐

Length (m) ______________________________

Position (latitude/longitude) ______________________________

Course ______________________________

Speed ______________________________

Intended port of destination ______________________________

Nearest port ______________________________

Other possible ports of call ______________________________

On-scene sea state ______________________________

Wind direction ______________________________

Wind speed ______________________________

Visibility ______________________________

Weather conditions ______________________________

Patient health status form

(To accompany patient being evacuated)

Surname and first name________________________________

Age (years)______________________________________

Sex________

Time (hour) and date____________________

Vital signs

Blood pressure (systolic/diastolic)________

Pulse (beats/min)____________________

Body temperature (oral), note F or C____________________

Presenting medical problem: symptoms, site(s) of pain or injury, time of onset, duration of problem, contributing factors.____

Treatment given (medication, dressings, etc.)______________________________

Telemedical advice received____

Other current medical problems______________________________________

Past history of significant medical problems ______________________________

Current medication being taken (generic **and** brand names; dosage; time of last dose)

Primary physician's report form

(For use by an on-shore physician caring for a sick or injured seafarer)

Administrative information

Patient

Surname____________________ First name____________________

Sex________

Date of birth (dd-mm-yyyy)________________

Nationality________________

Occupation____________________

Seafarer registration number____________________

Insurance claims administrator/Ship's agent

Name____

Claims reference No.________________________

Telephone No.____________________________

Fax No._________________________________

E-mail address_________________________________

Employer

Name____

Telephone No.____________________________

Fax No._________________________________

E-mail address_________________________________

Medical information

Key dates

- Date of injury or of onset of illness (dd-mm-yyyy)____________________
- Dates of previous medical consultations (dd-mm-yyyy)_______________
- Date of current consultation (dd-mm-yyyy)________________________

History

- Symptoms or (in the case of injury) circumstances ____________________________

____

- Personal history pertinent to current illness ____________________
- Clinical examination ____________________
- Findings of diagnostic tests (X-ray, CT or MRI scans, lab. tests, etc.)____________________
- Diagnoses
  - 1____________________
  - 2____________________
  - 3____________________

Summary notes of contact with telemedical service____________________

- Treatment prescribed____________________
- Reasons for stopping treatment ____________________
- Suggested follow-up action (examinations, tests, treatment, etc.)____________________
- Fitness to work and restrictions on shipboard activities____________________

Physician's professional identity

Name____________________

Issued by____________________

Date issued____________________

Speciality____________________

Telephone No.____________________

Fax No.____________________

E-mail address____________________

Office address____________________

Signature____________________

Index

Abandoning ship, 339–340
Abdominal injuries
  blunt abdominal injuries, 59–61
  penetrating abdominal injuries, 61
Abdominal pain, 149–152
  red flags, 151–152
Abdominal pain, severe
  appendicitis, 152–153
  bowel obstruction, 155–156
  pancreatitis, 153–155
Abscess (see Skin abscess)
Acne, 211
Acquired immunodeficiency syndrome (AIDS)
  later stages of HIV and AIDS, 206
  post-exposure prophylaxis, 207
  treatment of HIV Infection, 206
Acute pain in the scrotum
  epididymitis, 200
  testicular torsion, 200–201
  testicular inflammation (orchitis), 201
  trauma to the scrotum, 201
Alcohol intoxication
  alcohol withdrawal, 235
  delirium tremens, DTs, 235–238
  "the shakes", 235
Amphetamines, 243–244
Anatomical terms and descriptions, 375–376
Angina pectoris
  blocked arteries in the legs, 137–138
  complications of myocardial infarction
    abnormal heart rhythm (cardiac arrhythmia), 135–136
    congestive heart failure, 136
  deep vein thrombosis, 138
  palpitations, 136–137
Asthma, 145–147

Bacterial skin infections
  carbuncles and furuncles (furunculosis), 216
  impetigo, 215–216
Balanitis, 201–202
Barber's rash
  folliculitis, 210
  pseudofolliculitis, 210
  tinea barbae, 211
Basic life support
  mouth-to-mouth rescue breathing, 3–4
  mouth-to-nose rescue breathing, 4
  use of automatic external defibrillators, 7–9
  using a bag and mask resuscitator, 4–7
Bell's palsy, 125–126
Bites and stings
  jellyfish stings, 102
  rat bites, 101
  scorpions and spiders, 103–104
  sea urchins, 103
  snake bites, 101–102
  venomous fish, 102–103
Bleeding
  bleeding from the nose, 11–12
  bleeding wounds, 11
Bleeding from the gastrointestinal tract (gastrointestinal haemorrhage)
  anal fissure, 168
  anal pruritis (anal itch), 169
  haemorrhoids (piles), 168–169
  heavy lower gastrointestinal bleeding, 167–168
  heavy upper gastrointestinal bleeding, 165–167
Blood
  blood and anaemia, 388–389
Bronchitis
  bronchitis due to cigarette smoking, 139–140
  bronchitis due to infection, 139
Bronchiectasis, 140
Burial at sea, 336–337

Cannabis intoxication, 238–239
Cells, 375
Cellulitis and erysipelas
  cellulitis, 221–222
  erysipelas, 221–223
  cellulitis arising from wounds exposed to estuary or seawater, 222–223
Chaps, 211–212
Charges
  charges for baggage, cargo, containers, conveyances, goods or postal parcels, 408
  charges for health measures regarding travellers, 407–408
Chemical splashes, 85
  flash burns (arc eye), 38
Chest injuries
  flail chest, 63–64
  penetrating chest wounds, 65–66
  pneumothorax, 64
  simple rib fracture, 62–63
  spontaneous pneumothorax, 64
  tension pneumothorax, 64–65
Childbirth
  caring for the baby after delivery, 191–192
  caring for the mother after delivery, 192–193
  managing the birth, 190–191
  managing the early stages of childbirth, 190
  problems after childbirth
    after pains, 194
    difficulty passing urine, 194
    discharge of the lochia, 193
    post-partum chills, 193

Index

puerperal sepsis (puerperal fever or childbirth fever), 194
post-partum haemorrhage, 193
preparing for the birth, 188–190
Choking, abdominal thrusts
in a conscious patient, 10
in an unconscious patient, 10
on yourself, 10
Circulatory system, 379
Clothing on fire, 79
Cocaine ("coke", "snow", etc.), 242–243
Common cold, 140–141
Consent, of the patient, 105–106

Death, signs of, 333–334
Dermatitis
allergic contact dermatitis, 213–214
eczema (atopic dermatitis), 213
irritant contact dermatitis, 212–213
Definitions, purpose and scope, principles and responsible authorities
definitions, 393–397
purpose and scope, 397–398
Dental problems
a bleeding socket, 288–289
lost fillings and broken teeth, 288
lost teeth, 289
pericoronitis, 287–288
periodontal disease (gum inflammation), 287
pulpitis and peri-apical abscess, 287
red flags, 288
tooth decay (caries), 287
Diarrhoea
antibiotic-associated colitis, 162–163
Crohn's disease, 161–162
dysentery, 158
foodborne illness
diarrhoea with blood in the stools, 156–158
symptom, 156–158
vomiting, 156
watery diarrhoea, 156
food poisoning from marine toxins
ciguatera fish, 159–160
scombroid fish, 160
inflammatory bowel disease (colitis), 160
traveller's diarrhoea, 158–159
ulcerative colitis, 160–161
Digestive system, 381–386
Disposal of liquid and solid wastes, 360
Disposal of the body, 335–336
Dressing wounds that cannot be closed, 77

Ectopic pregnancy, 186
Electrical burns and electrocution
electrical burns, 84
electrical shocks from electronic weapons, 85
electrocution, 84–85
Endocrine system, 387–388
Evacuation by helicopter, 293–295
Examining a dead body, 334–335
Eye diseases, noninfectious
subconjunctival haemorrhage, 39
cataract, 39
glaucoma
acute angle closure glaucoma (or acute congestive glaucoma), 40
primary open angle glaucoma, 40
Eye injuries
a blow on or near the eye, 35–36
arc eyes ("welder's flash"), 38
chemical burns, 38
corneal abrasion, 36
foreign bodies embedded in the eye, 37
loose foreign bodies, 36–37
red flags, 34–35
wounds of the eyelids and eyeball, 37–38

First aid on board
abc sequence of basic life support, 1–2
airway, 2
breathing, 2–3
circulation, 3
shake and shout, 2
"Flashbacks", 245–246
Food and water for rescued survivors, 348–349
Food hygiene
food-handlers, 353
food service facilities, 354
food storage
non-refrigerated items, 354–355
refrigerated items, 355–356
the galley (ship's kitchen), 356–357
toilet and washing facilities, 357
Fungal skin infections
tinea corporis (ringworm), 214
tinea cruris (jock itch, dhobie itch), 215
tinea pedis (athlete's foot), 214

Genital ulcers, 198–200
Gonococcal pharyngitis, 198
Gonococcal proctitis, 198
Gout, 225–226

Hallucinogen intoxication
lysergic acid diethylamide (LSD), 245
phencyclidine ("PCP", "angel dust"), 245
plant hallucinogens, 245
Hay fever, 144–145
Headache
common causes of headache, 116
uncommon causes or forms of headache, 117
red flags, 117–118
Head injuries
general note on head injuries, 27–28
post-concussion syndrome, 30–31
skull fractures, 28
traumatic brain injury (brain damage), 28–30
Health documents
certificates of vaccination or other prophylaxis, 406
general rule, 405
maritime declaration of health, 406
ship sanitation certificates, 406–407
Heat burns and scalds, 79–83
infection of a burn, 83
respiratory tract burns, 83
Heat stroke, 87–88
Heat stroke, how to prevent, 88–89
heat exhaustion (or "heat collapse"), 89
stoker's cramps, 89
Hernia
inguinal (groin) hernia, 170–171
complications, 170–171

Immune system, 389–391
allergy, 390–391
Indigestion and pain related to meals
gastro-oesophageal reflux disease, 163
peptic ulcer, 163–164
complications, 163–164
red flags, 164–165
Infections, common terms
fever, 250
onset, 249
rash, 250
Infections, how they spread, 247–249
Infections (see also Preventing communicable diseases)
anthrax, 254
chickenpox and shingles (varicella-zoster virus)
chickenpox, 255
complications, 255–256
shingles (herpes zoster), 256
complications, 256–257
cholera, 257–258
dengue, 258–259
complications, 259
diphtheria, 259–260
ear infections
complications, 261–262
infection of the outer ear (otitis externa), 260–261
infection of the middle ear (otitis media), 261
hand infections in seafarers and fishers, 262
infectious mononucleosis (glandular fever), 262–263
influenza
avian influenza (H5N1, "bird flu"), 264–265
human influenza, 263–264
complications, 264
malaria, 265–269
complications, 266–267
meningitis and meningococcal infection, 269–270
mumps, 270–271
plague, 271–272
complications, 271–272
rabies, 272–273
rubella (German measles), 273
SARS (severe acute respiratory syndrome), 273–274
precautions in cases of possible SARS, 273–274
sore throat, 274
red flags, 274
tetanus (lockjaw), 275
tuberculosis, 275–276
typhoid and paratyphoid fever, 277–278
viral hepatitis (hepatitis a, b, and c)
hepatitis a virus infection, 278
complications, 278–279
hepatitis b virus infection, 279–280
complications, 279–280
hepatitis c virus infection, 280
whooping cough (pertussis), 280–281
worms
beef and pork tapeworm, 282–283
fish tapeworm, 283
hookworm, 282
pinworm (or "threadworm"), 281
roundworm and whipworm, 281–282
tapeworm, 282–283
trichinellosis (or trichinosis), 283–284
yellow fever, 284–285
Infectious agents, 247
Infectious diseases, managing
isolation, 251
needle-stick injuries, 252–253
Infectious diseases, treating, 253
food, 253
Infectious eye diseases
blepharitis, 40–41
conjunctivitis, 41–42
hordeolum, 42
keratitis, 42

Injuries, bone, joint, and muscle
ankle injuries
ankle injuries caused by a fall from a height, 55
trip-and-fall ankle injuries, 54–55
collar bone (clavicle) injury, 46
compound fractures, 44
fractures of the foot and toes, 56
fractures of the pelvis, hip, and femur, 52
injury to the upper arm (humerus) and elbow
elbow fracture or dislocation, 48–49
fracture of the mid-shaft of the humerus, 48
fracture of the upper end of the humerus, 48
hand and finger injuries
cuts on the hands and fingers, 51–52
metacarpal fractures, 50–51
scaphoid fractures, 50
thumb fractures, 51
knee injuries, 52–54
neck (cervical spine) injuries, 45–46
nose, jaw, and face fractures
the lower jaw (mandible), 44–45
the nose, 44
the upper jaw (maxilla) and face, 45
rib fractures (see chest injuries)
shin (tibia and fibula) fractures, 54
shoulder injury
shoulder dislocation, 47
shoulder sprain, 47–48
skull fractures (see head injuries)
strains and sprains, 43
complications, 54
wrist and forearm fractures, 49
Injuries, general treatment, 43
International Health Regulations (2005)

Joint inflammation, 225
Joints, problems
the back, 229–230
red flags, 230
the knee, 227–228
the neck, 230–231
red flags, 231
the shoulder, 228–229

Kava kava, 246
Kidney disorders
acute renal (kidney) failure, 177–179
chronic renal failure (Bright's disease), 179
kidney stones (renal colic), 179–180

Lighting, ship's, 352
Liquid transport and potable water
liquid transport systems, 357–358
disinfection of potable water, 359–360
potable water sources, 358
potable water storage, 359
potable water transport system, 358
taking water on board, 359
Liver and biliary disease
alcoholic liver disease
alcoholic hepatitis, 172–173
cirrhosis of the liver, 173
complications, 174
gallstones, 174–175
jaundice, 171–172
liver failure, 172
Local anaesthesia, 74
Loss of consciousness
diabetic ketoacidosis, 124
diabetes mellitus and coma, 123–124
finding an unconscious person, 122–123
hypoglycaemia, 125
sudden loss of consciousness (syncope)
micturition syncope, 122
postural syncope, 122
vaso-vagal syncope (fainting), 122
Lymph node swelling in the groin, 202

Medical advice, external assistance, 291–293
Medical resources on a lifeboat, 349
Medical procedures
administering medicines, 323
applying cold
cold eye compresses, 317
cooling a patient with a very high temperature, 317–318
applying heat, 318–319
catheterizing the urinary bladder, 319–322
ear medication
infection control, 330–331
eye medication, 329–330
injections
after you have given an injection, 324–329
routes of administration
intramuscular, 324
intravenous, 324
oral, 323
rectal, 324
subcutaneous, 324
sublingual, 323
surgical dressings, 322–323
Medicines
analgesics, 427–428
antibiotics, 427
antimalarial medicines, 427

fluids for intravenous infusion
flow rate, 428
nasal cannula, 429
oxygen cylinders, 429
oxygen masks, 429
oxygen, 428–429
parenteral solutions, 428
quantities, 428
quantities and flow rate, 429–430
Medicine chest, management of
drug allergy, 424
expiry date, 424
identification of medicines, 424
keeping records, 423
pregnancy, 424
responsibility, 423
storage, 424
unwanted effects and drug interactions, 424
anaphylaxis, 425
controlled drugs, 426–427
drug rash and other drug-related skin problems, 425–426
ships carrying dangerous goods, 427
Medicines and equipment
order of listing, 430
recommended medicine, 430
storage, 430
Mental illness
after an unsuccessful suicide attempt, 131–132
depression, 129
forms of psychosis
bipolar affective disorder (or manic depressive psychosis), 127
brief reactive psychosis, 128
drug-induced psychosis, 128
organic psychosis, 128
schizophrenia, 127
post-traumatic stress disorder, 132
psychosis
symptoms of psychosis, 126–127
schizophrenia, 127
suicide, 130–131
violent or threatening behaviour
signs of potential danger to others, 130
Miscarriage, 186–188
Muscular system, 377–379

Nursing care
basic principles, 298–299
bodily functions
fluid balance, 309–310
urinary and intestinal excretion, 308–309
bed-bound patient
bed baths, 300
bedsores, 301
breathing difficulties, 301
feeding, 300
mouth care, 300–301
the bed, 299–300
examining faeces, urine, sputum, and vomited matter
faeces, 311
sputum, 312–313
urine, 311–312
vomited matter, 313
mentally disturbed patients, 313–314
monitoring the vital signs, 302–307
preparing sick-quarters, 397
the unconscious patient, 314–316
Nervous system, 386–387

Opioids, opiates, and related drugs
heroin intoxication, 239–240
heroin overdose, 240
heroin withdrawal, 241–242
infection in heroin users, 240–241
Organs, 375
Osteoarthritis, 227
Other opioids, 242

Pain, management of, 17–25
Pediculosis (lice infestation), 219–220
head and body lice, 219
pubic lice, 220
Pelvic inflammatory disease, 204
Physical examination, 109–112
Pleurisy, 141
pneumothorax (see also chest injuries), 141
Pneumonia
aspiration pneumonia and lung abscess, 143–144
empyema, 143
lobar pneumonia, 141–143
Points of entry
airports and ports, 398–399
general obligations, 398
role of competent authorities, 399–400
Poisoning agents
acetylsalicylic acid (Aspirin®), 94
anticoagulants (warfarin, rat poison), 96
caustics, 97
dangerous prescription drugs, 97–98
disinfectants and bleach, 97
methanol and ethylene glycol, 94–95
organophosphate and carbamate insecticides, 95–96
paracetamol (acetaminophen), 93–94
petroleum products, 96–97

Index

Poisoning from exposure to common gases or vapours
- carbon dioxide, 100
- carbon monoxide, 98–99
- cyanide, 99
- flammable liquid vapours, 100
- Freons, 100
- hydrogen sulphide ("rotten egg gas", "sewer gas"), 100–101
- irritant gases – phosgene, chlorine, ammonia, 99

Poisoning with ingested drugs and chemicals, 91–93
Pregnancy, 185
- drugs in pregnancy, 185

Preventing communicable diseases (see also infectious agents)
- hepatitis a and hepatitis b, 367
- immunization
  - diphtheria and tetanus, 367
- other infections, 367

Preventing ill-health from seafaring work, 371
Preventing other diseases
- a balanced diet, 369
- foot injuries, 371
- lack of exercise and boredom, 371
- lifting heavy weights, 370
- preventing illness from exposure to extremes of temperature, 87–89, 341–348, 370
- sleep, 370
- stopping smoking, 368
- sunburn and skin cancer, 370

Privacy and confidentiality, 107–109
Pruritus vulvae (external genital itching) (see also vaginal discharge), 188
Public health measures
- affected conveyances, 402
- container and container loading areas, 405
- conveyance operators, 401
- goods in transit, 405
- health measures on arrival and departure, 400–401
- ships and aircraft at points of entry, 402–403
- ships and aircraft in transit, 401
- travellers under public health observation, 404
- treatment of travellers, 404–405

Pubic lice (see Pediculosis)

Referral information to accompany evacuated patients, 296
Respiratory system, 379–381
Rheumatoid arthritis, 226
Safety on board ship
- briefing for new tasks, 372
- provision of good medical care, 373
- seafarers' lifestyles, 373
- the health and safety committee, 372
- work place assessment, 373

Salpingitis (inflammation of a fallopian tube) (see Pelvic inflammatory disease), 188
Sanitary inspection, 365
Scabies, 220–221
Seizures and epilepsy
- drugs that can precipitate seizures, 121
- types of epileptic seizure
  - generalized seizures, 119–120
  - partial seizures, 118–119
- red flags
  - status epilepticus, 120–121

Septic arthritis, 226
Shingles (herpes zoster and varicella zoster), 254–257
Ship-to-ship transfer of doctor or patient, 295–296
Shock, 13
Sinusitis, 144
Skeletal system, 376–377
Skin abscess, 216–219
Smoke inhalation, 86
Splints and slings
- complications of splinting, 58
- splints, 56–58

Stroke, 113–116
- transient ischaemic attack (TIA), 115–116

Surviving in a survival craft
- cold exposure injuries, 344–345
- contamination with oil, 348
- dehydration and malnutrition, 347–348
- frostbite, 345–346
- frostnip, 345
- heat exposure (see also Heat stroke), 348
- hypothermia due to cold water immersion, 343–344
- immersion foot (trench foot), 346
- near-drowning, 341–343
- other medical problems aboard survival craft, 347
- seasickness, 347
- sunburn, 347

Tissues, 375

Urethritis, 196–197
Urethritis in women, 197–198
Urinary disorders
- acute urinary retention, 183
- benign prostatic hyperplasia (bph, enlarged prostate), 182–183
- chronic pelvic pain in men, 182
- prostatitis, 181–182
- red urine, 180
- urinary tract infection, 181

Index

urinary tract infection in men, 181
urinary tract infection in women, 181
Urinary system, 386
Urticaria (hives), 221

Vaginal bleeding during pregnancy or suspected pregnancy, 185–186
Vaginal discharge
bacterial vaginosis, 203
trichomoniasis, 203–204
vaginal candidiasis, 203
Vectors
bedbugs, 364–365
cockroaches, 364
flies, 363
insects, 362–363
mosquitoes, 363–364
rodents, 360–362
Ventilation, 351–352
Vision, loss of, 42

Warts, ano-genital, 205
Wound healing, 67–69
red flags 68-69
Wound, how to close
suturing a wound, 71–74
using adhesive skin closures, 69–70
using skin adhesive (liquid stitches), 70–71
Wound infection, 76–77
Wounds
ears and nose, 75
eyelids, 75–76
feet, 76
lips, 74–75
tongue, 75